Vaccines and Viruses: Design and Development of Vaccines

Vaccines and Viruses: Design and Development of Vaccines

Editor: Abrianna Bentley

AMERICAN
MEDICAL PUBLISHERS
www.americanmedicalpublishers.com

AMERICAN
MEDICAL PUBLISHERS
www.americanmedicalpublishers.com

Cataloging-in-Publication Data

Vaccines and viruses : design and development of vaccines / edited by Abrianna Bentley.
p. cm.
Includes bibliographical references and index.
ISBN 979-8-88740-551-3
1. Vaccines. 2. Vaccines--Design. 3. Vaccines--Development. 4. Vaccines--Biotechnology.
5. Vaccination. 6. Viruses I. Bentley, Abrianna.
RM281 .V33 2023
615.372--dc23

American Medical Publishers,
41 Flatbush Avenue,
1st Floor, New York,
NY 11217, USA

ISBN 979-8-88740-551-3 (Hardback)

Contents

Preface

A virus is a microorganism that functions and replicates only inside the living cells of other organisms known as host cells. It causes damage to the host cells and often kills the host cell in the process. Some common examples of human diseases caused by viruses are common cold, SARS, influenza, chickenpox, cold sores, rabies, Ebola virus disease, AIDS (HIV), avian influenza, etc. Vaccinations are the most effective method for preventing viral diseases as they provide immunity against infections. Another method of dealing with viruses is the use of antiviral drugs that selectively interfere with the replication of virus. There are multiple types of vaccines based on how they are prepared; and these include live-attenuated vaccines, inactivated vaccines, toxoid vaccines, mRNA vaccines, and viral vector vaccines. Due to large-scale vaccination drives, there has been a considerable decline in morbidity and mortality associated with viral infections, such as polio, measles, mumps, and rubella. This book provides a comprehensive understanding of the role of vaccines in the treatment of viral infections. It will serve as a valuable source of reference to students, virologists, public health experts, and clinicians.

This book unites the global concepts and researches in an organized manner for a comprehensive understanding of the subject. It is a ripe text for all researchers, students, scientists or anyone else who is interested in acquiring a better knowledge of this dynamic field.

I extend my sincere thanks to the contributors for such eloquent research chapters. Finally, I thank my family for being a source of support and help.

Editor

1

Effects of the Japanese Encephalitis Virus Genotype V-Derived Sub-Viral Particles on the Immunogenicity of the Vaccine Characterized by a Novel Virus-Like Particle-Based Assay

Sarah Honjo, Michiaki Masuda and Tomohiro Ishikawa *

Department of Microbiology, Dokkyo Medical University School of Medicine, 880 Kita-kobayashi, Mibu-machi, Shimotsuga-gun, Tochigi 321-0293, Japan

* Correspondence: toishika@dokkyomed.ac.jp

Abstract: Japanese encephalitis virus (JEV) is classified into five genotypes labelled I through V. Although the genotype V (GV) JEV was originally found and had apparently been limited in Malaysia for more than 50 years, its emergence in Korea and China has recently been reported. Therefore, the GV JEV might be spreading over new geographical regions as a cause of potential public health problems. However, it is unknown whether the currently available JEV vaccines are effective against the emerging GV strains. To investigate this issue, a novel virus-like particle-based neutralizing assay was developed in this study. By using this assay, the inactivated JEV vaccine used in Japan and the recombinant sub-viral particles (SVPs) bearing the E protein of the GV Muar strain were characterized for the immunogenicity against the GV JEV. Although the inactivated vaccine alone failed to elicit a detectable level of neutralizing antibodies against the GV JEV, the vaccine added with the Muar-derived SVPs induced relatively high titers of neutralizing antibodies, associated with the efficient Th1 immune responses, against the GV JEV. The results indicate that addition of the GV JEV-derived antigens may be useful for developing the vaccine that is universally effective against JEV including the emerging GV strains.

Keywords: Japanese encephalitis virus; genotype V; vaccine; virus-like particle; sub-viral particle; immunogenicity

1. Introduction

The Japanese encephalitis virus (JEV), which belongs to the genus *flavivirus* of the family of *Flaviviridae*, is a major cause of viral encephalitis in Asia. Although most JEV infection is asymptomatic [1], symptomatic cases range from mild manifestations, such as diarrhea, headache, and vomiting, to severe forms including seizure, polio-like flaccid paralysis, meningitis, or encephalitis [2]. The typical fatality rate of the symptomatic cases is considered to be 20–30% [3]. Moreover, 30–50% of the cases with severe symptoms result in psychoneurological sequelae.

JEV is maintained in the mosquito—bird/swine cycle in nature and is transmitted to humans by the vector mosquito, *Culex tritaeniorhynchus* [4]. JEV possesses an approximately 11 kb-long positive-stranded RNA as a genome, which encodes three structural proteins, capsid (C), precursor membrane (prM), and the envelope (E), as well as seven non-structural (NS) proteins, NS1, NS2A, NS2B, NS3, NS4A, NS4B, and NS5 [5]. Based on the nucleotide sequences of the structural protein genes, JEV is classified into five distinct genotypes, which is labelled I through V [6]. Until the 1990s, the genotype III (GIII) JEV had been widely spread and most frequently isolated in the southern, southeastern, and eastern Asia. However, it was replaced by genotype I (GI) in many countries including Japan, South

Korea, Vietnam, and Thailand [7]. The Muar strain of JEV was originally isolated from an encephalitis patient in Malaysia in 1952 [8] and later classified as genotype V (GV) [9]. Although the GV JEV had long been found only in Malaysia, isolation in China of a new GV strain designated as XZ0934 from the mosquito was reported in 2009 [10]. In Korea, the RNA molecules corresponding to the GV JEV genome were detected in mosquitoes in 2010 [11] and in 2012 [12]. Although the GV JEV has not extensively been characterized, recent studies revealed its potent virulence and neuro-invasiveness in mice [13,14]. These previous studies suggest that the GV JEV, which may already have colonized in Eastern Asia, could cause public health problems.

To prevent JEV infection, several vaccines are currently licensed in the world, including the cell-culture derived inactivated vaccine, the live-attenuated vaccine, and the chimeric vaccine [15]. All of these currently available vaccines contain antigens derived from the GIII JEV. These vaccines have been shown to elicit high titers of neutralizing antibodies against JEV of GI through genotype IV (GIV) [16]. On the other hand, it has been reported that the JEV vaccine currently used in Japan elicits lower titers of neutralizing antibodies against the Muar strain, which is the prototype GV JEV, than against GI and GIII strains [14].

In this study, immunogenicity of the JEV vaccine against the GV strains emerging in Eastern Asia was examined. For this purpose, a novel neutralization assay was developed by using the virus-like particles (VLPs) carrying a reporter gene-expressing sub-genomic replicon. By using the assay, effects of the sub-viral particle (SVP) antigens derived from the GV JEV on the immunogenicity of the vaccine against the emerging GV strains were also examined. The results indicated that, while the immunogenicity of the JEV vaccine currently used in Japan against the emerging GV JEV was relatively poor, addition of the GV-derived SVP antigens led to abundant production of the neutralizing antibodies, as well as the Th1 immune responses, against the emerging GV JEV. Therefore, addition of the GV JEV-derived antigens may be useful for the development of the vaccine that is universally effective against JEV including the emerging GV strains.

2. Materials and Methods

2.1. Cells and Viruses

Vero and BHK cells were grown at 37 °C with 5% CO_2 in Eagle's minimum essential media (MEM) and Dulbecco's modified MEM, respectively, which was supplemented with 10% fetal bovine serum (FBS), 10 mM nonessential amino acid (NEAA, Thermo Fisher Scientific, Waltham, MA, USA), and penicillin (1000 unit/mL)-streptomycin (100 μg/mL) (PS). Mosquito-derived C6/36 cells were grown at 30 °C with 5% CO_2 in MEM supplement with 10% FBS, 10 mM NEAA, and PS. Nakayama and Muar strains of JEV were prepared in C6/36 cells and Vero cells, respectively, as described previously [17]. After inoculation with the virus or VLPs, cells were maintained in MEM supplemented with 1% FBS, 10 mM NEAA, and 10 mM 2- [4- (2-Hydroxyethyl) -1-piperazinyl] ethanesulfonic acid (HEPES) (MEM-1%FBS). To collect SVPs and VLPs, cells were maintained after electroporation in 10% VP-SFM (Thermo Fisher Scientific)-90% MEM supplemented with 10 mM HEPES and 10mM NEAA (VPSFM-MEM).

2.2. Preparation of VLPs and SVPs

Cloned DNA of the replicon, MuarLucrep, derived from the JEV Muar strain [17] was modified by substituting the firefly luciferase gene and the partially deleted C gene with the deep sea shrimp-derived smaller luciferase (NanoLuc) [18] of pNLVF1-N (Promega, Madison, WI, USA) and the full-length C gene to construct MuarfullCnLucrep (Figure 1). Plasmid DNA of MuarfullCnLucrep was linearized with *Swa*I digestion and then subjected to in vitro transcription by using a MEGAscript T7 Kit (Thermo Fisher Scientific, Waltham, MA, USA).

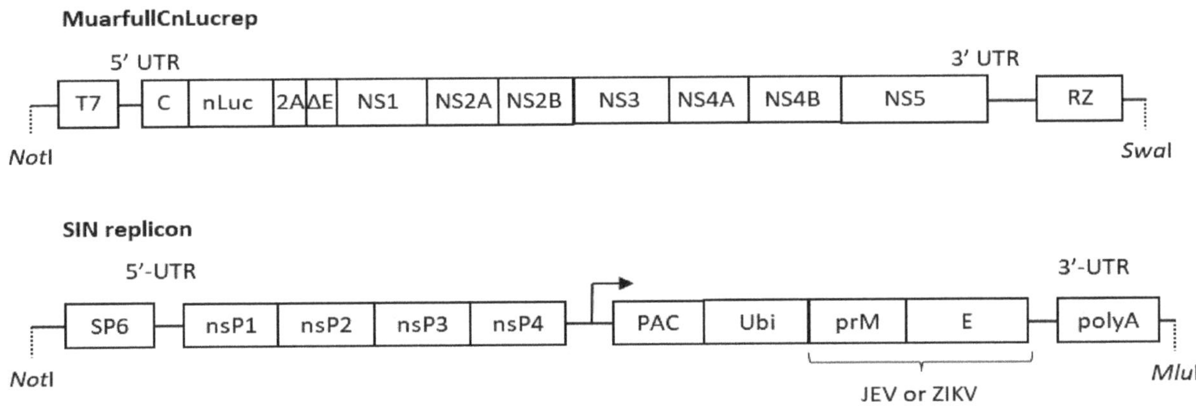

Figure 1. Structure of MuarfullCnLucrep and the Sindbis virus replicon (SIN replicon). MuarfullCnLucrep and the SIN replicon were constructed into a pACYC177-based plasmid and a pToto1101-based plasmid, respectively. The backbone structures of these plasmids were omitted in this figure. NS—non-structural protein of Japanese encephalitis virus. 2A—foot-and-mouse disease virus derived 2A protein. RZ; hepatitis delta virus ribozyme. nsP—non-structural protein of sindbis virus. PAC—puromycin N-acetyl-transferase. Ubi—ubiquitin. Arrow indicates secondary promotor of the sindbis virus genome.

The DNA clone of the Sindbis virus sub-genomic replicon (SIN replicon) was constructed by inserting the Sindbis virus nonstructural protein genes under the SP6 promoter. In the downstream of the secondary promoter for the sub-genomic viral RNA, the fragment of the fusion protein consisting of puromycin N-acetyl-transferase, ubiquitin, as well as the C-terminal 20 amino acids of the C protein, and the prM-E protein of JEV and Zika virus (ZKV) strains, was inserted (Figure 1). The JEV strains from which the prM-E gene was derived were Nakayama and Muar strains, and the emerging GV strains with amino acid substitution (R84K, V186I, P171L or A343V; Table 1) in the E protein, which was compared to Muar strain. The PRVABC59 strain was used for ZKV. Each replicon plasmid was linearized by *Mlu*I digestion and then used as a template for in vitro transcription with a MEGAscript SP6 kit (Thermo Fisher Scientific, Waltham, MA, USA).

Table 1. Amino acid substitutions among JEV GV strains.

Strain	Accession number *	Designation **	Amino Acid Position in E Protein										
			52	58	84	129	156	171	186	208	240	292	343
Muar	HM596272	Muar	Q	T	R	I	S	P	V	T	L	D	A***
K12AS1148	KJ420590	R84K	E	T	K	I	T	P	V	S	M	E	A
K12AS1151	KJ420591	R84K	E	T	K	I	T	P	V	S	M	E	A
10-1827	JN587258	R84K	E	T	K	I	T	P	V	S	M	E	A
XZ0934	JF915894	V186I	E	T	R	I	T	P	I	S	M	E	A
K12YJ1203	KJ420592	P171L	E	T	K	I	T	L	V	S	M	E	A
K12HC959	KJ420589	A343V	E	A	K	T	T	P	V	S	M	E	V
Beijing 1	AB920347	-	Q	S	K	T	S	P	V	S	M	D	A
Nakayama	AB920348	-	Q	S	K	T	S	P	V	S	M	D	A

* Gene bank accession number was shown. ** These designations were used hereinafter. ***Q: glutamine, E: glutamic acid, T: threonine, A: alanine, S: serine, R: arginine, K: lysine, I: isoleucine, P: proline, L: leucine, V: valine, M: methionine, D: aspartic acid.

For preparation of VLPs, C6/36 cells were introduced by electroporation [17] with a mixture of the RNA samples derived from MuarfullCnLucrep (8 μg) and one of the SIN replicons (8 μg). Then, the cells were maintained in VPSFM-MEM, and culture fluids were collected every 24 h for 4 days and pooled. The VLPs in the pooled samples were concentrated by using Amicon Ultra-15, 100K (Merck, Darmstadt, Germany), according to the manufacturer's instruction.

The SVPs were prepared similarly except that BHK cells were introduced with in vitro-transcribed SIN replicon RNA alone (16 μg). An aliquot of the SVP samples was subjected to polyacrylamide gel electrophoresis and silver staining, and the amount of the proteins in SVPs was estimated by comparing the band densities with those of known amounts of proteins.

2.3. *Immunization of Mice*

Four-week-old ICR mice (5–6 mice/immunogen) were immunized twice via the intraperitoneal route with a two-week interval. As immunogens, Vero cell-derived inactivated JE Beijing-1 vaccine (JEVAX, BIKEN, Osaka, Japan) approved and currently used in Japan (1/10 of the normal adult dose in 200 μL of saline), Muar-derived SVP (Mu-SVP, 800 ng), or a mixture of JEVAX (1/10 dose) and Mu-SVP (400 ng) were used. Saline alone was used as the control. Three weeks after the secondary immunization, mice were euthanized, and whole blood was collected from each mouse. Collected blood samples were incubated at 37 °C for 30 min and then centrifuged at 3000 rpm for 10 min to obtain serum samples, which were stored at −30 °C until further use. All of the animal experiments were conducted in accordance with the guidelines of the Laboratory Animal Research Center, Dokkyo Medical University, by using the approved protocol (no. 1028).

2.4. *Neutralization Test*

Neutralization tests by using the infectious JEV were conducted as described previously [19] with minor modifications. Pooled mouse sera were heat inactivated at 56 °C for 30 min, serially diluted by two-fold and incubated with JEV at 37 °C for 1 h. Then, the mixture was inoculated onto Vero cells seeded in a 96-well plate. After absorption for 2 h, cells were overlaid with 1% methylcellulose in MEM supplemented with 1% FBS. Forty-eight hours later, the cells were fixed with the mixture of 50 *v/v*% acetone- 50 *v/v*% methanol, and the foci of virus-infected cells were visualized by immunostaining with an anti-JEV E monoclonal antibody 10B4 [19]. The neutralizing antibody titer was expressed as the highest serum dilution yielding 70% reduction in the number of foci.

The neutralizing tests by using VLPs were performed similarly except that, after absorption, inoculum was removed, and the cells were grown in MEM-1% FBS for 48 h, rinsed with phosphate buffer saline (PBS), and used for the luciferase assay. The luciferase activities of the cell lysates were measured by using the Nano-Glo Luciferase Assay System (Promega, Madison, WI, USA), according to the manufacturer's instructions. Briefly, 25 μl of the cell lysate was mixed with 25 μl of substrate, and the mixture was incubated for 3 min. Then, the luminescence was measured for 10 s by Lumat LB9501 (Berthold Technologies, Bad Wilbad, Germany). The neutralization titer was expressed as the highest serum dilution yielding 70% reduction in the relative light unit.

2.5. *Enzyme-Linked ImmunoSorbent Assay (ELISA)*

A 96-well EIA plate (Corning Inc., Corning, NY, USA) was sensitized with concentrated SVPs (approximately 2 μg protein/well) in carbonate buffer (pH 9.6) at 4 °C overnight. After rinsing with PBS-0.05% Tween-20, each well was blocked with PBS containing 0.05% Tween-20 and 1% bovine serum albumin for 20 min and then added with individual sera diluted at 1:100. Following incubation at room temperature for 2 h, the plate was incubated with HRP-labeled anti-mouse IgG (GE Healthcare, Chicago, IL, USA). Prior to incubation with the substrate from an ELISA POD Substrate TMB Kit (Nacalai Tesque, Kyoto, Japan), the plate was rinsed with PBS-0.05% Tween-20 and then with water. The reaction was stopped by adding 1N H2SO4. The optical density (OD) was measured on the iMark Microplate Reader (Bio Rad, Hercules, CA, USA).

For Th1/Th2 profiling, a 96-well plate was sensitized as described above, and pooled mouse serum samples serially diluted by two-fold were added to each well and incubated at room temperature for 2 h. Then, the plate was reacted with the HRP-labeled anti-mouse IgG1 or IgG2a antibody (Southern Biotechnology Associates, Birmingham, UK) and then the substrate was added after a rinse with PBS-0.05% Tween-20 and water. The optical density (OD) was measured as described above. The IgG1 and IgG2a antibody titers were expressed as the highest serum dilution exhibiting OD greater than the average plus three times the standard deviation obtained for the serum sample of the saline-inoculated mouse.

3. Results

3.1. Preparation of the Luciferase Gene-Transducing VLP Bearing the E Protein of JEV and ZKV

The luciferase-expressing replicon (MuarfullCnLucrep) RNA was introduced into C6/36 cells with the SIN replicon RNA bearing the prME gene derived from the GIII Nakayama strain or various GV strains (Muar, R84K, V186I, P171L or A343V) of JEV, or ZKV. Then, the pooled culture fluids corresponding to respective SIN replicons were inoculated onto Vero cells, and luciferase activities of the cell lysates were measured at 48 h post-inoculation. As shown in Figure 2, high levels of luciferase activity were detected for all of the seven SIN replicons, but not the control MuarfullCnLucrep or SIN replicon alone. The data indicate the successful transduction of luciferase gene mediated by the VLPs bearing the E protein expressed by the SIN replicon.

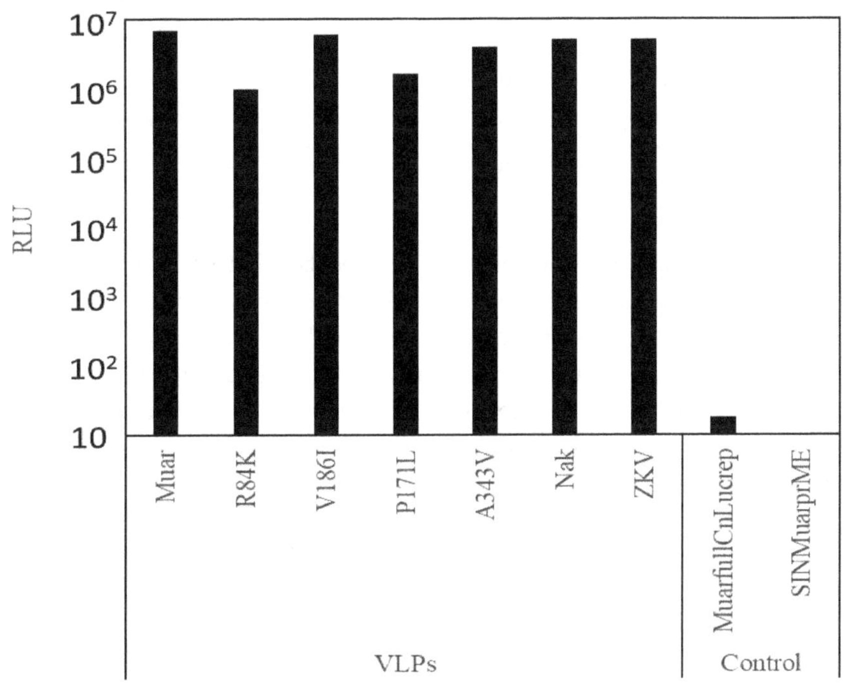

Figure 2. Production of nLuc-expressing virus like particles (VLPs). The nLuc-expressing VLP obtained from C6/36 cells electroporated with MuarfullCnLucrep RNA and sindbis virus replicon expressing prM-E genes were inoculated to Vero cells. Cells were lysed at 48 h post inoculation and then nano-luciferase activities were measured.

3.2. Evaluation of the VLP for Application in the Neutralization Test

Mice were immunized with 1/10 dose of JEVAX, and the sera obtained from these mice were tested for the neutralization titers by using infectious JEV (Nakayama strain) and the VLP bearing the E protein derived from the Nakayama strain. As expected, JEVAX was able to elicit antibody production (1:20) against the Nakayama strain, which belongs to GIII. Similarly, neutralization antibodies (1:10) were detected against the VLP bearing the E protein of the Nakayama strain. When the VLP bearing the ZKV E protein was used, the neutralization titer was shown to be <1:10. Therefore, the VLP bearing the JEV E protein appeared to serve as a useful tool for measuring the virus-specific neutralization antibody titer even though the sensitivity might be slightly lower than the infectious virus.

3.3. Immunogenicity of JEVAX and JEV Muar Strain-Derived SVP Against JEV GV

Mice were immunized with JEVAX (1/10 dose), the Muar strain-derived SVP (Mu-SVP), or the mixture of these two, and the sera obtained from these mice were examined for the neutralization titers by the VLP-based assay described above. Whereas mice immunized with JEVAX alone did not elicit a detectable level of antibody production against any of the JEV GV strains examined, immunization with Mu-SVP alone developed neutralizing antibodies (1:10) against most of the JEV GV strains examined except R84K (Table 2). Unexpectedly, the Mu-SVP-induced neutralization titer (1:20) against Nakayama strain, which belongs to GIII, was higher (Table 2). Immunization with the mixture of JEVAX with Mu-SVP led to considerably higher neutralization titers against JEV GV (1:40), as well as GIII (1:80) (Table 2). No detectable levels of neutralization antibody production against ZKV were induced by any of these immunization protocols.

Table 2. Immunogenicity of JEVAX and Mu-SVP.

Immunogen	Virus like particles Used in the Neutralization Test *						
	Muar	**R84K**	**V186I**	**P171L**	**A343V**	**Nak**	**ZKV**
1/10 dose of JEVAX	<1:10	<1:10	<1:10	<1:10	<1:10	1:10	<1:10
Mu-SVP** (800 ng)	1:10	<1:10	1:10	1:10	1:10	1:20	<1:10
1/10 dose of JEVAX and Mu-SVP (400 ng)	1:40	1:40	1:40	1:40	1:40	1:80	<1:10
Saline	<1:10	<1:10	<1:10	<1:10	<1:10	<1:10	<1:10

* Neut titers were expressed as the highest serum dilution yielding 70% reduction in a relative light unit.
** Muar-derived sub-viral particle.

The levels of antibody production were also measured by ELISA (Figure 3). The results appeared to be correlated with those of the neutralization test. The highest antibody levels were observed in the sera from mice immunized with the mixture of JEVAX and Mu-SVP, which was followed by Mu-SVP alone and JEVAX alone (Figure 3). Intriguingly, the antibody level in the sera from Mu-SVP-immunized mice against the Nakayama strain tended to be higher than against most of the GV strains except A343V. In most cases, no significant levels of antibody production against ZKV were observed with any of the immunization protocols (Figure 3).

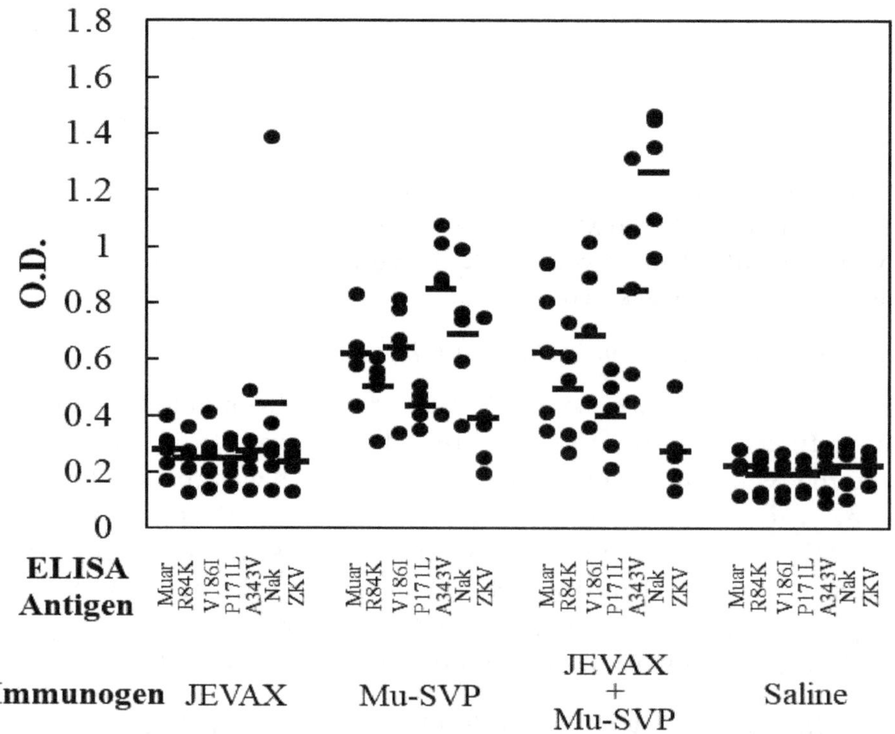

Figure 3. ELISA antibody levels induced by JEVAX and/or Muar-derived sub-viral particle (Mu-SVP). Antibody levels of individual mouse sera were examined on the antigen-sensitized plates. SVPs (Muar, R84K, V186I, P171L, A343V, Nak, and ZKV) were used as antigens. The individual sera were analyzed and bars represent the average of each group.

3.4. Th1/Th2 Immune Profile Induced by JEVAX and Mu-SVP

Th1 cells are known to promote cellular immune responses while Th2 cells promote humoral immune responses. In mice, the degrees of Th1 and Th2 immune responses are represented by the levels of IgG2a and IgG1 antibodies, respectively [20]. The isotype-specific ELISA revealed that production of IgG1, but not IgG2a, was elicited by immunization with JEVAX against the GV strains except P171L against which neither IgG1 nor IgG2a were detected (Figure 4). Similarly, the IgG1 titers were markedly higher than the IgG2a titers when Mu-SVP alone or the mixture of JEVAX and Mu-SVP was used as immunogen. The results indicate that the Th2-dominant immune responses were generally elicited by all of the immunogens tested. However, it should be noted that Th1 immune responses represented by production of IgG2a against the Nakayama strain and most of the GV strains examined were also observed when the mixture of JEVAX and Mu-SVP was used (Figure 4).

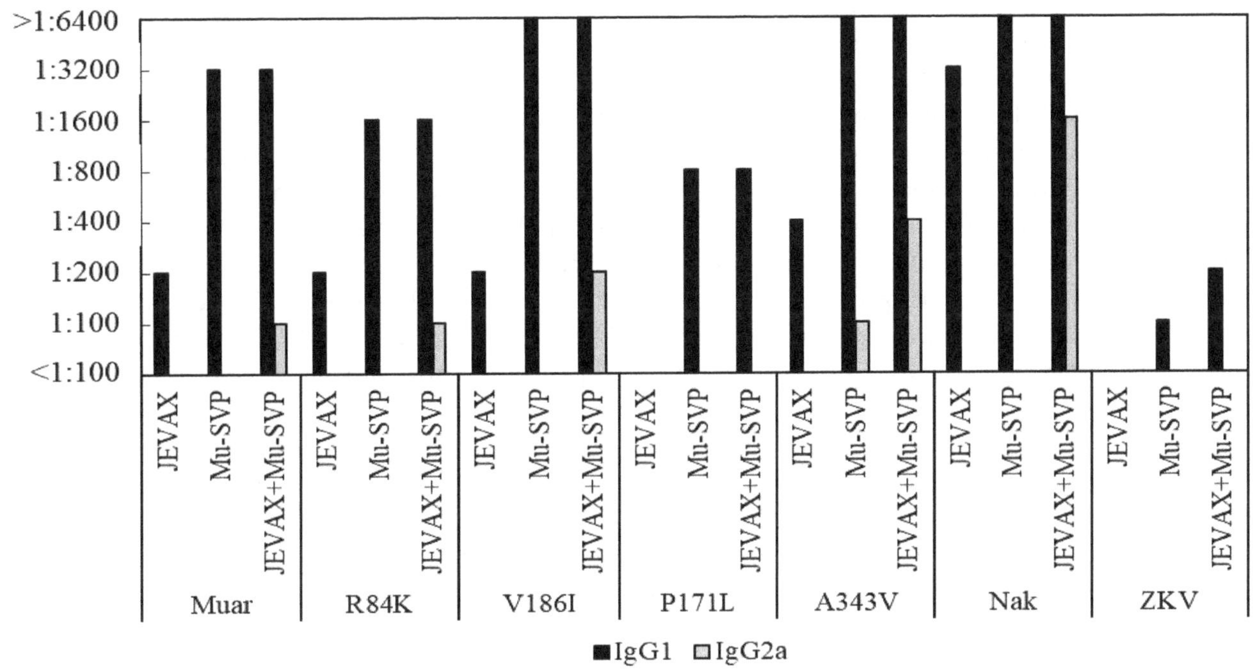

Figure 4. The Th1/Th2 immune profile induced by JEVAX and/or Muar-derived subviral particle (Mu-SVP). The serial two-fold diluted pooled mouse sera (start from 1:100) were examined on the antigen-sensitized plates. SVPs (Muar, R84K, V186I, P171L, A343V, Nak, and ZKV) were used as antigens. Antibody titers of IgG1 (Th2) and IgG2a (Th1) of each group were determined as the highest serum dilution exhibiting optical density (O.D.) greater than average O.D. plus three times the standard deviation obtained by saline inoculated mouse sera.

4. Discussion

For prevention of the JEV infection, effective vaccines have been developed and utilized in the endemic areas. For evaluating the immunogenicity of the vaccines, the titers of the neutralizing antibodies in the immunized sera have usually been measured by the plaque reduction assay. However, this assay needs an infectious virus and generally takes at least a week to obtain the results. Recently, the neutralizing assays by using the VLPs, which carry the reporter gene-expressing sub-genomic replicon, have been developed for some flaviviruses [19,21–24]. These VLP-based assays for which infectious virus is unnecessary are thought to be safe. In addition, the reporter VLP assay can be performed in a few days and could be applicable for high throughput tests. In this study, a novel VLP-based neutralization assay was developed by modifying the previous system [19] and shown to be useful for measuring the anti-JEV antibody titers.

All of the currently approved JEV vaccines, which contain antigens derived from the GIII strains, are known to be effective against the GI through GIV viruses [16]. It has previously been reported that the inactivated JEV vaccine, which contains the antigens derived from the GIII Beijing-1 strain, is poorly immunogenic against the Muar strain, which is the prototype GV JEV isolated in Malaysia decades ago [14]. Our present study confirmed the previous results by using the VLP-based neutralization assay and demonstrated that the GIII-based vaccine was not effective against the emerging GV strains reported from Eastern Asia. Our results are consistent with the previous study showing that the live attenuated vaccine derived from the GIII SA14-14-2 strain induced only low titers of neutralizing antibodies against the GV XZ0934 strain recently isolated in China [25]. Relatively poor immune responses by JEVAX were observed in this study. The neutralizing antibody titers were determined in this study by a 70% reduction method, which is often used for evaluating a novel vaccine, whereas the 50% reduction method is quality assurance of existing vaccine evaluations. In addition, sensitivities of the VLP-based neutralization test might be slightly lower than the infectious virus-based test, as mentioned above. These might be a reason for the low neutralization titers by JEVAX. Regarding the ELISA assay, structural differences between immunogen (JEVAX) and antigens used in ELISA evaluation (SVPs), and differences in cells used to prepare JEVAX (Vero cells) and SVPs (BHK cells) might be reasons for lower ELISA values.

The envelope of the individual JEV particle is estimated to bear 180 molecules of E protein, which plays crucial roles in receptor binding and membrane fusion. The E protein is highly immunogenic, and, thus, most neutralizing antibodies against JEV react with the E protein [5]. The poor immunogenicity of the GIII-based vaccine against the GV viruses is most likely due to the lower amino acid identities of the E protein between GIII and GV. In fact, the amino acid sequence identities of the E protein between the GIII and GV strains are about 90%, whereas those between GIII and GI, GII, or GIV are 94% or higher [8]. Neutralizing monoclonal antibodies (mAbs) derived from the GIII JEV-infected mice have been shown to recognize specific amino acids in the E protein. For example, the 503 mAb recognized Q52, I126, K136, and S275 [26], and neutralization by the E3.3 mAb was shown to require S331 and D332 [27]. Among these critical residues, Q52 is substituted in all GV viruses except the Muar strain, and S331 is substituted to T in all GV viruses examined (Table 1). The amino acid at the positions 52 and 331 are located on the surface of the E protein, and their substitution might affect the accessibility and, thus, the neutralizing activity of the antibodies elicited by the GIII-based vaccine. The amino acid identities of the E protein between JEV and ZKV are only 54–55%. Reasonably, no significant levels of neutralizing antibodies were detected in mice immunized with the JEVAX or Mu-SVP.

As to flaviviruses, it is known that the cells expressing only prM-E gene can produce viral RNA-free SVPs, which bear E and M proteins in the envelope [28]. Our present study demonstrated that the Mu-SVP served as a potent immunogen for eliciting neutralizing antibodies against various strains of GV JEV except R84K. Unexpectedly, the neutralizing antibodies raised by Mu-SVP to Nak were higher than homologous GV viruses, even though the mechanism of this observation is unknown. For the West Nile virus, which also belongs to the genus flavivirus, it was reported that at least approximately 30 antibodies per single virion were required for neutralization [29]. Therefore, it is possible that the GV virus might require a larger number of antibodies to be neutralized compared to the GIII virus. Interestingly, a mixture of JEVAX and Mu-SVP exhibited the enhanced immunogenicity against not only the GV strains but also the GIII strain, which suggests the synergistic effects between the vaccine and the SVPs. For the protection from JEV, the neutralizing antibody titer at 1:10 has been accepted as immunological correlates [30]. Thus, the neutralizing antibodies induced particularly by the mixture of JEVAX and Mu-SVP were considered protective. Although the exact mechanism for the enhancement is unknown, it is possible that the SVPs may act as an adjuvant as well as antigens because the SVPs (about 30 nm in diameter) are smaller than the inactivated virus particles (50–70 nm) and could easily be drained into lymph nodes and recognized by the resident dendritic cells and macrophages [31]. These enhancements might result from a simple mixture of antigens derived from different genotypes. To investigate this possibility, a comparison of immunogenicity of Mu-SVP and a Muar-based inactivated vaccine will be valuable for further study.

In general, viral infection and immunization with live attenuated vaccines elicit the Th1-dominant immune responses [32,33], while immunization with inactivated or subunit vaccines usually induces the Th2-dominant immune responses [32]. Consistently, our data indicated that the Th2-dominant immune responses were elicited by JEVAX. Additionally, the Th2-dominant immune responses were induced when Mu-SVPs were injected alone, likely because the SVPs, unlike live attenuated vaccines, are replication-defective. Although IgG1 antibodies were elevated to GV viruses by JEVAX alone, no detectable neutralizing antibodies were observed. The IgG1 as well as IgG2a levels shown in Figure 4 contain total anti-JEV antibodies whether they have neutralizing activities or not, which is likely causing these differences. Intriguingly, a mixture of the vaccine and the SVPs were able to elicit notable levels of Th1 immune responses represented by the production of IgG2a. Although Th2 immune responses have been recognized as a major contributor for protection, Th1 immune responses were also reported to play supplementary roles in the protection of JEV [34]. Therefore, induction of both Th1 and Th2 immune responses by our vaccine is considered useful. Although the profile of the T cell responses are known to be affected by several factors, such as the route for vaccine inoculation and the adjuvant used with the immunogen [35–37], it is unknown how the Th1 immune responses were elicited when the two immunogens were mixed. Further studies are necessary to elucidate the mechanism.

Taken together, the new VLP-based neutralizing assay demonstrated that immunogenicity against the prototype and the emerging GV strains of the JEV vaccine currently used in Japan was relatively poor. However, the addition of Mu-SVP increased the vaccine's immunogenicity against the GV viruses apparently in a synergistic manner. Additionally, the vaccine added with Mu-SVP was able to elicit the Th1 immune responses more effectively than either immunogen alone. Therefore, the addition of the vaccine with the GV-derived antigens may be useful for developing the new JEV vaccine universally effective against a wide range of genotypes including GV.

Author Contributions: Conceptualization, T.I. Methodology, T.I. Investigation, S.H. and T.I. Resources, T.I. and M.M. Writing-Original Draft Preparation, S.H. and T.I. Writing-Review and Editing, T.I. and M.M. Supervision, M.M. Project Administration, T.I. Funding Acquisition, T.I.

Acknowledgments: We thank Takashi Namatame (Research Support Center, Dokkyo Medical University) for assistance in DNA sequencing, and Yuki Shinozaki and Satomi Yoshida (Department of Microbiology, Dokkyo Medical University School of Medicine) for technical and secretarial assistance.

References

1. Solomon, T.; Dung, N.M.; Kneen, R.; Gainsborough, M.; Vaughn, D.W.; Khanh, V.T. Japanese encephalitis. *J. Neurol. Neurosurg. Psychiatry* **2000**, *68*, 405–415. [CrossRef] [PubMed]
2. Pierson, T.C.; Diamond, M.S. Flaviviruses. In *Fields Virology*, 6th ed.; Knipe, D.M., Howley, P.M., Eds.; Lippincott Williams & Wilkins: Philadelphia, PA, USA, 2013; pp. 747–794.
3. Ishikawa, T.; Konishi, E. Combating Japanese encephalitis: Vero-cell derived inactivated vaccines and the situation in Japan. *Future Virol.* **2010**, *5*, 785–799. [CrossRef]
4. Van den Hurk, A.F.; Ritchie, S.A.; Mackenzie, J.S. Ecology and geographical expansion of Japanese encephalitis virus. *Annu. Rev. Entomol.* **2009**, *54*, 17–35. [CrossRef] [PubMed]
5. Lindenbach, B.D.; Murray, C.; Thiel, H.J.; Rice, C.M. Flaviviridae. In *Fields Virology*, 6th ed.; Knipe, D.M., Howley, P.M., Eds.; Lippincott Williams & Wilkins: Philadelphia, PA, USA, 2013; pp. 712–746.
6. Hasegawa, H.; Yoshida, M.; Fujita, S.; Kobayashi, Y. Comparison of structural proteins among antigenically different Japanese encephalitis virus strains. *Vaccine* **1994**, *12*, 841–844. [CrossRef]
7. Ishikawa, T.; Konishi, E. Japanese encephalitis: Epidemiology, prevention and current status of antiviral drug development. *Expert Opin. Orphan Drugs* **2014**, *2*, 923–936. [CrossRef]
8. Solomon, T.; Ni, H.; Beasley, D.W.; Ekkelenkamp, M.; Cardosa, M.J.; Barrett, A.D. Origin and evolution of Japanese encephalitis virus in southeast Asia. *J. Virol.* **2003**, *77*, 3091–3098. [CrossRef]

9. Mohammed, M.A.; Galbraith, S.E.; Radford, A.D.; Dove, W.; Takasaki, T.; Kurane, I.; Solomon, T. Molecular phylogenetic and evolutionary analyses of Muar strain of Japanese encephalitis virus reveal it is the missing fifth genotype. *Infect. Genet. Evol.* **2011**, *11*, 855–862. [CrossRef]
10. Li, M.H.; Fu, S.H.; Chen, W.X.; Wang, H.Y.; Guo, Y.H.; Liu, Q.Y.; Li, Y.X.; Luo, H.M.; Da, W.; Duo Ji, D.Z.; et al. Genotype v Japanese encephalitis virus is emerging. *PLoS Negl. Trop. Dis.* **2011**, *5*, e1231. [CrossRef]
11. Takhampunya, R.; Kim, H.C.; Tippayachai, B.; Kengluecha, A.; Klein, T.A.; Lee, W.J.; Grieco, J.; Evans, B.P. Emergence of Japanese encephalitis virus genotype V in the Republic of Korea. *Virol. J.* **2011**, *8*, 449. [CrossRef]
12. Kim, H.; Cha, G.W.; Jeong, Y.E.; Lee, W.G.; Chang, K.S.; Roh, J.Y.; Yang, S.C.; Park, M.Y.; Park, C.; Shin, E.H. Detection of Japanese encephalitis virus genotype V in *Culex orientalis* and *Culex pipiens* (Diptera: Culicidae) in Korea. *PLoS ONE* **2015**, *10*, e0116547. [CrossRef]
13. De Wispelaere, M.; Frenkiel, M.P.; Despres, P. A Japanese encephalitis virus genotype 5 molecular clone is highly neuropathogenic in a mouse model: Impact of the structural protein region on virulence. *J. Virol.* **2015**, *89*, 5862–5875. [CrossRef]
14. Tajima, S.; Yagasaki, K.; Kotaki, A.; Tomikawa, T.; Nakayama, E.; Moi, M.L.; Lim, C.K.; Saijo, M.; Kurane, I.; Takasaki, T. In vitro growth, pathogenicity and serological characteristics of the Japanese encephalitis virus genotype V Muar strain. *J. Gen. Virol.* **2015**, *96*, 2661–2669. [CrossRef]
15. Ishikawa, T.; Yamanaka, A.; Konishi, E. A review of successful flavivirus vaccines and the problems with those flaviviruses for which vaccines are not yet available. *Vaccine* **2014**, *32*, 1326–1337. [CrossRef]
16. Erra, E.O.; Askling, H.H.; Yoksan, S.; Rombo, L.; Riutta, J.; Vene, S.; Lindquist, L.; Vapalahti, O.; Kantele, A. Cross-protective capacity of Japanese encephalitis (JE) vaccines against circulating heterologous JE virus genotypes. *Clin. Infect. Dis.* **2013**, *56*, 267–270. [CrossRef]
17. Ishikawa, T.; Abe, M.; Masuda, M. Construction of an infectious molecular clone of Japanese encephalitis virus genotype V and its derivative subgenomic replicon capable of expressing a foreign gene. *Virus Res.* **2015**, *195*, 153–161. [CrossRef]
18. Hall, M.P.; Unch, J.; Binkowski, B.F.; Valley, M.P.; Butler, B.L.; Wood, M.G.; Otto, P.; Zimmerman, K.; Vidugiris, G.; Machleidt, T.; et al. Engineered luciferase reporter from a deep sea shrimp utilizing a novel imidazopyrazinone substrate. *ACS Chem. Biol.* **2012**, *7*, 1848–1857. [CrossRef]
19. Ishikawa, T.; Widman, D.G.; Bourne, N.; Konishi, E.; Mason, P.W. Construction and evaluation of a chimeric pseudoinfectious virus vaccine to prevent Japanese encephalitis. *Vaccine* **2008**, *26*, 2772–2781. [CrossRef]
20. Whitton, J.L.; Oldstone, M.B.A. The immune response to flaviviruses. In *Fields Virology*, 4th ed.; Knipe, D.M., Howley, P.M., Eds.; Lippincott-Raven Publisher: New York, NY, USA, 2001; pp. 285–320.
21. Yoshii, K.; Ikawa, A.; Chiba, Y.; Omori, Y.; Maeda, J.; Murata, R.; Kariwa, H.; Takashima, I. Establishment of a neutralization test involving reporter gene-expressing virus-like particles of tick-borne encephalitis virus. *J. Virol. Methods* **2009**, *161*, 173–176. [CrossRef]
22. Mercier-Delarue, S.; Durier, C.; de Verdiere, N.C.; Poveda, J.D.; Meiffredy, V.; Garcia, M.D.F.; Lastere, S.; Cesaire, R.; Manuggera, J.C.; Molina, J.M.; et al. Screening test for neutralizing antibodies against yellow fever virus, based on a flavivirus pseudotype. *PLoS ONE* **2017**, *12*, e0177882. [CrossRef]
23. Mattia, K.; Puffer, B.A.; Williams, K.L.; Gonzalez, R.; Murray, M.; Sluzas, E.; Pagano, D.; Ajith, S.; Bower, M.; Berdougo, E.; et al. Dengue reporter virus particles for measuring neutralizing antibodies against each of the four dengue serotypes. *PLoS ONE* **2011**, *6*, e27252. [CrossRef]
24. Garg, H.; Sedano, M.; Plata, G.; Punke, E.B.; Joshi, A. Development of Virus-Like-Particle Vaccine and Reporter Assay for Zika Virus. *J. Virol.* **2017**, *91*, e00834-17. [CrossRef]
25. Cao, L.; Fu, S.; Gao, X.; Li, M.; Cui, S.; Li, X.; Cao, Y.; Lei, W.; Lu, Z.; He, Y.; et al. Low Protective Efficacy of the Current Japanese Encephalitis Vaccine against the Emerging Genotype 5 Japanese Encephalitis Virus. *PLoS Negl. Trop. Dis.* **2016**, *10*, e0004686. [CrossRef]
26. Morita, K.; Tadano, M.; Nakaji, S.; Kosai, K.; Mathenge, E.G.; Pandey, B.D.; Hasebe, F.; Inoue, S.; Igarashi, A. Locus of a virus neutralization epitope on the Japanese encephalitis virus envelope protein determined by use of long PCR-based region-specific random mutagenesis. *Virology* **2001**, *287*, 417–426. [CrossRef]
27. Lin, C.W.; Wu, S.C. A functional epitope determinant on domain III of the Japanese encephalitis virus envelope protein interacted with neutralizing-antibody combining sites. *J. Virol.* **2003**, *77*, 2600–2606. [CrossRef]

28. Mason, P.W.; Pincus, S.; Fournier, M.J.; Mason, T.L.; Shope, R.E.; Paoletti, E. Japanese encephalitis virus-vaccinia recombinants produce particulate forms of the structural membrane proteins and induce high levels of protection against lethal JEV infection. *Virology* **1991**, *180*, 294–305. [CrossRef]
29. Pierson, T.C.; Xu, Q.; Nelson, S.; Oliphant, T.; Nybakken, G.E.; Fremont, D.H.; Diamond, M.S. The stoichiometry of antibody-mediated neutralization and enhancement of West Nile virus infection. *Cell Host Microbe* **2007**, *1*, 135–145. [CrossRef]
30. Kimura-Kuroda, J.; Yasui, K. Protection of mice against Japanese encephalitis virus by passive administration with monoclonal antibodies. *J. Immunol.* **1988**, *141*, 3606–3610.
31. Manolova, V.; Flace, A.; Bauer, M.; Schwarz, K.; Saudan, P.; Bachmann, M.F. Nanoparticles target distinct dendritic cell populations according to their size. *Eur. J. Immunol.* **2008**, *38*, 1404–1413. [CrossRef]
32. Aberle, J.H.; Aberle, S.W.; Kofler, R.M.; Mandl, C.W. Humoral and cellular immune response to RNA immunization with flavivirus replicons derived from tick-borne encephalitis virus. *J. Virol.* **2005**, *79*, 15107–15113. [CrossRef]
33. Coutelier, J.P.; van der Logt, J.T.; Heessen, F.W.; Warnier, G.; Van Snick, J. IgG2a restriction of murine antibodies elicited by viral infections. *J. Exp. Med.* **1987**, *165*, 64–69. [CrossRef]
34. Chen, H.W.; Huang, H.W.; Hu, H.M.; Chung, H.H.; Wu, S.H.; Chong, P.; Tao, M.H.; Pan, C.H. A poorly neutralizing IgG2a/c response elicited by a DNA vaccine protects mice against Japanese encephalitis virus. *J. Gen. Virol.* **2014**, *95*, 1983–1990. [CrossRef]
35. Kuroda, E.; Coban, C.; Ishii, K.J. Particulate adjuvant and innate immunity: Past achievements, present findings, and future prospects. *Int. Rev. Immunol.* **2013**, *32*, 209–220. [CrossRef]
36. Levast, B.; Awate, S.; Babiuk, L.; Mutwiri, G.; Gerdts, V.; van Drunen Littel-van den Hurk, S. Vaccine Potentiation by Combination Adjuvants. *Vaccines* **2014**, *2*, 297–322. [CrossRef]
37. Ramakrishna, C.; Ravi, V.; Desai, A.; Subbakrishna, D.K.; Shankar, S.K.; Chandramuki, A. T helper responses to Japanese encephalitis virus infection are dependent on the route of inoculation and the strain of mouse used. *J. Gen. Virol.* **2003**, *84*, 1559–1567. [CrossRef]

2

New Kids on the Block: RNA-Based Influenza Virus Vaccines

Francesco Berlanda Scorza [1] and Norbert Pardi [2,*]

1 PATH's Center for Vaccine Innovation and Access, 455 Massachusetts Ave. NW, Suite 1000, Washington, DC 20001, USA; fberlanda-scorza@path.org
2 Department of Medicine, University of Pennsylvania, Philadelphia, PA 19104, USA
* Correspondence: pnorbert@pennmedicine.upenn.edu

Abstract: RNA-based immunization strategies have emerged as promising alternatives to conventional vaccine approaches. A substantial body of published work demonstrates that RNA vaccines can elicit potent, protective immune responses against various pathogens. Consonant with its huge impact on public health, influenza virus is one of the best studied targets of RNA vaccine research. Currently licensed influenza vaccines show variable levels of protection against seasonal influenza virus strains but are inadequate against drifted and pandemic viruses. In recent years, several types of RNA vaccines demonstrated efficacy against influenza virus infections in preclinical models. Additionally, comparative studies demonstrated the superiority of some RNA vaccines over the currently used inactivated influenza virus vaccines in animal models. Based on these promising preclinical results, clinical trials have been initiated and should provide valuable information about the translatability of the impressive preclinical data to humans. This review briefly describes RNA-based vaccination strategies, summarizes published preclinical and clinical data, highlights the roadblocks that need to be overcome for clinical applications, discusses the landscape of industrial development, and shares the authors' personal perspectives about the future of RNA-based influenza virus vaccines.

Keywords: RNA vaccine; influenza virus; infectious disease; clinical trial

---

1. Introduction

Influenza virus causes millions of illnesses and up to 650,000 deaths worldwide every year [1]. Approved seasonal influenza vaccines protect from well-matched circulating strains but are not effective against drifted seasonal and pandemic viruses; thus, there is an urgent need for more broadly protective vaccines. Recent publications have discussed the challenges that need to be resolved by a broadly protective or universal influenza virus vaccine, such as: lack of protection from antigenically drifted or shifted viral strains, suboptimal epitope-specific antibody responses caused by pre-existing host immunity (original antigenic sin), short-lived protective immunity after vaccine administration, potential side effects of live virus vaccines, or inhibitory effects of maternal antibodies on vaccine immunogenicity in infants [2–6]. The data available to date suggest that RNA-based influenza vaccines have the potential to induce broadly protective immune responses and may address some of the above-mentioned challenges.

Vaccination with in vitro transcribed (IVT) messenger RNA (mRNA) was not widely considered as a viable approach until the early 2000s; however, several early studies using various types of mRNA vaccines demonstrated promising preclinical results [7–9]. Seminal publications from the past years made it clear that mRNA vaccines—targeting cancer and infectious diseases—have significant therapeutic potential and might represent the next generation of prophylactic and therapeutic vaccines (reviewed in [10]).

Early studies using naked (uncomplexed) unmodified RNA for immunization via the intramuscular route demonstrated some efficacy against various infectious pathogens [11] but substantial improvements were necessary to make mRNA into a potent vaccine. The major goals were to increase the in vivo half-life of mRNA and achieve high in vivo translatability to produce large amounts of immunogen for extended periods of time after vaccine administration. Apart from intranodally administered naked mRNA vaccines (discussed in [10]), most potent iterations of directly injectable mRNA vaccines have two major components: (1) a fairly stable, highly translatable, optimized mRNA and (2) a carrier molecule that encapsulates mRNA. (1) mRNA is transcribed by a bacteriophage RNA polymerase from a linear DNA template (linearized plasmid or PCR product) containing a T3, T7 or Sp6 phage promoter [12]. Introduction of naturally occurring modified nucleosides, optimization of the codon composition (replacing rare codons with frequently used synonymous codons) and purification of the in vitro transcribed mRNA can yield increases of many orders of magnitude in protein translation from mRNA via the silencing of various innate immune sensing pathways [13–18]. Further optimization steps, such as the incorporation of 5′ and 3′ UTR elements that increase mRNA stability and translatability, optimization of the length of poly(A) tail and addition of a 5′ cap structure also proved to be critical in achieving therapeutic potency [19–22]. (2) The vast majority of directly injectable mRNA vaccines have a component that protects mRNA from extracellular RNases, facilitates cellular uptake, and often serves as an adjuvant to improve immune responses. Lipid nanoparticles (LNPs) are probably the most frequently used mRNA carriers, but several natural and synthetic polymers have also proved to be efficacious mRNA delivery tools (reviewed in [23,24]).

Various formats of RNA vaccines against influenza virus have demonstrated potent immunogenicity in preclinical models (Table 1 and discussed in Section 2). Moreover, RNA-based influenza vaccines offer critical advantages over other approaches (detailed in Table 2) such as a favorable safety profile (RNA is a non-infectious, non-integrating molecule degraded by normal cellular processes), highly controllable immunogen production, the absence of anti-vector immunity that enables repeated administration, and, importantly, rapid, scalable production without the use of eggs or complex cell culture systems. The latter is particularly important because some viruses do not grow well in eggs or they can develop egg-adaptive mutations that can alter the antigenicity of the viral surface proteins [25–27]. Additionally, generation of FDA-approved conventional influenza virus vaccines can take several months, which can be too long to influence the outcome of an influenza virus pandemic [28]. In contrast, once the genetic sequences of the circulating influenza virus strains are known, RNA vaccines can be easily updated giving an adequate response to viral antigenic drift.

Table 1. RNA vaccines against influenza virus.*

Vaccine Platform	Immunogens and Route (s) of Administration	Species	Results and References
SAM (uncomplexed)	HA from A/Puerto Rico/8/34; i.m.	mouse	Partial protection from homologous virus [11]
SAM-LNP	NP and M1 from A/Puerto Rico/8/34; i.m.	mouse	Increased survival after homologous and heterosubtypic virus infection [29]
SAM-CNE	HA from A/California/7/2009; i.m.	mouse ferret	Increased survival after homologous and heterologous virus infection [30]
SAM-PEI and unmodified, uncomplexed mRNA	HA from A/California/07/2009, A/Hong Kong/1/68, B/Massachusetts/2/2012; i.m.	mouse	Protection from the homologous viruses [31]

Table 1. *Cont.*

SAM-MDNP	HA from A/WSN/33; i.m.	mouse	Protection from the homologous virus [32]
RNActive vaccine	HA from multiple antigenically distant influenza virus strains, NA and NP from A/Puerto Rico/8/34; i.d.	mouse ferret pig	Protection from homologous viruses and increased survival after heterologous virus challenge in mice, protection from heterologous virus in pigs [33]
Nucleoside-modified mRNA-LNP	HA from A/Jiangxi-Donghu/346/2013 (H10N8) and A/Anhui/1/2013 (H7N9); i.d., i.m.	mouse ferret NHP human	Protection from homologous virus in mice and ferrets, protective HAI titers in NHPs and humans [34]

* only studies where protective efficacy was reported are listed here. SAM: self-amplifying mRNA, LNP: lipid nanoparticle, CNE: cationic nanoemulsion, PEI: polyethylenimine, MDNP: modified dendrimer nanoparticle, NHP: non-human primate, HA: hemagglutinin, NP: nucleoprotein, NA: neuraminidase, M1: matrix protein 1, i.d.: intradermal, i.m.: intramuscular.

Table 2. Main characteristics of various influenza vaccine platforms.

Vaccine Platform against Influenza Virus	**Safety**	**Efficacy**	**Manufacturing**
mRNA vaccine	No risks of infection or integration of the vector. Controllable in vivo activity and degradation of mRNA by natural cellular processes. More human data is required to evaluate safety.	Limited efficacy data are available from clinical trials. mRNA vaccines induce immunological correlates of protection and protective effects similar or superior compared to licensed influenza vaccines in preclinical models.	mRNA vaccines are in vitro transcribed in a sterile process that does not require cell culture. The production time is short, the process is sequence-independent and potentially inexpensive and has been demonstrated to be scalable.
DNA vaccine	Good safety record in human studies. Theoretical risks of integration of the vector. Unable to revert to a pathogenic form.	Poor immunogenicity in humans when compared with traditional protein-based vaccines. Ability to induce both humoral and cellular responses. Provide immune priming but poor immune boosting.	Relatively inexpensive. Reproducible, large-scale production. Highly stable vaccines, and no cold chain is required. The production time is short, the process is sequence independent.
Virus-like particle	Influenza vaccines are in clinical development. Licensed vaccines exist for other targets (HBV, HPV) with excellent safety profile.	High effectiveness, and has the ability to induce long-lasting antibody responses.	The major challenge is to develop novel production platforms that overcome issues with current production systems to enable higher throughput at lower cost.
Inactivated virus vaccine	May require adjuvants (for example vaccines for avian strains) that can cause significant reactogenicity.	Cell-based inactivated vaccines are effective for seasonal strains. Pandemic vaccines require use of adjuvants. Good serum antibody responses, but less efficient in triggering mucosal IgA antibodies.	Currently, egg-derived vaccines are the most common in the influenza vaccine market. Cell-based vaccines have demonstrated improved immunogenicity against circulating strains, but manufacturing is challenging and expensive.
Live attenuated influenza virus vaccine	Theoretical risk of recombination with circulating wild-type influenza viruses. Risks of hospitalization and wheezing were increased in children younger than 2 years of age.	LAIV has the ability to induce both humoral and cellular responses. It provides immune priming but low antibody titers.	Only egg-derived vaccines are licensed for use in humans. Cell-based vaccine technologies are under development.

LAIV: live attenuated influenza vaccine

2. RNA Vaccines Against Influenza Virus—Vaccine Types, Preclinical and Clinical Data

Influenza virus infection is a major public health problem; thus, tremendous effort has been invested in improving current vaccines and creating new, more effective vaccines over the past decades. The need for a broadly protective/universal influenza virus vaccine, combined with the enormous infrastructure and research experience behind influenza virus research, and the relative ease of testing influenza virus vaccine efficacy in small animal models, have made it an optimal system for RNA vaccine development. Thus, influenza virus RNA vaccines (using IVT RNA) are among the most extensively studied infectious disease RNA vaccines, with studies dating back over 25 years (Table 1). Two major types of RNA vaccines have been developed against influenza virus: self-amplifying mRNA (SAM) vaccines and non-replicating mRNA vaccines (Table 3). SAM vaccines do not use modified nucleosides, while non-replicating mRNA vaccines can be made with or without the incorporation of various modified nucleosides. A great variety of lipid/carbohydrate-based carrier molecules have also been developed that enable highly efficacious in vivo RNA delivery.

Table 3. Advantages and disadvantages of non-replicating mRNA and SAM vaccines.

mRNA Vaccine Platform against Influenza Virus	Potency	Safety	Immunity against the Vector
Non-replicating mRNA	High level of protein translation requires a very efficient delivery system and relatively high doses.	Potent type I interferon response elicited by non-purified and unmodified mRNA can induce serious inflammation. Potential toxic effects may originate from the use of non-natural nucleotides and various delivery system components.	No theoretical risk of anti-vector immunity with non-viral delivery systems.
Self-amplifying mRNA	The auto-replicative ability of SAM enables the production of high levels of vaccine antigen in the host cells. Duration of protein expression from SAM molecules is enhanced.	Similarly to non-replicating unmodified and non-purified mRNA, SAM can induce high level of inflammation. Additionally, SAM-transfected cells likely die due to the continuous replication cycles. Use of a lower effective dose may be possible for SAM compared to non-replicating mRNA.	No anti-vector effect has been observed yet, but potential interactions between encoded non-structural proteins and host factors require additional investigation.

2.1. *Self-Amplifying Influenza Virus RNA Vaccines*

The majority of current SAM vaccines use a modified alphavirus genome that encodes the genes for the RNA replication machinery and the antigen of interest in the place of the viral structural protein-encoding genes [35,36]. The full-length RNA is ~9 kilobases long and can be synthetized by IVT from a DNA template. Importantly, the SAM platform enables a high level of immunogen production for extended duration from an exceptionally small dose of vaccine due to intracellular replication of the antigen-encoding RNA. An early study demonstrated that immunization with 10 μg of uncomplexed SAM vaccine encoding A/Puerto Rico/8/34 (H1N1) influenza virus hemagglutinin (HA) elicited antibody responses and partial protection from lethal homologous viral challenge in mice [11]. Hekele and colleagues developed SAM vaccines where the A/California/07/2009 (H1N1) or A/Shanghai/2/2013 (H7N9) influenza virus HA-encoding SAM was formulated in LNPs [37]. Small doses (0.1 or 1 μg) of HA SAM-LNPs induced protective levels of hemagglutination inhibition (HAI) titers after two intramuscular injections in mice. Magini and coworkers developed SAM-LNP vaccines encoding for the nucleoprotein (NP) and matrix protein 1 (M1) from the A/Puerto Rico/8/34 influenza virus [29]. Intramuscular administration of 0.1 or 0.2 μg of NP, M1 or combined NP+M1 SAM-LNP vaccine resulted in potent antigen-specific T cell responses and some level of protection from viral challenge. A seminal work demonstrated that intramuscular delivery of A/California/07/2009 HA-encoding SAM in an oil-in-water nanoemulsion elicited protection from homologous and heterologous (A/Puerto Rico/8/34) influenza virus challenge in mice and ferrets [30]. Influenza virus HA and NP replicon RNA complexed with chitosan-containing LNPs or polyethylenimine (PEI) has elicited T and B cell immune responses in mice after subcutaneous delivery [38,39]. Chahal and colleagues developed a delivery platform consisting of a chemically modified, ionizable dendrimer complexed into LNPs [32]. Using this platform, they demonstrated that intramuscular delivery of RNA replicons encoding A/WSN/33 (H1N1) influenza virus HA protected mice against lethal homologous virus challenge. In a recent study, Vogel and coworkers directly compared the immune responses and protective efficacy after SAM and non-replicating mRNA immunization in mice [31]. Animals were intramuscularly immunized two times with increasing doses of A/Puerto Rico/8/34 HA-encoding unformulated (naked) SAM or unmodified non-replicating mRNA and challenged eight weeks after the first vaccination. Both platforms induced protection against infection with the homologous virus. Of note, 64-fold lower dose (1.25 μg vs. 80 μg) of SAM than non-replicating mRNA generated an equal level of protection. Formulation of HA SAM with PEI significantly increased its efficacy and immunization with HA SAM from various influenza strains induced protection from matched viruses in mice. Immunization with a trivalent SAM vaccine containing HAs from A/California/07/2009 (H1N1), A/Hong Kong/1/68 (X31, H3N2) and B/Massachusetts/2/2012 protected animals from matched H1N1 and H3N2 virus infection. Protection from B/Massachusetts/2/2012 influenza virus was not tested because influenza B-specific antibody responses were inconsistent in mice. Finally, the authors demonstrated that a single immunization with 1.5 μg of PEI-formulated A/California/07/2009 HA SAM induced protection from the homologous virus.

In summary, several proof-of-concept studies have been published about the efficacy of SAM influenza virus vaccines in preclinical models (Table 1), but no published data from human trials using this vaccine format are available to date.

2.2. *Non-Replicating Influenza Virus mRNA Vaccines*

A substantial amount of research has been invested into the development of directly injectable non-replicating mRNA vaccines. The first study that demonstrated efficacy after vaccination with mRNA was published in 1993. This seminal work showed that administration of influenza virus NP-encoding mRNA complexed in liposomes induced cytotoxic T cell responses in mice [7]. Interestingly, the first publication that demonstrated protection from influenza virus challenge after mRNA vaccine delivery was published almost 20 years later [33]. Petsch and colleagues intradermally immunized mice, ferrets and pigs with various influenza virus HA, NP and NA-encoding RNActive vaccines (containing unmodified, purified, antigen-encoding and protamine-complexed mRNA [40]) that elicited protective immune responses even after a single immunization. The RNActive vaccine platform has demonstrated potency against various infectious pathogens in multiple preclinical models [33,41]. Kranz and colleagues took an unusual approach and performed intravenous immunizations in mice using A/Puerto Rico/8/34 influenza virus HA-encoding unmodified mRNA-lipid complexes and showed evidence of T cell activation after administration of a single dose [42].

Recently published, highly efficacious influenza virus mRNA vaccines use unmodified or nucleoside-modified full-length HA-encoding mRNAs encapsulated in a LNP carrier. The LNP component of the vaccine has previously been shown to be efficacious for siRNA delivery [43]. CureVac AG developed a sequence-engineered mRNA-LNP platform that enables a high level of in vivo protein translation without the use of modified nucleosides [44]. Using this platform, Lutz and colleagues demonstrated that a single intramuscular immunization with 10 μg of A/Netherlands/602/2009 (H1N1) HA-encoding mRNA-LNPs induced HAI titers in the protective range (≥1:40) in non-human primates (NHPs) [45]. Administration of a second dose potently boosted immune responses and resulted in HAI titers ≥1:160 for over a year in all vaccinated animals. Finally, they provided evidence that two immunizations (4 weeks apart) with mRNA-LNPs encoding for HA from A/Hong Kong/4801/2014 (H3N2) induced stronger T and B cell immune responses than the licensed MF59-adjuvanted trivalent inactivated influenza virus vaccine, Fluad.

Nucleoside-modified mRNA-LNP vaccines represent a new and highly efficacious category of RNA vaccines that can elicit protective immune responses against various pathogens [34,46–48]. Several recently published studies provided some insights into the mechanism of action of the nucleoside-modified mRNA-LNP vaccine platform and demonstrated its great ability to create a favorable cytokine/chemokine milieu that rapidly activates critical immune cells and induces potent immune responses after intramuscular or intradermal delivery [49–51]. A seminal study from Bahl and colleagues provided evidence that a single intradermal immunization with 10 µg of nucleoside-modified mRNA-LNPs encoding for HA from A/Jiangxi-Donghu/346/2013 (H10N8) or A/Anhui/1/2013 (H7N9) influenza viruses induced durable (>1 year) antibody responses in mice [34]. Furthermore, they showed that administration of a single dose of 0.4 µg of H7N9 HA mRNA-LNPs protected mice from a homologous lethal virus challenge and 10 µg of vaccine reduced lung viral titers in ferrets [34]. Both the H7 and H10 vaccine induced very high HAI titers (~1:10,000) in NHPs after two intradermal or intramuscular immunizations (three weeks apart) with 200–400 µg doses. Due to the promising preclinical results, a Phase I clinical trial (NCT03076385) using this platform was started and the interim analysis of a small cohort of subjects who received two intramuscular doses of LNP-formulated H10N8 HA-encoding nucleoside-modified mRNA was reported [34]. Thirty-one subjects were randomized into groups of 23 vaccinees and 8 saline placebo recipients. The vaccine regimen was 100 µg of mRNA-LNPs administered on day 1 and day 22 (same arm). The study is ongoing and will include a one-year post-vaccination follow up for safety and immunogenicity. In the interim analysis, 43 days after vaccination, no serious systemic adverse events were observed. Two of the subjects who received the vaccine had local reactions that were rated severe (erythema/induration >10 cm in diameter), while none were observed in the placebo group. Systemic reactogenicity was comparable in the vaccinee and placebo groups. Seroprotection (defined as percent of subjects that achieve a HAI titer ≥40 and MNT ≥20) was 100% by HAI and 87% by microneutralization titer (MNT) at day 43. Seroconversion by HAI was 78% (defined as percent of subjects with HAI baseline <10 and post-vaccination HAI ≥40) or 87% (defined as four-fold increase). The geometric mean HAI and MNT titers were increased by 10.6-fold and 7.7-fold, respectively. These results are encouraging in that a microgram-dose vaccine was consistently immunogenic and had an acceptable safety profile similar to other adjuvanted vaccines. Additionally, it is important to note that induction of antibodies for avian strains has proven to be very challenging in clinical trials with traditional protein antigen based vaccines as naïve individuals respond poorly to split virus vaccines containing H5 or H7 HAs [52–54].

3. Industrial Development of Influenza Virus RNA Vaccines—Global Players in the Field

RNA vaccines have recently received significant attention and attracted massive academic and industrial investment. A limited number of medium-size biotechnology companies have successfully raised capital to develop innovative RNA vaccines (Table 4 and discussed in [10]). Additionally, multiple Phase I and Phase II clinical trials with various RNA vaccines have been conducted to target cancer and infectious pathogens [10]. The first directly injectable infectious disease RNA vaccines that entered clinical trials were against rabies, Zika and influenza viruses [34,48,55]. Several other RNA vaccines are in preclinical development against a wide spectrum of pathogens, including HIV-1, RSV, HCMV and *Coxiella burnetii* [10,56]. Initiation of new clinical trials—including trials targeting influenza virus—is underway.

Table 4. Companies involved in RNA-based influenza virus vaccine development.

Company Name	Technology/Vaccine Platform	Development Phase
CureVac AG	Sequence-optimized, purified unmodified mRNA (RNActive, RNArt, RNAdjuvant)	Preclinical
Moderna Therapeutics	Nucleoside-modified mRNA	Phase 1
BioNTech Pharmaceuticals	Unspecified	Preclinical
eTheRNA Immunotherapies	Injectable TriMix-mRNA product	Preclinical
Vir Biotechnology	Unspecified	Unknown
EpiVax	T cell epitope vaccine	Preclinical

Currently, there is one ongoing influenza virus RNA vaccine trial reported on clinicaltrials.gov (NCT03076385) conducted by Moderna Therapeutics (Cambridge, MA, USA). Early results from this Phase I trial using nucleoside-modified mRNA-LNPs are discussed in Section 2.2. CureVac AG (Tübingen, Germany) has plans to initiate its first human seasonal influenza virus RNA vaccine trial, using unmodified mRNA-LNPs, in 2018. Moreover, they announced that an RNActive prophylactic vaccine for seasonal influenza virus will also be evaluated in a Phase I clinical trial in 2018 (www.curevac.com). Both CureVac and Moderna have invested in internal production capabilities. Expected in 2018, CureVac's "GMP III" facility will have the capacity to produce 10 million doses of GMP mRNA per year, while the commercial scale "GMP IV" facility is currently under construction and will be able to produce up to 30 million mRNA doses per year (www.curevac.com). The company envisions a "GMP V" facility that will be able to increase the capacity to 400 million doses per year (presented at the 5th mRNA Health Conference, Berlin, Germany). Other companies have also announced investments in developing RNA-based influenza virus vaccines; however, little is currently known about their research strategies (Table 4).

4. Considerations for Developing a Highly Effective Influenza Virus RNA Vaccine

Companies focused on developing RNA-based influenza vaccines aim to create a product that is superior to the currently available split (inactivated) or LAIV vaccines. Requirements for innovative, broadly protective influenza virus vaccines have been extensively discussed in the influenza vaccine scientific community [57] and the World Health Organization (WHO) has summarized the guidelines in a recent publication, titled Preferred Product Characteristics (PPCs) for Next-Generation Influenza Vaccine [58]. PPCs describe WHO's preferences for vaccine parameters, including the indications, target groups, immunization strategies, and clinical data for assessment of safety and efficacy. PPCs provide early guidance for the improvement of current influenza virus vaccines and the development of new vaccines, with five and ten-year time horizons (Table 5). The Target Product Profile (TPP) for each RNA vaccine should reflect these PPCs so that the corresponding development plan will meaningfully demonstrate the vaccine candidate's superior value. The PPC advisory group defined two strategic goals and preferred vaccine characteristics based on WHO's evaluation of the possible impact on public health. The first goal includes incremental vaccine improvements, such as greater protection against vaccine-matched or drifted influenza virus strains. The second goal aims at greater research and development advances towards vaccines providing broader protection against influenza virus disease (protection across groups or universal influenza virus vaccines) and increased duration of protection (at least five years).

Table 5. Summary of the WHO PPC document on next-generation influenza vaccines and relevant considerations for RNA vaccines.

Preferred Characteristics	Goal 1 (2022)	Goal 2 (2027)	RNA Vaccines
Indication	Prevention of severe influenza illness.	Prevention of severe laboratory-confirmed influenza illness caused by human influenza A virus infection.	Prevention of severe laboratory-confirmed influenza illness caused by human influenza A and B virus infection.
Target population	Children aged 6 weeks through 59 months.	Persons aged 6 weeks and older belonging to a group at high risk for severe influenza illness.	Age de-escalation studies need to be performed to demonstrate safety (for RNA and the formulating agent) in very young children.
Safety	Low level of reactogenicity may be acceptable if the vaccine prevents severe influenza illness.		Low level of reactogenicity can be accepted based on efficacy. Initial studies in humans have shown some reactogenicity.
Co-administration	Documented absence of clinically important interference with concomitantly administered vaccines.		Lack of interference with other vaccines must be demonstrated. Potentially achievable with RNA vaccines.
Duration of protection	>1 full year	>5 years	No human data is available but durable immune responses were observed in animal models, including non-human primates.
Outcome measure and efficacy	Better than standard efficacy (severe laboratory-confirmed influenza illness) for matched or drifted strains.	Better than standard efficacy (severe laboratory-confirmed influenza illness) for matched and drifted strains.	Expression of conserved or engineered antigens and potent, durable T and B cell immunity could lead to broadly protective vaccines.
Immunogenicity	Based on correlates of protection (if the correlates of protection against severe laboratory-confirmed influenza illness is identified for a specific class of influenza vaccine).		A correlate of protection for RNA vaccines has not been established yet, but they have the potential to generate superior cellular and humoral immune responses compared to licensed vaccines.

Currently used seasonal influenza vaccines show some level of protection against matched viruses but they offer little protection against drifted seasonal or pandemic viruses. A critical requirement for a new class of vaccine is to greatly improve efficacy and breadth of protection. Prophylactic RNA vaccines demonstrated heterologous protection in preclinical models (Table 1), but translation of this benefit to humans is uncertain and needs to be demonstrated with clinical data. Additionally, individual variations in immune responses to RNA vaccines need to be carefully investigated. The only candidate that has entered clinical development induced protective levels of HAI titers against the homologous virus strain [34], but evaluation of broad protection will require multi-year clinical-endpoint trials. A potential requirement for licensure of a novel RNA influenza vaccine could be the ability to prevent influenza virus disease over several years regardless of antigenic drift in a large-scale field trial. To demonstrate superiority over the conventional vaccine platforms, RNA vaccine candidates will need to be tested in head to head trials, and may be considered to be superior if they protect for longer durations and/or show protection against mismatched strains.

Large-scale efficacy trials are expensive, and thus, an early indication of the level of protection and cross-protection against drifted strains could be provided by Controlled Human Influenza Virus Infection Models (CHIVIM). The utility of such a challenge system for predicting vaccine effectiveness depends on the nature of the challenge virus, its infectious dose, and route of administration. Currently available challenge viruses (influenza H1N1 [59,60] and H3N2 [61]) were isolated four to eight years ago; therefore, finding highly susceptible adult subjects is difficult because of prior exposure.

Moreover, the challenge virus dose is large (e.g., $10^{5–7}$ PFU or $TCID_{50}$) and it is in a liquid suspension or large droplet spray that induce only an upper respiratory tract infection after administration into the nares [59–61]. This does not model the typical natural infection, in which an inhaled virus inoculum reaches the upper and lower respiratory tracts. These attributes of the current CHIVIM limit the generalizability of challenge trial outcomes, and restrict its suitability for testing broadly protective influenza countermeasures that are now entering early phase clinical development. Improved CHIVIM are needed to support the development of broadly protective influenza vaccines, including potent RNA vaccines. Ideal CHIVIM would use influenza virus strains to which young adults are susceptible and a suitable but low challenge dose to better mimic natural exposure.

Immune correlates of protection are invaluable in vaccine development as they minimize complexity, size and cost of clinical trials. While HAI titers are used as a correlate of protection against laboratory-confirmed influenza viruses, no correlates are available for severe disease outcome (or even for lower respiratory tract infection). Non-HA based vaccines or LAIV do not have a known correlate and need to rely on large-scale field efficacy trials. The most potent RNA vaccines induce very high HAI titers in small and large animals and HAI titers in the protective range in humans (discussed in Section 2). Some RNA vaccines have been shown to increase survival in a lethal challenge preclinical model, even in the absence of protective antibodies [34], which suggests that both the cellular and humoral immune responses contribute to RNA vaccine protection. CHIVIM that induce lower respiratory tract disease could be used to explore the correlation of pre-challenge immune measures with reduced risk of illness. This could be an approach to reduce the risk of large trials, and perhaps a pathway for accelerated approval of improved influenza vaccines.

Durability of protective immunity is also a critical consideration for influenza vaccines. The results of non-human primate studies [34,45] raise the possibility that RNA-based influenza vaccines may elicit more durable immune responses in humans compared to split virus or recombinant protein vaccines. Clinical studies have demonstrated that when naïve subjects are immunized with a vaccine that induces potent cellular immune responses such as LAIV, antibody titers could be boosted with an inactivated virus vaccine up to five years after the original LAIV prime [62]. Since some RNA vaccines have been shown to confer protection before antibodies reached protective titers [34], it would be tempting to test if prime-boost regimens using RNA as a prime would give similar results in preclinical models and humans.

The ultimate goal of an improved and broadly protective influenza virus vaccine is the prevention of influenza virus disease, especially among infants who are at increased risk for severe disease because their respiratory system is immature and they have little to no anti-influenza virus immune memory. This implies that improved vaccines should be indicated for children soon after birth, or not later than three to four months of age if maternal immunization is used to provide passive protection for the first three to four months of life. The lack of an indication for LAIV below two years of age due to increased risk of hospitalization and wheezing is a major limitation of LAIV [63]. RNA vaccines could potentially be evaluated in this patient population, particularly if they are shown to be well-tolerated with an acceptable safety profile in children age two and older. Of note, if RNA vaccines proved to be superior to currently licensed vaccines, a benefit-risk balance could be favorable despite some level of adverse events.

A high level of safety is a critical requirement for vaccines, particularly for those that are administered prophylactically to healthy individuals. RNA vaccine production does not require toxic materials or cell cultures that could be contaminated with viruses; thus, it circumvents the major risk factors associated with manufacturing of live virus, inactivated virus, protein subunit or viral vector-based platforms. Additionally, RNA does not have the ability to integrate into the host cell DNA, thus avoiding the risk of insertional mutagenesis. Potential adverse events such as fever can arise from the potent induction of type I interferons and proinflammatory cytokines by some RNA vaccines [64,65]. Moreover, the presence of extracellular RNA following vaccine administration could potentially raise safety concerns by contributing to formation of pathological thrombus or oedema [66,67]. Although various mRNA vaccine formats have proved to be safe and well tolerated in clinical trials (reviewed in [10]), continuous evaluation of safety of this new platform is critically important.

Due to the limitations of egg-based influenza vaccine production, new manufacturing technologies that do not use eggs to grow viruses have been actively investigated [68]. Vaccines that are produced in cell lines have several advantages, such as a lower risk of adverse events after vaccine administration to people with egg allergies, a sterile manufacturing process that eliminates the use of antibiotics, the absence of egg-adapted mutations, and most importantly, a potentially higher effectiveness [68]. Egg-adapted mutations in the sequence of HA have been associated with low vaccine effectiveness during the 2016–17 influenza season in the United States [26,27]. Zost and colleagues demonstrated that the loss of a glycosylation site by a mutation in the HA of the egg-adapted H3N2 vaccine strain resulted in poor neutralization of the circulating H3N2 viruses in vaccinated humans and ferrets [26]. On the contrary, H3 antigens expressed in the baculovirus-insect cell system did not contain the mutation, and, therefore humans vaccinated with these antigens generated potent neutralizing antibodies against the circulating H3N2 virus [26]. While recombinant protein production by the baculovirus-insect cell system has several critical advantages over egg-based vaccine production, improper glycosylation of HA antigens made by insect cells can be a potential limitation of this approach as reported in a recent study [69]. Vaccine production in mammalian cell lines such as Madin-Darby Canine Kidney (MDCK) cells or Vero cells resolves potential glycosylation issues and allows the production of large amounts of influenza vaccines under carefully controlled conditions, but they require complex and expensive infrastructure [68]. As a comparison, RNA vaccines are produced without the use of eggs or cell culture systems and properly folded and glycosylated mRNA-encoded proteins (vaccine antigens) are made by the host cells after vaccine administration, thus avoiding the risk of the production of incorrect antigens.

Finally, additional characteristics for a potent RNA vaccine would include considerations on WHO programmatic suitability. Optimal presentation, packaging, thermostability, formulation and disposal are some of the parameters that need to be achieved. WHO has published several documents on programmatic suitability [70] and these requirements should be considered early on during development. In principle, there are no barriers for an RNA influenza vaccine to meet these criteria, and could even be superior to existing vaccines, if, for example, needle-free administration and vaccine stability at ambient temperature could be achieved.

5. Conclusions and Future Directions

The past six to eight years brought a clear breakthrough in the fields of cancer and infectious disease RNA vaccines, demonstrating proof-of-concept in both preclinical and clinical settings [10]. Influenza virus RNA vaccines comprise the best-studied RNA vaccines to date. As discussed above, multiple vaccine formats have elicited potent influenza-virus specific, protective immune responses in various preclinical models (Table 1).

One of the biggest uncertainties of the field is the translatability of the promising animal data to humans. Encouraging early results from the first influenza virus RNA vaccine trial have been published [34]. Long term safety and immunogenicity data from this and other future trials are required to confidently judge the impact of RNA vaccines on the influenza virus vaccine field; thus the coming years will be critical for this new vaccine approach. The authors are optimistic and believe that one or more influenza virus RNA vaccine platform(s) will enter the clinic; however, it is possible that further significant optimization of the current vaccines will be required to decrease the cost of production and increase potency and safety.

There are multiple ways to improve the current influenza virus RNA vaccines. Here, we consider some of the possibilities. As discussed above, most influenza virus RNA vaccine studies used a single full-length HA as an immunogen. Immunization with antibody-accessible conserved influenza virus proteins such as the stalk domain of HA, various domains of NA, and the ectodomain of matrix protein 2 (M2e) has been shown to correlate well with protection in preclinical [71,72] and clinical settings [72,73]; thus it would be intriguing to include these antigens encoded as RNAs in multivalent RNA vaccines. Similarly to the conventional tri- and quadrivalent vaccines, RNA-encoded HAs from various antigenically distant influenza virus strains could be included in a single vaccine regimen to increase neutralization breadth (similarly to the recent study by Vogel and colleagues [31]). In fact, multivalency of RNA vaccines could be easily increased due to the simple manufacturing process and the same supply chain for each coding sequence. The use of optimized RNA-encoded influenza virus immunogens or more efficient immunization schemes (prime-boost) that can elicit favorable immune responses could also lead to more protective vaccines. Finally, addition of various adjuvants (traditional small molecules or RNAs encoding immune modulatory proteins) to RNA vaccines could also increase efficacy.

As discussed in several recent publications [4,57], an optimal broadly protective/universal influenza vaccine would confer durable protection from various antigenically distant (for example group 1 and group 2 influenza A and influenza B) viruses without causing severe adverse events after vaccine administration. Some RNA vaccines elicit durable influenza virus-specific immune responses in preclinical models, including non-human primates [34,45], and induce protection from heterologous influenza viruses [29,30,33] but protective efficacy across groups has not yet been reported. The production time of broadly protective/universal influenza vaccines should be relatively short (several weeks) which would allow for the protection of the majority of the population from disease caused by a newly emerging seasonal or pandemic virus. The flexibility of RNA vaccine immunogen design and short production time (without the use of eggs and cell culture) are critical advantages over currently approved influenza vaccines. Additionally, storage of all licensed influenza vaccines requires cold chain, while RNActive vaccines have been reported to be active after lyophilization and storage at 5–25 °C for 3 years and at 40 °C for six months [55] and development of mRNA-LNP vaccines that are stable at ambient temperature is underway (Arbutus Biopharma, personal communications).

Collectively, RNA-based vaccines represent a new vaccine class that can be used to effectively combat influenza virus. As noted, more data from clinical trials, including improved controlled human influenza virus infection models, and large-scale field efficacy trials will be critical to demonstrate the viability of this vaccine technology.

Acknowledgments: The authors thank Bruce Innis, Drew Weissman, Katalin Karikó, Michael J Hogan, Elinor Willis and Istvan Tombacz for valuable feedback on the manuscript.

Author Contributions: F.B.S. and N.P. wrote the manuscript and created the tables.

References

1. World Health Organization (WHO). Up to 650 000 People Die of Respiratory Diseases Linked to Seasonal Flu Each Year. Available online: http://www.who.int/mediacentre/news/releases/2017/seasonal-flu/en/ (accessed on 20 February 2018).
2. Andrews, S.F.; Graham, B.S.; Mascola, J.R.; McDermott, A.B. Is It Possible to Develop a "Universal" Influenza Virus Vaccine? Immunogenetic Considerations Underlying B-Cell Biology in the Development of a Pan-Subtype Influenza A Vaccine Targeting the Hemagglutinin Stem. *Cold Spring Harb. Perspect. Biol.* **2017**. [CrossRef] [PubMed]
3. Henry, C.; Palm, A.E.; Krammer, F.; Wilson, P.C. From Original Antigenic Sin to the Universal Influenza Virus Vaccine. *Trends Immunol.* **2018**, *39*, 70–79. [CrossRef] [PubMed]
4. Krammer, F.; Garcia-Sastre, A.; Palese, P. Is It Possible to Develop a "Universal" Influenza Virus Vaccine? Toward a Universal Influenza Virus Vaccine: Potential Target Antigens and Critical Aspects for Vaccine Development. *Cold Spring Harb. Perspect. Biol.* **2017**. [CrossRef] [PubMed]
5. Altman, M.O.; Angeletti, D.; Yewdell, J.W. Antibody Immunodominance: The Key to Understanding Influenza Virus Antigenic Drift. *Viral Immunol.* **2018**. [CrossRef] [PubMed]

6. Halasa, N.B.; Gerber, M.A.; Chen, Q.; Wright, P.F.; Edwards, K.M. Safety and immunogenicity of trivalent inactivated influenza vaccine in infants. *J. Infect. Dis.* **2008**, *197*, 1448–1454. [CrossRef] [PubMed]
7. Martinon, F.; Krishnan, S.; Lenzen, G.; Magné, R.; Gomard, E.; Guillet, J.G.; Lévy, J.P.; Meulien, P. Induction of virus-specific cytotoxic T lymphocytes in vivo by liposome-entrapped mRNA. *Eur. J. Immunol.* **1993**, *23*, 1719–1722. [CrossRef] [PubMed]
8. Boczkowski, D.; Nair, S.K.; Snyder, D.; Gilboa, E. Dendritic cells pulsed with RNA are potent antigen-presenting cells in vitro and in vivo. *J. Exp. Med.* **1996**, *184*, 465–472. [CrossRef] [PubMed]
9. Hoerr, I.; Obst, R.; Rammensee, H.G.; Jung, G. In vivo application of RNA leads to induction of specific cytotoxic T lymphocytes and antibodies. *Eur. J. Immunol.* **2000**, *30*, 1–7. [CrossRef]
10. Pardi, N.; Hogan, M.J.; Porter, F.W.; Weissman, D. mRNA vaccines—A new era in vaccinology. *Nat. Rev. Drug Discov.* **2018**, *17*, 261–279. [CrossRef] [PubMed]
11. Fleeton, M.N.; Chen, M.; Berglund, P.; Rhodes, G.; Parker, S.E.; Murphy, M.; Atkins, G.J.; Liljeström, P. Self-replicative RNA vaccines elicit protection against influenza A virus, respiratory syncytial virus, and a tickborne encephalitis virus. *J. Infect. Dis.* **2001**, *183*, 1395–1398. [CrossRef] [PubMed]
12. Pardi, N.; Muramatsu, H.; Weissman, D.; Kariko, K. In vitro transcription of long RNA containing modified nucleosides. *Methods Mol. Biol.* **2013**, *969*, 29–42. [PubMed]
13. Kariko, K.; Muramatsu, H.; Welsh, F.A.; Ludwig, J.; Kato, H.; Akira, S.; Weissman, D. Incorporation of pseudouridine into mRNA yields superior nonimmunogenic vector with increased translational capacity and biological stability. *Mol. Ther.* **2008**, *16*, 1833–1840. [CrossRef] [PubMed]
14. Gustafsson, C.; Govindarajan, S.; Minshull, J. Codon bias and heterologous protein expression. *Trends Biotechnol.* **2004**, *22*, 346–353. [CrossRef] [PubMed]
15. Weissman, D.; Pardi, N.; Muramatsu, H.; Kariko, K. HPLC purification of in vitro transcribed long RNA. *Methods Mol. Biol.* **2013**, *969*, 43–54. [PubMed]
16. Andries, O.; Mc Cafferty, S.; De Smedt, S.C.; Weiss, R.; Sanders, N.N.; Kitada, T. N(1)-methylpseudouridine-incorporated mRNA outperforms pseudouridine-incorporated mRNA by providing enhanced protein expression and reduced immunogenicity in mammalian cell lines and mice. *J. Control. Release* **2015**, *217*, 337–344. [CrossRef] [PubMed]
17. Kariko, K.; Buckstein, M.; Ni, H.; Weissman, D. Suppression of RNA recognition by Toll-like receptors: The impact of nucleoside modification and the evolutionary origin of RNA. *Immunity* **2005**, *23*, 165–175. [CrossRef] [PubMed]
18. Kariko, K.; Muramatsu, H.; Ludwig, J.; Weissman, D. Generating the optimal mRNA for therapy: HPLC purification eliminates immune activation and improves translation of nucleoside-modified, protein-encoding mRNA. *Nucleic Acids Res.* **2011**, *39*, e142. [CrossRef] [PubMed]
19. Ross, J.; Sullivan, T.D. Half-lives of beta and gamma globin messenger RNAs and of protein synthetic capacity in cultured human reticulocytes. *Blood* **1985**, *66*, 1149–1154. [PubMed]
20. Holtkamp, S.; Kreiter, S.; Selmi, A.; Simon, P.; Koslowski, M.; Huber, C.; Türeci, Ö.; Sahin, U. Modification of antigen-encoding RNA increases stability, translational efficacy, and T-cell stimulatory capacity of dendritic cells. *Blood* **2006**, *108*, 4009–4017. [CrossRef] [PubMed]
21. Martin, S.A.; Paoletti, E.; Moss, B. Purification of mRNA guanylyltransferase and mRNA (guanine-7-) methyltransferase from vaccinia virions. *J. Biol. Chem.* **1975**, *250*, 9322–9329. [PubMed]
22. Stepinski, J.; Waddell, C.; Stolarski, R.; Darzynkiewicz, E.; Rhoads, R.E. Synthesis and properties of mRNAs containing the novel "anti-reverse" cap analogs 7-methyl(3′-O-methyl)GpppG and 7-methyl (3′-deoxy)GpppG. *RNA* **2001**, *7*, 1486–1495. [PubMed]
23. Kauffman, K.J.; Webber, M.J.; Anderson, D.G. Materials for non-viral intracellular delivery of messenger RNA therapeutics. *J. Control. Release* **2016**, *240*, 227–234. [CrossRef] [PubMed]
24. Midoux, P.; Pichon, C. Lipid-based mRNA vaccine delivery systems. *Expert Rev. Vaccines* **2015**, *14*, 221–234. [CrossRef] [PubMed]
25. Medina, J.; Boukhebza, H.; De Saint Jean, A.; Sodoyer, R.; Legastelois, I.; Moste, C. Optimization of influenza A vaccine virus by reverse genetic using chimeric HA and NA genes with an extended PR8 backbone. *Vaccine* **2015**, *33*, 4221–4227. [CrossRef] [PubMed]

26. Zost, S.J.; Parkhouse, K.; Gumina, M.E.; Kim, K.; Perez, S.D.; Wilson, P.C.; Treanor, J.J.; Sant, A.J.; Cobey, S.; Hensley, S.E. Contemporary H3N2 influenza viruses have a glycosylation site that alters binding of antibodies elicited by egg-adapted vaccine strains. *Proc. Natl. Acad. Sci. USA* **2017**, *114*, 12578–12583. [CrossRef] [PubMed]
27. Wu, N.C.; Zost, S.J.; Thompson, A.J.; Oyen, D.; Nycholat, C.M.; McBride, R.; Paulson, J.C.; Hensley, S.E.; Wilson, I.A. A structural explanation for the low effectiveness of the seasonal influenza H3N2 vaccine. *PLoS Pathog.* **2017**, *13*, e1006682. [CrossRef] [PubMed]
28. Krammer, F.; Palese, P. Advances in the development of influenza virus vaccines. *Nat. Rev. Drug Discov.* **2015**, *14*, 167–182. [CrossRef] [PubMed]
29. Magini, D.; Giovani, C.; Mangiavacchi, S.; Maccari, S.; Cecchi, R.; Ulmer, J.B.; De Gregorio, E.; Geall, A.J.; Brazzoli, M.; Bertholet, S. Self-Amplifying mRNA Vaccines Expressing Multiple Conserved Influenza Antigens Confer Protection against Homologous and Heterosubtypic Viral Challenge. *PLoS ONE* **2016**, *11*, e0161193. [CrossRef] [PubMed]
30. Brazzoli, M.; Magini, D.; Bonci, A.; Buccato, S.; Giovani, C.; Kratzer, R.; Zurli, V.; Mangiavacchi, S.; Casini, D.; Brito, L.M.; et al. Induction of Broad-Based Immunity and Protective Efficacy by Self-amplifying mRNA Vaccines Encoding Influenza Virus Hemagglutinin. *J. Virol.* **2015**, *90*, 332–344. [CrossRef] [PubMed]
31. Vogel, A.B.; Lambert, L.; Kinnear, E.; Busse, D.; Erbar, S.; Reuter, K.C.; Wicke, L.; Perkovic, M.; Beissert, T.; Haas, H.; et al. Self-Amplifying RNA Vaccines Give Equivalent Protection against Influenza to mRNA Vaccines but at Much Lower Doses. *Mol. Ther.* **2017**, *26*, 446–455. [CrossRef] [PubMed]
32. Chahal, J.S.; Khan, O.F.; Cooper, C.L.; McPartlan, J.S.; Tsosie, J.K.; Tilley, L.D.; Sidik, S.M.; Lourido, S.; Langer, R.; Bavari, S.; et al. Dendrimer-RNA nanoparticles generate protective immunity against lethal Ebola, H1N1 influenza, and Toxoplasma gondii challenges with a single dose. *Proc. Natl. Acad. Sci. USA* **2016**, *113*, E4133–E4142. [CrossRef] [PubMed]
33. Petsch, B.; Schnee, M.; Vogel, A.B.; Lange, E.; Hoffmann, B.; Voss, D.; Schlake, T.; Thess, A.; Kallen, K.J.; Stitz, L.; et al. Protective efficacy of in vitro synthesized, specific mRNA vaccines against influenza A virus infection. *Nat. Biotechnol.* **2012**, *30*, 1210–1216. [CrossRef] [PubMed]
34. Bahl, K.; Senn, J.J.; Yuzhakov, O.; Bulychev, A.; Brito, L.A.; Hassett, K.J.; Laska, M.E.; Smith, M.; Almarsson, Ö.; Thompson, J.; et al. Preclinical and Clinical Demonstration of Immunogenicity by mRNA Vaccines against H10N8 and H7N9 Influenza Viruses. *Mol. Ther.* **2017**, *25*, 1316–1327. [CrossRef] [PubMed]
35. Perri, S.; Greer, C.E.; Thudium, K.; Doe, B.; Legg, H.; Liu, H.; Romero, R.E.; Tang, Z.; Bin, Q.; Dubensky, T.W.; et al. An alphavirus replicon particle chimera derived from venezuelan equine encephalitis and sindbis viruses is a potent gene-based vaccine delivery vector. *J. Virol.* **2003**, *77*, 10394–10403. [CrossRef] [PubMed]
36. Brito, L.A.; Kommareddy, S.; Maione, D.; Uematsu, Y.; Giovani, C.; Scorza, F.B.; Otten, G.R.; Yu, D.; Mandl, C.W.; Mason, P.W.; et al. Self-amplifying mRNA vaccines. *Adv. Genet.* **2015**, *89*, 179–233. [PubMed]
37. Hekele, A.; Bertholet, S.; Archer, J.; Gibson, D.G.; Palladino, G.; Brito, L.A.; Otten, G.R.; Brazzoli, M.; Buccato, S.; Bonci, A.; et al. Rapidly produced SAM® vaccine against H7N9 influenza is immunogenic in mice. *Emerg. Microbes Infect.* **2013**, *2*, e52. [CrossRef] [PubMed]
38. McCullough, K.C.; Bassi, I.; Milona, P.; Suter, R.; Thomann-Harwood, L.; Englezou, P.; Démoulins, T.; Ruggli, N. Self-replicating Replicon-RNA Delivery to Dendritic Cells by Chitosan-nanoparticles for Translation In Vitro and In Vivo. *Mol. Ther. Nucleic Acids* **2014**, *3*, e173. [CrossRef] [PubMed]
39. Démoulins, T.; Milona, P.; Englezou, P.C.; Ebensen, T.; Schulze, K.; Suter, R.; Pichon, C.; Midoux, P.; Guzmán, C.A.; Ruggli, N.; et al. Polyethylenimine-based polyplex delivery of self-replicating RNA vaccines. *Nanomedicine* **2016**, *12*, 711–722. [CrossRef] [PubMed]
40. Kallen, K.J.; Heidenreich, R.; Schnee, M.; Petsch, B.; Schlake, T.; Thess, A.; Baumhof, P.; Scheel, B.; Koch, S.D.; Fotin-Mleczek, M. A novel, disruptive vaccination technology: Self-adjuvanted RNActive® vaccines. *Hum. Vaccines Immunother.* **2013**, *9*, 2263–2276. [CrossRef] [PubMed]
41. Schnee, M.; Vogel, A.B.; Voss, D.; Petsch, B.; Baumhof, P.; Kramps, T.; Stitz, L. An mRNA Vaccine Encoding Rabies Virus Glycoprotein Induces Protection against Lethal Infection in Mice and Correlates of Protection in Adult and Newborn Pigs. *PLoS Negl. Trop. Dis.* **2016**, *10*, e0004746. [CrossRef] [PubMed]
42. Kranz, L.M.; Diken, M.; Haas, H.; Kreiter, S.; Loquai, C.; Reuter, K.C.; Meng, M.; Fritz, D.; Vascotto, F.; Hefesha, H.; et al. Systemic RNA delivery to dendritic cells exploits antiviral defence for cancer immunotherapy. *Nature* **2016**, *534*, 396–401. [CrossRef] [PubMed]

43. Kanasty, R.; Dorkin, J.R.; Vegas, A.; Anderson, D. Delivery materials for siRNA therapeutics. *Nat. Mater.* **2013**, *12*, 967–977. [CrossRef] [PubMed]
44. Thess, A.; Grund, S.; Mui, B.L.; Hope, M.J.; Baumhof, P.; Fotin-Mleczek, M.; Schlake, T. Sequence-engineered mRNA Without Chemical Nucleoside Modifications Enables an Effective Protein Therapy in Large Animals. *Mol. Ther.* **2015**, *23*, 1456–1464. [CrossRef] [PubMed]
45. Lutz, J.; Lazzaro, S.; Habbeddine, M.; Schmidt, K.E.; Baumhof, P.; Mui, B.L.; Tam, Y.K.; Madden, T.D.; Hope, M.J.; Heidenreich, R.; et al. Unmodified mRNA in LNPs constitutes a competitive technology for prophylactic vaccines. *NPJ Vaccines* **2017**, *2*, 29. [CrossRef] [PubMed]
46. Meyer, M.; Huang, E.; Yuzhakov, O.; Ramanathan, P.; Ciaramella, G.; Bukreyev, A. Modified mRNA-Based Vaccines Elicit Robust Immune Responses and Protect Guinea Pigs From Ebola Virus Disease. *J. Infect. Dis.* **2018**, *217*, 451–455. [CrossRef] [PubMed]
47. Pardi, N.; Hogan, M.J.; Pelc, R.S.; Muramatsu, H.; Andersen, H.; DeMaso, C.R.; Dowd, K.A.; Sutherland, L.L.; Scearce, R.M.; Parks, R.; et al. Zika virus protection by a single low-dose nucleoside-modified mRNA vaccination. *Nature* **2017**, *543*, 248–251. [CrossRef] [PubMed]
48. Richner, J.M.; Himansu, S.; Dowd, K.A.; Butler, S.L.; Salazar, V.; Fox, J.M.; Julander, J.G.; Tang, W.W.; Shresta, S.; Pierson, T.C.; et al. Modified mRNA Vaccines Protect against Zika Virus Infection. *Cell* **2017**, *168*, 1114–1125. [CrossRef] [PubMed]
49. Liang, F.; Lindgren, G.; Lin, A.; Thompson, E.A.; Ols, S.; Röhss, J.; John, S.; Hassett, K.; Yuzhakov, O.; Bahl, K.; et al. Efficient Targeting and Activation of Antigen-Presenting Cells In Vivo after Modified mRNA Vaccine Administration in Rhesus Macaques. *Mol. Ther.* **2017**, *25*, 2635–2647. [CrossRef] [PubMed]
50. Lin, A.; Liang, F.; Thompson, E.A.; Vono, M.; Ols, S.; Lindgren, G.; Hassett, K.; Salter, H.; Ciaramella, G.; Loré, K. Rhesus Macaque Myeloid-Derived Suppressor Cells Demonstrate T Cell Inhibitory Functions and Are Transiently Increased after Vaccination. *J. Immunol.* **2018**, *200*, 286–294. [CrossRef] [PubMed]
51. Lindgren, G.; Ols, S.; Liang, F.; Thompson, E.; Lin, A.; Hellgren, F.; Bahl, K.; John, S.; Yuzhakov, O.; Hassett, K.; et al. Induction of Robust B Cell Responses after Influenza mRNA Vaccination Is Accompanied by Circulating Hemagglutinin-Specific ICOS+ PD-1+ CXCR3+ T Follicular Helper Cells. *Front. Immunol.* **2017**, *8*, 1539. [CrossRef] [PubMed]
52. Berlanda Scorza, F. Advancing new vaccines against pandemic influenza in low-resource countries. *Vaccine* **2017**, *35*, 5397–5402. [CrossRef] [PubMed]
53. Keitel, W.A.; Campbell, J.D.; Treanor, J.J.; Walter, E.B.; Patel, S.M.; He, F.; Noah, D.L.; Hill, H. Safety and immunogenicity of an inactivated influenza A/H5N1 vaccine given with or without aluminum hydroxide to healthy adults: Results of a phase I-II randomized clinical trial. *J. Infect. Dis.* **2008**, *198*, 1309–1316. [CrossRef] [PubMed]
54. Wong, S.S.; DeBeauchamp, J.; Zanin, M.; Sun, Y.; Tang, L.; Webby, R. H5N1 influenza vaccine induces a less robust neutralizing antibody response than seasonal trivalent and H7N9 influenza vaccines. *NPJ Vaccines* **2017**, *2*, 16. [CrossRef] [PubMed]
55. Alberer, M.; Gnad-Vogt, U.; Hong, H.S.; Mehr, K.T.; Backert, L.; Finak, G.; Gottardo, R.; Bica, M.A.; Garofano, A.; Koch, S.D.; et al. Safety and immunogenicity of a mRNA rabies vaccine in healthy adults: An open-label, non-randomised, prospective, first-in-human phase 1 clinical trial. *Lancet* **2017**, *390*, 1511–1520. [CrossRef]
56. Mass General News. Mass. Available online: http://www.massgeneral.org/News/pressrelease.aspx?id=1816 (accessed on 20 February 2018).
57. Paules, C.I.; Marston, H.D.; Eisinger, R.W.; Baltimore, D.; Fauci, A.S. The Pathway to a Universal Influenza Vaccine. *Immunity* **2017**, *47*, 599–603. [CrossRef] [PubMed]
58. World Health Organization (WHO). *WHO Preferred Product Characteristics for Next-Generation Influenza Vaccines*. Available online: http://www.who.int/immunization/documents/ISBN_978-92-4-151246-6/en/ (accessed on February 20 2018).
59. Memoli, M.J.; Czajkowski, L.; Reed, S.; Athota, R.; Bristol, T.; Proudfoot, K.; Fargis, S.; Stein, M.; Dunfee, R.L.; Shaw, P.A.; et al. Validation of the wild-type influenza A human challenge model H1N1pdMIST: An A(H1N1)pdm09 dose-finding investigational new drug study. *Clin. Infect. Dis.* **2015**, *60*, 693–702. [CrossRef] [PubMed]

60. Watson, J.M.; Francis, J.N.; Mesens, S.; Faiman, G.A.; Makin, J.; Patriarca, P.; Treanor, J.J.; Georges, B.; Bunce, C.J. Characterisation of a wild-type influenza (A/H1N1) virus strain as an experimental challenge agent in humans. *Virol. J.* **2015**, *12*, 13. [CrossRef] [PubMed]
61. Fullen, D.J.; Noulin, N.; Catchpole, A.; Fathi, H.; Murray, E.J.; Mann, A.; Eze, K.; Balaratnam, G.; Borley, D.W.; Gilbert, A.; et al. Accelerating Influenza Research: Vaccines, Antivirals, Immunomodulators and Monoclonal Antibodies. The Manufacture of a New Wild-Type H3N2 Virus for the Human Viral Challenge Model. *PLoS ONE* **2016**, *11*, e0145902.
62. Talaat, K.R.; Luke, C.J.; Khurana, S.; Manischewitz, J.; King, L.R.; McMahon, B.A.; Karron, R.A.; Lewis, K.D.; Qin, J.; Follmann, D.A.; et al. A live attenuated influenza A(H5N1) vaccine induces long-term immunity in the absence of a primary antibody response. *J. Infect. Dis.* **2014**, *209*, 1860–1869. [CrossRef] [PubMed]
63. U.S. Food and Drug Administration (FDA). Available online: https://www.fda.gov/downloads/biologicsbloodvaccines/vaccines/approvedproducts/ucm294307.pdf (accessed on 20 February 2018).
64. Edwards, D.K.; Jasny, E.; Yoon, H.; Horscroft, N.; Schanen, B.; Geter, T.; Fotin-Mleczek, M.; Petsch, B.; Wittman, V. Adjuvant effects of a sequence-engineered mRNA vaccine: Translational profiling demonstrates similar human and murine innate response. *J. Transl. Med.* **2017**, *15*, 1. [CrossRef] [PubMed]
65. Pepini, T.; Pulichino, A.M.; Carsillo, T.; Carlson, A.L.; Sari-Sarraf, F.; Ramsauer, K.; Debasitis, J.C.; Maruggi, G.; Otten, G.R.; Geall, A.J.; et al. Induction of an IFN-mediated antiviral response by a self-amplifying RNA vaccine: Implications for vaccine design. *J. Immunol.* **2017**, *198*, 4012–4024. [CrossRef] [PubMed]
66. Kannemeier, C.; Shibamiya, A.; Nakazawa, F.; Trusheim, H.; Ruppert, C.; Markart, P.; Song, Y.; Tzima, E.; Kennerknecht, E.; Niepmann, M.; et al. Extracellular RNA constitutes a natural procoagulant cofactor in blood coagulation. *Proc. Natl. Acad. Sci. USA* **2007**, *104*, 6388–6393. [CrossRef] [PubMed]
67. Fischer, S.; Gerriets, T.; Wessels, C.; Walberer, M.; Kostin, S.; Stolz, E.; Zheleva, K.; Hocke, A.; Hippenstiel, S.; Preissner, K.T. Extracellular RNA mediates endothelial-cell permeability via vascular endothelial growth factor. *Blood* **2007**, *110*, 2457–2465. [CrossRef] [PubMed]
68. Settembre, E.C.; Dormitzer, P.R.; Rappuoli, R. Bringing influenza vaccines into the 21st century. *Hum. Vaccines Immunother.* **2014**, *10*, 600–604. [CrossRef]
69. An, Y.; Rininger, J.A.; Jarvis, D.L.; Jing, X.; Ye, Z.; Aumiller, J.J.; Eichelberger, M.; Cipollo, J.F. Comparative Glycomics Analysis of Influenza Hemagglutinin (H5N1) Produced in Vaccine Relevant Cell Platforms. *J. Proteome Res.* **2013**, *12*, 3707–3720. [CrossRef] [PubMed]
70. World Health Organization (WHO). Assessing the Programmatic Suitability of Vaccine Candidates for WHO Prequalification. Available online: http://apps.who.int/iris/handle/10665/76537 (accessed on 20 February 2018).
71. Schotsaert, M.; Ysenbaert, T.; Smet, A.; Schepens, B.; Vanderschaeghe, D.; Stegalkina, S.; Vogel, T.U.; Callewaert, N.; Fiers, W.; Saelens, X. Long-Lasting Cross-Protection Against Influenza A by Neuraminidase and M2e-based immunization strategies. *Sci. Rep.* **2016**, *6*, 24402. [CrossRef] [PubMed]
72. Krammer, F. Novel universal influenza virus vaccine approaches. *Curr. Opin. Virol.* **2016**, *17*, 95–103. [CrossRef] [PubMed]
73. Monto, A.S.; Petrie, J.G.; Cross, R.T.; Johnson, E.; Liu, M.; Zhong, W.; Levine, M.; Katz, J.M.; Ohmit, S.E. Antibody to Influenza Virus Neuraminidase: An Independent Correlate of Protection. *J. Infect. Dis.* **2015**, *212*, 1191–1199. [CrossRef] [PubMed]

3

MicroRNA-Attenuated Virus Vaccines

Elizabeth J. Fay [1,2] **and Ryan A. Langlois** [1,2,3,*]

1 Biochemistry, Molecular Biology, and Biophysics Graduate Program, University of Minnesota, Minneapolis, MN 55455, USA; fayxx084@umn.edu
2 Center for Immunology, University of Minnesota, Minneapolis, MN 55455, USA
3 Department of Microbiology and Immunology, University of Minnesota, Minneapolis, MN 55455, USA
* Correspondence: langlois@umn.edu

Abstract: Live-attenuated vaccines are the most effective way to establish robust, long-lasting immunity against viruses. However, the possibility of reversion to wild type replication and pathogenicity raises concerns over the safety of these vaccines. The use of host-derived microRNAs (miRNAs) to attenuate viruses has been accomplished in an array of biological contexts. The broad assortment of effective tissue- and species-specific miRNAs, and the ability to target a virus with multiple miRNAs, allow for targeting to be tailored to the virus of interest. While escape is always a concern, effective strategies have been developed to improve the safety and stability of miRNA-attenuated viruses. In this review, we discuss the various approaches that have been used to engineer miRNA-attenuated viruses, the steps that have been taken to improve their safety, and the potential use of these viruses as vaccines.

Keywords: live-attenuated vaccine; RNAi; siRNA

---

1. Introduction

MicroRNAs (miRNAs) are short RNAs that bind with partial complementarity to mRNAs to inhibit translation of their target. miRNAs are transcribed by Pol II and form a secondary hairpin structure that is initially processed in the nucleus by the RNase III enzyme Drosha. Following nuclear export, additional processing is completed by a second RNase III enzyme, Dicer. The miRNA is then loaded into the multi-protein RNA-induced silencing complex (RISC), which mediates mRNA decay and translational inhibition. miRNA bind to target mRNAs through the seed sequence, nucleotides 2–8 on the 5′ end of the miRNA, resulting in translation repression of ~2 fold. However, perfect complementarity can result in target mRNA cleavage and significant enhancement of repression. In rare cases of binding with perfect complementarity between miRNA-mRNA sequences, mRNA cleavage will be induced. In eukaryotes, miRNAs are essential regulators of mRNA expression during development and fine tune translation to control other diverse cellular processes [1].

Plants and invertebrates use miRNAs for gene regulation, but also have a separate, partially overlapping antiviral defense mechanism, RNA interference (RNAi). Similar to miRNAs, small interfering RNA (siRNA) processing is carried out by Dicer and siRNAs are loaded into RISC, although in many organisms, there are generally separate versions of these proteins for each pathway. In these species, the processing of long, double-stranded viral RNA and miRNA processing are carried out by separate Dicer proteins, but share components of other steps of the RNAi pathway [2,3]. As an antiviral mechanism, silencing through RNAi is achieved by producing virus-derived siRNAs that bind with perfect complementarity to the target viral sequence. While small virus-derived RNAs have been identified in mammalian cells following infection [4], siRNAs are not the primary antiviral mechanism in mammals [5,6]. However, while not naturally antiviral, the miRNA pathway can be experimentally coopted to repress virus replication. Importantly, miRNA and siRNA function through the same mechanisms in mammalian cells, suggesting that miRNAs could be exploited to be antiviral [7]. This has been achieved by inserting perfectly complementary target sites for the miRNA into the viral gene of interest, effectively turning the miRNA into an siRNA. Tissue- and species-specific miRNAs have been exploited to control virus replication in a myriad of biological contexts, including to improve the safety of oncolytic viruses by attenuating the virus in non-tumor tissues [8–11] and to attain tissue-specific expression of virus-derived transgenes or to limit the immune response against the transgene for gene therapy [12–14]. These studies have demonstrated the ability of engineered miRNA targeting to control virus replication in vitro and in vivo.

Vaccines have been highly successful at limiting viral infections and have led to the elimination of smallpox from the human population [15]. There are four main classes of viral vaccines: killed, subunit, mRNA, and live-attenuated. Live-attenuated vaccines have several advantages, including providing more robust, long-lasting immunity compared to inactivated vaccines [16]. Viruses can be attenuated through several different mechanisms, including altering the temperature of the optimal polymerase function and deleting or mutating viral immune antagonists. However, some effective attenuation strategies result in poor immunogenicity, limiting their use as a vaccine. Mechanisms of attenuation may not be identical across viral species. For example, the mechanism of temperature sensitivity will vary from virus to virus. Additionally, safety is a major concern when developing any live-attenuated vaccine, where reversion to wild type replication could be devastating [16]. miRNAs have been used as a platform to develop live-attenuated vaccines for DNA and both positive and negative sense RNA viruses by exploiting host endogenous miRNAs. The broad array of cell- and species-specific miRNAs, as well as the ability to target using multiple miRNAs, allow for customizable attenuation for different viruses. A major advantage of this strategy is that this provides a known mechanism of attenuation, which can be applied across a diverse range of viruses. In this review, we will discuss the approaches for generating miRNA-targeted viruses and several strategies for improving the safety and efficacy of miRNA-attenuated vaccines.

2. MicroRNA-Attenuated Vaccines

2.1. Mechanisms of MicroRNA Targeting of Viruses

Endogenous miRNA targeting primarily occurs at the three prime untranslated region (3′ UTR) of host mRNA transcripts [17]. However, many viral RNAs contain short 3′ UTRs, potentially as an evolutionary mechanism to evade miRNA regulation. There are two ways that viruses can be engineered to be sensitive to miRNAs: through the generation of silent mutations in the open reading frame to be complementary to the cognate miRNA or by inserting complete target sites into the endogenous or engineered UTRs. Some locations in the viral genome may not be amenable to miRNA machinery access due to the secondary RNA structure or binding of viral proteins, and therefore cannot be used to attenuate virus replication [18]. West Nile virus has been engineered to encode miRNA target sites between RNA secondary structures in the 3′ UTR to allow miRNA access and to prevent disruption of the important RNA structures [19]. These results demonstrate that care must be taken in choosing genomic sites for miRNA targeting. In addition to the location within a gene, engineered miRNA-mediated repression can be affected by the choice of viral gene being silenced. Targeting an essential gene can completely disrupt virus replication, while the targeting of a non-essential gene can prevent pathology but allow for the expression of some viral products, which may be necessary to produce a robust adaptive immune response. Reversion to virulence is a concern for all live-attenuated vaccines, including miRNA-targeted vaccines. Escape from miRNA targeting, as well as strategies to mitigate this risk, are discussed in a later section of this review.

Some DNA viruses naturally encode miRNAs to regulate the viral replication life cycle and control host gene expression [20–22]. RNA viruses have thus far been found to be devoid of this regulatory mechanism (with the notable exception of some retroviruses [23–26]). However, both positive and negative sense RNA viruses can be engineered to express a functional miRNA [27–31], which can be further exploited to generate self-attenuating viruses. Inserting an artificial miRNA with perfect sequence complementarity to nucleoprotein as an intron in the nonstructural gene segment created a self-attenuating influenza virus [32]. This strategy resulted in highly attenuated replication in vivo, even in the absence of a type I interferon response. Work from another group demonstrated that this self-attenuating virus could be used as a protective influenza virus vaccine [33]. However, as discussed in more detail below, the major drawback to this strategy is rapid escape from attenuation through loss of the artificial miRNA [32].

2.2. Species-, Tissue-, and Cell-Specific MicroRNA Targeting of Viruses

In a landmark study, Landgraf et al. developed an atlas of miRNA expression in a variety of cell types and tissues from mice and humans [34]. This study demonstrated that while the majority of miRNAs are broadly expressed, there are several whose expression is restricted to particular cell types, lineages, or tissues [34]. However, different tissue- or host-specific miRNAs may not repress viral gene expression equally, and the level of attenuation is of critical importance when designing a miRNA-attenuated vaccine. For example, three different central nervous system (CNS)-specific miRNAs effectively attenuated a targeted flavivirus in vitro, but only two were able to prevent pathogenesis and death in vivo [35]. This suggests that the presence of a miRNA alone cannot always predict target efficacy. One potential explanation for this is that endogenous targets for a miRNA can act as sponges, reducing the functional amount of a miRNA within a cell. Furthermore, it has been suggested that 100–1000 miRNAs need to be present in the cell for at least 6 h after infection to repress engineered miRNA sensitive virus replication [32]. Using a fluorescence-based screening approach, Mullokandov et al. were able to determine the functional repression capacity of endogenous miRNAs in a variety of cell types [36], and this platform can be used to screen for effective miRNAs for attenuated vaccines. One potential area of concern is altered miRNA expression during virus infection. Many acute RNA viruses replicate rapidly and the life cycle may be shorter than the time needed to upregulate sufficient quantities of antiviral miRNAs [37]. However, infections with a number of viruses have demonstrated changes in the overall pattern of miRNA expression. Therefore, infection-specific changes in miRNA expression should be considered, particularly for viruses with the capacity for latency. Overall, the capacity of a miRNA to repress targeted virus replication is difficult to predict based on small RNA abundance alone. Consideration of other factors and experimental validation in the relevant cells and systems are critical.

One strategy for the generation of a live-attenuated vaccine using miRNAs is to target the virus only in cells or tissues that underlie pathogenesis for that infection. Targeting tick-borne encephalitis virus or dengue virus using a CNS-specific miRNA limited neuropathogenesis in mice, while preserving immunogenicity [38]. Importantly, neutralizing antibodies could be generated following the inoculation of non-human primates with the targeted virus [38]. Similar results were obtained for Japanese encephalitis virus [39] and West Nile virus [19]. Muscle-specific miRNA-targeted Coxsackie B virus displayed reduced cardiopathology and generated a strong protective immune response [40]. In these examples, viral infection could still occur peripherally, including in antigen presenting cells, which potentially allows for the increased generation of adaptive immune responses. Influenza virus has a broad tropism and is able to replicate in both epithelial and immune cells [41]. Using a hematopoietic-specific miRNA to block influenza virus replication in immune cells still resulted in robust activation of CD8 T cells [42]. Because antigen presenting cells could not be directly infected, these data suggest that exogenous antigen acquisition and cross-presentation are sufficient to generate anti-influenza cell-mediated immunity. These studies suggest that blocking pathogenic replication, but allowing replication in other cells, is sufficient to generate robust antiviral immunity.

Many viruses that cause disease in humans also replicate in or are transmitted through non-human species. Continued replication or recombination of miRNA-attenuated vaccine strains in these species could result in the loss of miRNA target sites and reversion to a wild type strain, which could lead to the spread of the pathogenic virus to other hosts. It is therefore critical that vaccines that are attenuated in humans are also blunted in these zoonotic reservoirs. Attenuation of viruses using multiple species-specific miRNAs can improve the safety of live-attenuated vaccines. Mosquito-specific and tick-specific miRNAs have been used in combination with CNS-specific miRNAs to attenuate flaviviruses in the natural vectors and prevent the escape of vaccine strains [19,35,43] (Figure 1A). While there is a diverse array of tissue- and host-specific miRNAs, patterns of miRNA expression are not always perfectly tailored to the desired application. To circumvent this, Waring et al. eliminated a eukaryotic ubiquitously expressed miRNA, miR-21, from MDCK cells to allow for the growth of a targeted influenza virus [44]. This virus was attenuated in eukaryotic hosts, including avian and human cells and in mice [44] (Figure 1B). This approach allowed for a species universal attenuated vaccine, which provided robust protection upon lethal challenge in mice. This study also provides a platform for molecular biocontainment to prevent the spread of engineered influenza virus into human or zoonotic reservoirs, while still allowing for experimental analyses in cell lines lacking the cognate miRNA.

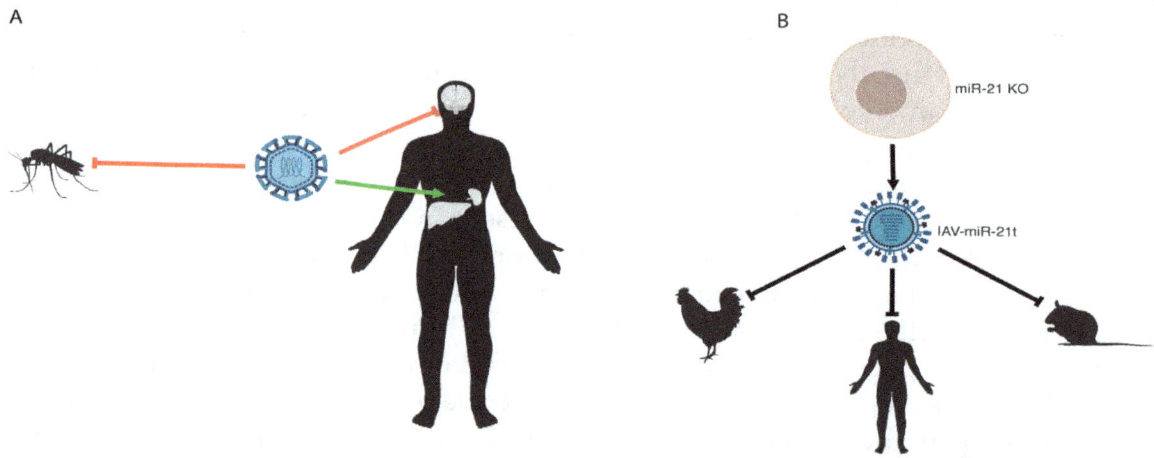

Figure 1. Tissue- and species-specific microRNA-attenuated viruses. (**A**) Model of tissue-specific attenuation of a flavivirus combined with attenuation in an insect vector. (**B**) Model depicting generation of a miRNA-attenuated influenza A virus in miRNA knock out cells to generate a species-universal attenuated vaccine. Created with BioRender (Toronto, ON, Canada).

As discussed above, miRNA targeting can be used to restrict a virus such that it can only replicate in the necessary viral amplification platform. Influenza viruses, including those used for vaccines, are grown to a high titer in embryonated chicken eggs. To generate influenza virus vaccines that could be grown in eggs but would be attenuated in mammals, Perez et al. screened the small miRNAs in avian and mammalian cells and found several that were absent in eggs but present in mammals. Using one of these, miR-93, they generated a vaccine that could replicate in eggs but was attenuated in mice [45]. Importantly, this vaccine provided robust protection upon challenge with lethal influenza strains. Species-specific attenuation can also be used to enhance safety when working with pathogenic viruses in the laboratory through molecular biocontainment. miR-192 is present in human lung, but absent from ferret lung. Targeting the influenza virus with miR-192 allowed for experimentation in ferrets without the concern for human infection [46]. Together, these studies demonstrate the plasticity in using cell- and species-specific miRNAs to control virus replication for the generation of live-attenuated vaccines.

2.3. *Immunogenicity of MicroRNA-Attenuated Viruses*

One concern with any live attenuated vaccine strategy is that replication will be reduced to a point where the immune response to the virus is severely compromised, resulting in insufficient protection from secondary infection. It is therefore important to characterize the innate and adaptive immune responses to miRNA-attenuated viruses. Benitez et al. found that a miRNA-targeted influenza virus induced the expression of a myriad of interferon-stimulated genes in mice, suggesting that the robust attenuation of the virus still allowed activation of the innate immune response [32]. In another influenza study, a miRNA-attenuated vaccine generated high anti-influenza A virus antibody titers in mice, despite the lack of detectable virus replication, and an equivalent dose of UV-killed virus failed to induce protection [44]. Similar results have been shown for attenuated flavivirus and enterovirus, where miRNA-mediated attenuation prevented disease, but still allowed for the generation of a protective adaptive immune response [38–40,44]. In the event that a virus is attenuated to the point where it is poorly immunogenic, there are strategies to improve immunogenicity. For example, increasing the starting inoculum can raise antibody titers while still preventing pathogenesis [19]. miRNA-mediated attenuation could potentially allow for increased inoculums compared to other live attenuated vaccine strategies as a strategy to increase immunogenicity. As has been shown for influenza virus, targeting different genes can result in differential attenuation, and targeting multiple genes can improve attenuation over targeting single genes [44]. If targeting an essential gene fails to induce sufficient immunity, this strategy of customizable attenuation using miRNAs can be employed to achieve appropriate levels of replication to generate an immune response without causing disease. Altogether, these studies demonstrate that miRNA-attenuation can prevent pathogenesis of the virus while still initiating an immune response that results in protection from secondary infections.

2.4. Escape from MicroRNA Targeting

Replication in the presence of the cognate miRNA applies selective pressure for the potential mutation or complete loss of miRNA target sites. Reduced targeting is a major concern when designing miRNA-attenuated vaccines. A single let-7 target site in poliovirus can accumulate escape mutations as early as 24 h post infection, restoring the full replicative potential of the virus [47]. Additionally, a single nucleotide mutation in a miRNA target site can restore the neurovirulence of a targeted flavivirus [38]. One way to mitigate escape is to engineer multiple target sites into the virus. Targeting only the 3′ UTR of Langat virus resulted in escape after multiple replication cycles due to the deletion of miRNA target sites, but when multiple genomic loci were targeted, miRNA target sites were retained and the virus did not escape [35]. Another study using influenza virus demonstrated that even reducing perfect complementarity from 20 base pairs to 16 base pairs did not result in escape when two target sites were inserted [32], further illustrating the benefit of multiple sites. Additionally, targeting multiple segments of influenza virus increased attenuation from segments that resulted in poor attenuation individually [44], demonstrating the power of combinatorial targeting. In addition to using multiple target sites for the same miRNA, enhanced viral repression can be achieved using multiple different miRNAs, and this strategy can be more effective at attenuating than multiple sites for the same miRNA [43]. However, studies still need to be done to determine how the order of miRNA target sites impacts the efficiency of each individual site within a multi-targeting cassette. A self-attenuating influenza virus engineered to express an artificial miRNA targeting its own genome also demonstrated escape. However, this occurred through deletions in the hairpin, not in the miRNA target site [32], indicating that endogenous target sites are not readily amenable to escape mutations, likely because viral genomic sequences are highly conserved. This is in contrast to engineered target sites where, for example, Dengue virus completely lost miRNA target sequences after infection in vivo [48]. While multiple target sites can improve safety and are likely necessary for designing safe miRNA-attenuated vaccines, additional strategies may be required to overcome viral escape through the loss of target sites.

Several alterations in the viral genome have improved the stability and efficacy of miRNA-mediated attenuation of flaviviruses and other viruses. One way that this has been achieved is by targeting only the artificially duplicated 5′ regulatory region of the Langat virus capsid RNA, leaving the optimized coding region intact. This method of targeting was more effective than targeting the viral 3′ UTR. Additionally, insertions in the duplicated 5′ region mitigated the risk of homologous recombination between the duplicated region and the coding region, improving the stability of the miRNA target sites [49]. This group also combined this strategy with insertion of the encephalomyocarditis virus internal ribosomal entry site (IRES) upstream of the capsid gene. This reduced the abundance of the capsid protein and caused general attenuation of the virus. Combining IRES-mediated attenuation with miRNA targeting improved the stability and effectiveness of miRNA attenuation compared to miRNA targeting alone [50]. This clever strategy also mitigated the risk of mutation in insect vectors, as RNA translation from the encephalomyocarditis virus IRES is inhibited in insect cells and the virus was therefore unable to replicate [51] (Figure 2A). While targeting the 3′ UTR is effective, the secondary RNA structure in this region may block miRNA targeting. Additionally, some viral UTRs contain packaging signals that need to remain intact to successfully incorporate viral genomes into the virion. Duplicating the 3′ UTR, which was done to insert miRNA target sites into influenza virus genes [42,44,46], retains the necessary packaging information and may allow for a linear single stranded targeting region, enhancing the efficiency of repression (Figure 2B). Dengue virus completely lost miRNA target sequences after infection in vivo [48], suggesting that genomic alterations may be necessary to produce a safe, stable miRNA-attenuated Dengue virus vaccine. While the strategies described above have been successful, genomic changes may need to be tailored for use in other viruses. Together, these data illustrate that increasing the number of target sites and engineering alterations to the virus genome can improve miRNA-mediated repression and mitigate the risk of escape.

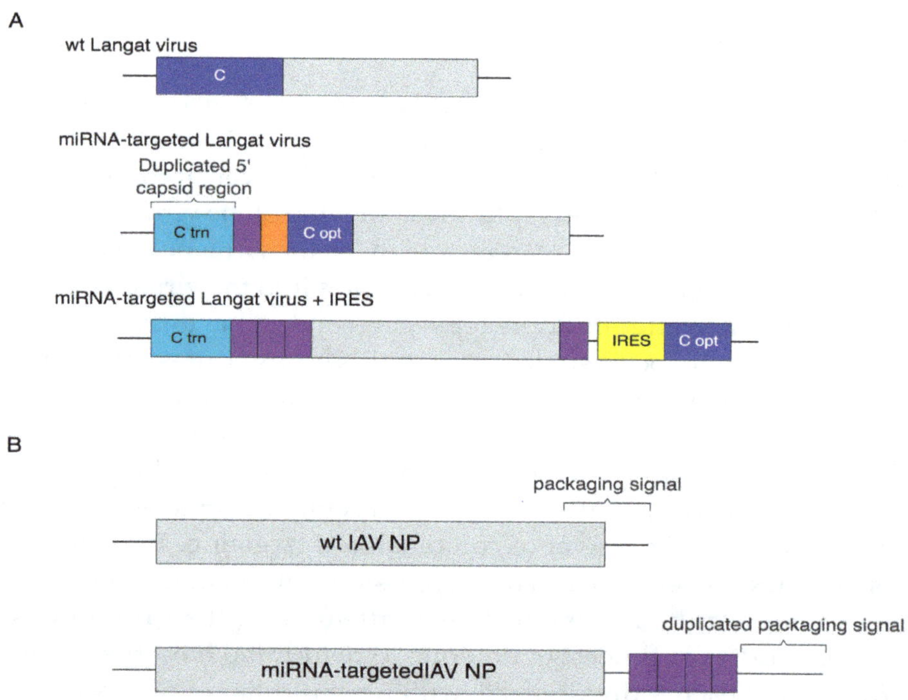

Figure 2. Altered viral genome structures to improve miRNA targeting. (**A**) Model of the wild type Langat virus genome, highlighting the capsid gene (top), the miRNA-targeted (purple) duplicated 5′ region followed by a 2A site (orange) to allow for expression of the codon-optimized capsid protein (middle), and the insertion of an IRES to regulate the expression of the capsid protein (bottom). (**B**) The wild type influenza virus NP gene (top) and the miRNA-targeted (purple) NP gene with a duplicated packaging signal (bottom). Created with BioRender (Toronto, ON, Canada).

2.5. Viral Suppressors of MicroRNAs

RNAi is the primary antiviral defense mechanism in many non-vertebrate species. Therefore, viruses that infect these hosts have evolved mechanisms to evade this response. Most plant viruses encode a protein that inhibits some component of the antiviral RNAi pathway [2]. Similarly, many invertebrate viruses encode a suppressor of RNAi, including suppressors of Dicer and RISC proteins [52–56]. Viruses that infect both invertebrates and mammals may possess these immune evasion mechanisms, and because the miRNA and RNAi pathways share many of the same components, virus proteins that target common elements would impact miRNA-mediated attenuation. Strikingly, arboviruses, which infect arthropods and mammals, do not appear to express viral suppressors of RNAi, despite being susceptible to the arthropod antiviral RNAi response [57]. However, West Nile virus may evade RNAi by positive selection for point mutations that prevent targeting [58]. Several DNA viruses are capable of suppressing miRNAs. For example, the poxvirus protein VP55, an essential component of the viral polyA polymerase, can additionally non-specifically polyadenylate miRNAs, resulting in their eventual destruction [59]. Adenoviruses inhibit both the nuclear export of miRNAs, as well as Dicer function [60]. There are several reports of influenza NS1 blocking RNAi. However we, and others, have shown that miRNAs can attenuate targeted influenza, even in the presence of increased NS1 expression [32,42,45,46,61,62]. These studies indicate that not all viruses can be candidates for miRNA-mediated attenuation unless steps are taken to cripple miRNA suppressive viral genes.

While mammalian viruses do not appear to express suppressors of RNAi, there may be mechanisms that indirectly inhibit the miRNA targeting of viruses. Induction of the interferon response in the presence of virus replication has been shown to inhibit miRNA function via poly-ADP-ribosylation of Ago2, an essential component of RISC [63]. This could reduce miRNA-mediated attenuation during vaccination/infection and provide a window for escape. The inhibition of RNAi by the interferon response suggests that these are not compatible systems and that miRNAs are not an effective intrinsic antiviral strategy in mammals. Furthermore, the absence of miRNAs from a cell did not hinder the replication of a variety of viruses, suggesting that miRNAs are not a potent natural antiviral defense mechanism for the host [64,65]. The lack of a mammalian antiviral RNAi system suggests that mammalian viruses would not need to evolve suppressors of this pathway, further supporting the ability to experimentally coopt miRNA targeting for safe and effective virus attenuation.

3. Conclusions

miRNA-mediated attenuation has been achieved for many viruses in many hosts. Several strategies have been employed that have improved the safety, stability, and efficacy of miRNA-mediated attenuation for the purpose of generating live-attenuated vaccines. The utility of miRNA targeting of viruses extends beyond vaccines and can be used for gene therapy and oncolytic virotherapy, and this strategy could be extended to non-viral pathogens by using viral vectors. Overall, miRNA targeting is a promising platform for developing safe, effective vaccines and provides increased plasticity over traditional live-attenuated vaccine strategies.

Author Contributions: E.J.F. and R.A.L. performed literature searches and wrote the manuscript. E.J.F. designed the models. R.A.L. edited the final version of the manuscript.

Acknowledgments: We wish to thank Stephen Rice for critical reading of this manuscript.

References

1. Bartel, D.P. Metazoan MicroRNAs. *Cell* **2018**, *173*, 20–51. [CrossRef] [PubMed]
2. Szittya, G.; Burgyan, J. RNA interference-mediated intrinsic antiviral immunity in plants. In *Intrinsic Immunity*; Cullen, B., Ed.; Springer: Berlin/Heidelberg, Germany, 2013; Volume 371, pp. 153–181.
3. Nayak, A.; Tassetto, M.; Kunitomi, M.; Andino, R. RNA interference-mediated intrinsic antiviral immunity in invertebrates. In *Intrinsic Immunity*; Cullen, B., Ed.; Springer: Berlin/Heidelberg, Germany, 2013; Volume 371, pp. 183–200.
4. Parameswaran, P.; Sklan, E.; Wilkins, C.; Burgon, T.; Samuel, M.A.; Lu, R.; Ansel, K.M.; Heissmeyer, V.; Einav, S.; Jackson, W.; et al. Six RNA viruses and forty-one hosts: Viral small RNAs and modulation of small RNA repertoires in vertebrate and invertebrate systems. *PLoS Pathog.* **2010**, *6*, e1000764. [CrossRef] [PubMed]
5. tenOever, B.R. Questioning antiviral RNAi in mammals. *Nat. Microbiol.* **2017**, *2*, 17052. [CrossRef] [PubMed]
6. Cullen, B.R.; Cherry, S.; tenOever, B.R. Is RNA interference a physiologically relevant innate antiviral immune response in mammals? *Cell Host Microbe* **2013**, *14*, 374–378. [CrossRef] [PubMed]

7. Zeng, Y.; Yi, R.; Cullen, B.R. MicroRNAs and small interfering RNAs can inhibit mRNA expression by similar mechanisms. *Proc. Natl. Acad. Sci. USA* **2003**, *100*, 9779–9784. [CrossRef] [PubMed]
8. Kelly, E.J.; Hadac, E.M.; Greiner, S.; Russell, S.J. Engineering microRNA responsiveness to decrease virus pathogenicity. *Nat. Med.* **2008**, *14*, 1278–1283. [CrossRef] [PubMed]
9. Kelly, E.J.; Nace, R.; Barber, G.N.; Russell, S.J. Attenuation of vesicular stomatitis virus encephalitis through microRNA targeting. *J. Virol.* **2010**, *84*, 1550–1562. [CrossRef] [PubMed]
10. Ruiz, A.J.; Hadac, E.M.; Nace, R.A.; Russell, S.J. MicroRNA-detargeted mengovirus for oncolytic virotherapy. *J. Virol.* **2016**, *90*, 4078–4092. [CrossRef] [PubMed]
11. Edge, R.E.; Falls, T.J.; Brown, C.W.; Lichty, B.D.; Atkins, H.; Bell, J.C. A let-7 MicroRNA-sensitive vesicular stomatitis virus demonstrates tumor-specific replication. *Mol. Ther.* **2008**, *16*, 1437–1443. [CrossRef] [PubMed]
12. Brown, B.D.; Venneri, M.A.; Zingale, A.; Sergi Sergi, L.; Naldini, L. Endogenous microRNA regulation suppresses transgene expression in hematopoietic lineages and enables stable gene transfer. *Nat. Med.* **2006**, *12*, 585–591. [CrossRef] [PubMed]
13. Suzuki, T.; Sakurai, F.; Nakamura, S.; Kouyama, E.; Kawabata, K.; Kondoh, M.; Yagi, K.; Mizuguchi, H. miR-122a-regulated expression of a suicide gene prevents hepatotoxicity without altering antitumor effects in suicide gene therapy. *Mol. Ther.* **2008**, *16*, 1719–1726. [CrossRef] [PubMed]
14. Xie, J.; Xie, Q.; Zhang, H.; Ameres, S.L.; Hung, J.H.; Su, Q.; He, R.; Mu, X.; Seher Ahmed, S.; Park, S.; et al. MicroRNA-regulated, systemically delivered rAAV9: A step closer to CNS-restricted transgene expression. *Mol. Ther.* **2011**, *19*, 526–535. [CrossRef] [PubMed]
15. Henderson, D.A. Smallpox eradication. *Public Health Rep.* **1980**, *95*, 422–426. [PubMed]
16. Lauring, A.S.; Jones, J.O.; Andino, R. Rationalizing the development of live attenuated virus vaccines. *Nat. Biotechnol.* **2010**, *28*, 573–579. [CrossRef] [PubMed]
17. Bartel, D.P. MicroRNAs: Target recognition and regulatory functions. *Cell* **2009**, *136*, 215–233. [CrossRef] [PubMed]
18. Gismondi, M.I.; Ortiz, X.P.; Curra, A.P.; Asurmendi, S.; Taboga, O. Artificial microRNAs as antiviral strategy to FMDV: Structural implications of target selection. *J. Virol. Methods* **2014**, *199*, 1–10. [CrossRef] [PubMed]
19. Brostoff, T.; Pesavento, P.A.; Barker, C.M.; Kenney, J.L.; Dietrich, E.A.; Duggal, N.K.; Bosco-Lauth, A.M.; Brault, A.C. MicroRNA reduction of neuronal West Nile virus replication attenuates and affords a protective immune response in mice. *Vaccine* **2016**, *34*, 5366–5375. [CrossRef] [PubMed]
20. Sullivan, C.S.; Grundhoff, A.T.; Tevethia, S.; Pipas, J.M.; Ganem, D. SV40-encoded microRNAs regulate viral gene expression and reduce susceptibility to cytotoxic T cells. *Nature* **2005**, *435*, 682–686. [CrossRef] [PubMed]
21. Umbach, J.L.; Kramer, M.F.; Jurak, I.; Karnowski, H.W.; Coen, D.M.; Cullen, B.R. MicroRNAs expressed by herpes simplex virus 1 during latent infection regulate viral mRNAs. *Nature* **2008**, *454*, 780–783. [CrossRef] [PubMed]
22. Gottwein, E.; Mukherjee, N.; Sachse, C.; Frenzel, C.; Majoros, W.H.; Chi, J.T.; Braich, R.; Manoharan, M.; Soutschek, J.; Ohler, U.; et al. A viral microRNA functions as an orthologue of cellular miR-155. *Nature* **2007**, *450*, 1096–1099. [CrossRef] [PubMed]
23. Kincaid, R.P.; Burke, J.M.; Sullivan, C.S. RNA virus microRNA that mimics a B-cell oncomiR. *Proc. Natl. Acad. Sci. USA* **2012**, *109*, 3077–3082. [CrossRef] [PubMed]
24. Burke, J.M.; Bass, C.R.; Kincaid, R.P.; Sullivan, C.S. Identification of tri-phosphatase activity in the biogenesis of retroviral microRNAs and RNAP III-generated shRNAs. *Nucleic Acids Res.* **2014**, *42*, 13949–13962. [CrossRef] [PubMed]
25. Whisnant, A.W.; Kehl, T.; Bao, Q.; Materniak, M.; Kuzmak, J.; Lochelt, M.; Cullen, B.R. Identification of novel, highly expressed retroviral microRNAs in cells infected by bovine foamy virus. *J. Virol.* **2014**, *88*, 4679–4686. [CrossRef] [PubMed]
26. Kincaid, R.P.; Chen, Y.; Cox, J.E.; Rethwilm, A.; Sullivan, C.S. Noncanonical microRNA (miRNA) biogenesis gives rise to retroviral mimics of lymphoproliferative and immunosuppressive host miRNAs. *mBio* **2014**, *5*, e00074. [CrossRef] [PubMed]
27. Shapiro, J.S.; Langlois, R.A.; Pham, A.M.; tenOever, B.R. Evidence for a cytoplasmic microprocessor of pri-miRNAs. *RNA* **2012**, *18*, 1338–1346. [CrossRef] [PubMed]

28. Langlois, R.A.; Shapiro, J.S.; Pham, A.M.; tenOever, B.R. In vivo delivery of cytoplasmic RNA virus-derived miRNAs. *Mol. Ther.* **2012**, *20*, 367–375. [CrossRef] [PubMed]
29. Rouha, H.; Thurner, C.; Mandl, C.W. Functional microRNA generated from a cytoplasmic RNA virus. *Nucleic Acids Res.* **2010**, *38*, 8328–8337. [CrossRef] [PubMed]
30. Shapiro, J.S.; Varble, A.; Pham, A.M.; tenOever, B.R. Noncanonical cytoplasmic processing of viral microRNAs. *RNA* **2010**, *16*, 2068–2074. [CrossRef] [PubMed]
31. Varble, A.; Chua, M.A.; Perez, J.T.; Manicassamy, B.; Garcia-Sastre, A.; tenOever, B.R. Engineered RNA viral synthesis of microRNAs. *Proc. Natl. Acad. Sci. USA* **2010**, *107*, 11519–11524. [CrossRef] [PubMed]
32. Benitez, A.A.; Spanko, L.A.; Bouhaddou, M.; Sachs, D.; tenOever, B.R. Engineered Mammalian RNAi Can Elicit Antiviral Protection that Negates the Requirement for the Interferon Response. *Cell Rep.* **2015**, *13*, 1456–1466. [CrossRef] [PubMed]
33. Li, J.; Arevalo, M.T.; Diaz-Arevalo, D.; Chen, Y.; Choi, J.G.; Zeng, M. Generation of a safe and effective live viral vaccine by virus self-attenuation using species-specific artificial microRNA. *J. Control. Release* **2015**, *207*, 70–76. [CrossRef] [PubMed]
34. Landgraf, P.; Rusu, M.; Sheridan, R.; Sewer, A.; Iovino, N.; Aravin, A.; Pfeffer, S.; Rice, A.; Kamphorst, A.O.; Landthaler, M.; et al. A mammalian microRNA expression atlas based on small RNA library sequencing. *Cell* **2007**, *129*, 1401–1414. [CrossRef] [PubMed]
35. Tsetsarkin, K.A.; Liu, G.; Kenney, H.; Hermance, M.; Thangamani, S.; Pletnev, A.G. Concurrent micro-RNA mediated silencing of tick-borne flavivirus replication in tick vector and in the brain of vertebrate host. *Sci. Rep.* **2016**, *6*, 33088. [CrossRef] [PubMed]
36. Mullokandov, G.; Baccarini, A.; Ruzo, A.; Jayaprakash, A.D.; Tung, N.; Israelow, B.; Evans, M.J.; Sachidanandam, R.; Brown, B.D. High-throughput assessment of microRNA activity and function using microRNA sensor and decoy libraries. *Nat. Methods* **2012**, *9*, 840–846. [CrossRef] [PubMed]
37. Tenoever, B.R. RNA viruses and the host microRNA machinery. *Nat. Rev. Microbiol.* **2013**, *11*, 169–180. [CrossRef] [PubMed]
38. Heiss, B.L.; Maximova, O.A.; Pletnev, A.G. Insertion of microRNA targets into the flavivirus genome alters its highly neurovirulent phenotype. *J. Virol.* **2011**, *85*, 1464–1472. [CrossRef] [PubMed]
39. Yen, L.C.; Lin, Y.L.; Sung, H.H.; Liao, J.T.; Tsao, C.H.; Su, C.M.; Lin, C.K.; Liao, C.L. Neurovirulent flavivirus can be attenuated in mice by incorporation of neuron-specific microRNA recognition elements into viral genome. *Vaccine* **2013**, *31*, 5915–5922. [CrossRef] [PubMed]
40. He, F.; Yao, H.; Wang, J.; Xiao, Z.; Xin, L.; Liu, Z.; Ma, X.; Sun, J.; Jin, Q.; Liu, Z. Coxsackievirus B3 engineered to contain microRNA targets for muscle-specific microRNAs displays attenuated cardiotropic virulence in mice. *J. Virol.* **2015**, *89*, 908–916. [CrossRef] [PubMed]
41. Fiege, J.K.; Langlois, R.A. Investigating influenza a virus infection: Tools to track infection and limit tropism. *J. Virol.* **2015**, *89*, 6167–6170. [CrossRef] [PubMed]
42. Langlois, R.A.; Varble, A.; Chua, M.A.; Garcia-Sastre, A.; tenOever, B.R. Hematopoietic-specific targeting of influenza A virus reveals replication requirements for induction of antiviral immune responses. *Proc. Natl. Acad. Sci. USA* **2012**, *109*, 12117–12122. [CrossRef] [PubMed]
43. Tsetsarkin, K.A.; Liu, G.; Kenney, H.; Bustos-Arriaga, J.; Hanson, C.T.; Whitehead, S.S.; Pletnev, A.G. Dual miRNA targeting restricts host range and attenuates neurovirulence of flaviviruses. *PLoS Pathog.* **2015**, *11*, e1004852. [CrossRef] [PubMed]
44. Waring, B.M.; Sjaastad, L.E.; Fiege, J.K.; Fay, E.J.; Reyes, I.; Moriarity, B.; Langlois, R.A. MicroRNA-based attenuation of influenza virus across susceptible hosts. *J. Virol.* **2017**, *92*, e01741-17. [CrossRef]
45. Perez, J.T.; Pham, A.M.; Lorini, M.H.; Chua, M.A.; Steel, J.; tenOever, B.R. MicroRNA-mediated species-specific attenuation of influenza A virus. *Nat. Biotechnol.* **2009**, *27*, 572–576. [CrossRef] [PubMed]
46. Langlois, R.A.; Albrecht, R.A.; Kimble, B.; Sutton, T.; Shapiro, J.S.; Finch, C.; Angel, M.; Chua, M.A.; Gonzalez-Reiche, A.S.; Xu, K.; et al. MicroRNA-based strategy to mitigate the risk of gain-of-function influenza studies. *Nat. Biotechnol.* **2013**, *31*, 844–847. [CrossRef] [PubMed]
47. Vignuzzi, M.; Wendt, E.; Andino, R. Engineering attenuated virus vaccines by controlling replication fidelity. *Nat. Med.* **2008**, *14*, 154–161. [CrossRef] [PubMed]
48. Pham, A.M.; Langlois, R.A.; Tenoever, B.R. Replication in cells of hematopoietic origin is necessary for Dengue virus dissemination. *PLoS Pathog.* **2012**, *8*, e1002465. [CrossRef] [PubMed]

49. Tsetsarkin, K.A.; Liu, G.; Shen, K.; Pletnev, A.G. Kissing-loop interaction between 5′ and 3′ ends of tick-borne Langat virus genome 'bridges the gap' between mosquito- and tick-borne flaviviruses in mechanisms of viral RNA cyclization: Applications for virus attenuation and vaccine development. *Nucleic Acids Res.* **2016**, *44*, 3330–3350. [CrossRef] [PubMed]
50. Tsetsarkin, K.A.; Liu, G.; Volkova, E.; Pletnev, A.G. Synergistic Internal Ribosome Entry Site/MicroRNA-Based Approach for Flavivirus Attenuation and Live Vaccine Development. *mBio* **2017**, *8*, e02326-16. [CrossRef] [PubMed]
51. Woolaway, K.E.; Lazaridis, K.; Belsham, G.J.; Carter, M.J.; Roberts, L.O. The 5′ untranslated region of Rhopalosiphum padi virus contains an internal ribosome entry site which functions efficiently in mammalian, plant, and insect translation systems. *J. Virol.* **2001**, *75*, 10244–10249. [CrossRef] [PubMed]
52. Chao, J.A.; Lee, J.H.; Chapados, B.R.; Debler, E.W.; Schneemann, A.; Williamson, J.R. Dual modes of RNA-silencing suppression by Flock House virus protein B2. *Nat. Struct. Mol. Biol.* **2005**, *12*, 952–957. [CrossRef] [PubMed]
53. Van Rij, R.P.; Saleh, M.C.; Berry, B.; Foo, C.; Houk, A.; Antoniewski, C.; Andino, R. The RNA silencing endonuclease Argonaute 2 mediates specific antiviral immunity in Drosophila melanogaster. *Genes Dev.* **2006**, *20*, 2985–2995. [CrossRef] [PubMed]
54. Nayak, A.; Berry, B.; Tassetto, M.; Kunitomi, M.; Acevedo, A.; Deng, C.; Krutchinsky, A.; Gross, J.; Antoniewski, C.; Andino, R. Cricket paralysis virus antagonizes Argonaute 2 to modulate antiviral defense in Drosophila. *Nat. Struct. Mol. Biol.* **2010**, *17*, 547–554. [CrossRef] [PubMed]
55. Qi, N.; Zhang, L.; Qiu, Y.; Wang, Z.; Si, J.; Liu, Y.; Xiang, X.; Xie, J.; Qin, C.F.; Zhou, X.; et al. Targeting of dicer-2 and RNA by a viral RNA silencing suppressor in Drosophila cells. *J. Virol.* **2012**, *86*, 5763–5773. [CrossRef] [PubMed]
56. van Mierlo, J.T.; Bronkhorst, A.W.; Overheul, G.J.; Sadanandan, S.A.; Ekstrom, J.O.; Heestermans, M.; Hultmark, D.; Antoniewski, C.; van Rij, R.P. Convergent evolution of argonaute-2 slicer antagonism in two distinct insect RNA viruses. *PLoS Pathog.* **2012**, *8*, e1002872. [CrossRef] [PubMed]
57. Blair, C.D. Mosquito RNAi is the major innate immune pathway controlling arbovirus infection and transmission. *Future Microbiol.* **2011**, *6*, 265–277. [CrossRef] [PubMed]
58. Brackney, D.E.; Beane, J.E.; Ebel, G.D. RNAi targeting of West Nile virus in mosquito midguts promotes virus diversification. *PLoS Pathog.* **2009**, *5*, e1000502. [CrossRef] [PubMed]
59. Backes, S.; Shapiro, J.S.; Sabin, L.R.; Pham, A.M.; Reyes, I.; Moss, B.; Cherry, S.; tenOever, B.R. Degradation of host microRNAs by poxvirus poly(A) polymerase reveals terminal RNA methylation as a protective antiviral mechanism. *Cell Host Microbe* **2012**, *12*, 200–210. [CrossRef] [PubMed]
60. Lu, S.; Cullen, B.R. Adenovirus VA1 noncoding RNA can inhibit small interfering RNA and MicroRNA biogenesis. *J. Virol.* **2004**, *78*, 12868–12876. [CrossRef] [PubMed]
61. Li, H.; Bradley, K.C.; Long, J.S.; Frise, R.; Ashcroft, J.W.; Hartgroves, L.C.; Shelton, H.; Makris, S.; Johansson, C.; Cao, B.; et al. Internal genes of a highly pathogenic H5N1 influenza virus determine high viral replication in myeloid cells and severe outcome of infection in mice. *PLoS Pathog.* **2018**, *14*, e1006821. [CrossRef] [PubMed]
62. Tundup, S.; Kandasamy, M.; Perez, J.T.; Mena, N.; Steel, J.; Nagy, T.; Albrecht, R.A.; Manicassamy, B. Endothelial cell tropism is a determinant of H5N1 pathogenesis in mammalian species. *PLoS Pathog.* **2017**, *13*, e1006270. [CrossRef] [PubMed]
63. Seo, G.J.; Kincaid, R.P.; Phanaksri, T.; Burke, J.M.; Pare, J.M.; Cox, J.E.; Hsiang, T.Y.; Krug, R.M.; Sullivan, C.S. Reciprocal inhibition between intracellular antiviral signaling and the RNAi machinery in mammalian cells. *Cell Host Microbe* **2013**, *14*, 435–445. [CrossRef] [PubMed]
64. Bogerd, H.P.; Whisnant, A.W.; Kennedy, E.M.; Flores, O.; Cullen, B.R. Derivation and characterization of Dicer- and microRNA-deficient human cells. *RNA* **2014**, *20*, 923–937. [CrossRef] [PubMed]
65. Backes, S.; Langlois, R.A.; Schmid, S.; Varble, A.; Shim, J.V.; Sachs, D.; Tenoever, B.R. The Mammalian response to virus infection is independent of small RNA silencing. *Cell Rep.* **2014**, *8*, 114–125. [CrossRef] [PubMed]

4

Virus-Like Particles and Nanoparticles for Vaccine Development against HCMV

Michela Perotti [1,2] and Laurent Perez [1,3,*]

1 Faculty of Biomedical Sciences, Institute for Research in Biomedicine, Università della Svizzera Italiana, 6500 Bellinzona, Switzerland; michela.perotti@irb.usi.ch
2 Institute of Microbiology, ETH Zürich, 8093 Zürich, Switzerland
3 European Virus Bioinformatics Center, 07743 Jena, Germany
* Correspondence: laurent.perez@irb.usi.ch

Abstract: Human cytomegalovirus (HCMV) infects more than 70% of the human population worldwide. HCMV is responsible for high morbidity and mortality in immunocompromised patients and remains the leading viral cause of congenital birth defects. Despite considerable efforts in vaccine and therapeutic development, HCMV infection still represents an unmet clinical need and a life-threatening disease in immunocompromised individuals and newborns. Immune repertoire interrogation of HCMV seropositive patients allowed the identification of several potential antigens for vaccine design. However, recent HCMV vaccine clinical trials did not lead to a satisfactory outcome in term of efficacy. Therefore, combining antigens with orthogonal technologies to further increase the induction of neutralizing antibodies could improve the likelihood of a vaccine to reach protective efficacy in humans. Indeed, presentation of multiple copies of an antigen in a repetitive array is known to drive a more robust humoral immune response than its soluble counterpart. Virus-like particles (VLPs) and nanoparticles (NPs) are powerful platforms for multivalent antigen presentation. Several self-assembling proteins have been successfully used as scaffolds to present complex glycoprotein antigens on their surface. In this review, we describe some key aspects of the immune response to HCMV and discuss the scaffolds that were successfully used to increase vaccine efficacy against viruses with unmet medical need.

Keywords: HCMV; cytomegalovirus; VLP; nanoparticle; vaccine; immune response

---

1. Introduction

Human cytomegalovirus (HCMV) is a ubiquitously distributed member of the *Herpesviridae* family belonging to the *Betaherpesvirinae* sub-family; it infects 70% of the human adult population worldwide [1,2] and primary infection is usually asymptomatic in immunocompetent individuals. Nevertheless, the virus establishes a lifelong latency of the host after a primary infection and viral reactivation is common, also it does not necessarily imply clinical symptoms [1,3]. However, infection or viral reactivation in immunodeficient individuals such as AIDS patients, solid organ (SOT) or hematopoietic stem cells (HSCT) transplant patients causes morbidity and mortality [4,5]. Furthermore, HCMV is the most common viral cause of congenital birth defects affecting 0.7% of the newborns with permanent sequelae such as sensorineural hearing loss, growth restriction, and cognitive disabilities [6]. Current antiviral therapies and transfusion with hyper-immune globulins to control viremia are not efficient [7]. Therefore, given the severity and importance of these diseases, as well as the associated socioeconomic cost, the need for an HCMV vaccine has been assigned in the highest priority category by the Institute of Medicine and it represents the second highest priority target after HIV by the Centers for Disease Control [8,9]. Over the last decades, considerable efforts were deployed to develop a vaccine capable of preventing HCMV infection, congenital transmission and viral spreading after SOT or HSCT from seropositive donors to seronegative recipients [10]. The potential vaccine included live virus, attenuated or vectored viral vaccines expressing HCMV immunogens as well as purified recombinant protein vaccines that have been evaluated in clinical trials [11,12]. The abundant virion envelope glycoprotein B (gB) was shown to elicit vigorous T cell and antibody responses and represents the basis of most vaccines developed so far [13]. In a recent phase II clinical trial the recombinant gB vaccine formulated in MF59 adjuvant (gB/MF59), an oil-in-water emulsion, generated antibody titers comparable to natural infection. However, the vaccine demonstrated only modest efficacy in preventing primary HCMV infections in seronegative women and in the reduction of viremia in transplant recipients [14,15]. Surprisingly, a recent study demonstrated that seronegative patients vaccinated with the gB/MF59 vaccine developed a faster humoral response against gB after solid organ transplantation from seropositive donors [16]. Still, it is of the utmost importance to evaluate possible strategies for HCMV next generation vaccines. In this review, we will summarize the current findings on the adaptive immune response to HCMV and provide an update on the new methodologies available to boost the immune response against infectious diseases using virus-like particles (VLPs) and nanoparticles (NPs).

2. Immune Response against HCMV

The establishment of a long-lasting immunity in response to a primary HCMV infection is required to control subsequent HCMV reactivation and prevent uncontrolled viral replication or serious HCMV diseases [17,18]. HCMV infection activates both humoral and cellular immune responses. It is commonly believed that cellular immunity controls most of HCMV replication. Nonetheless, HCMV-specific antibodies have been associated with the prevention and protection from reinfection as well as the congenital transmission of HCMV [6,19,20]. Despite this, it is clear that the humoral response on its own is not able to clear the virus and prevent viral reactivation [21,22]. Nevertheless, the two arms of the adaptive immune response appear to be necessary for protection and resolution of HCMV infection [23].

2.1. Cellular Immune Response against HCMV

The primary cellular response to HCMV infection arises from natural killer (NK) cells, which trigger the release of inflammatory cytokines and cause lysis or apoptosis of infected cells [24]. Secondly, T cells restrict HCMV viral replication and viral spreading, although they are not able to definitively clear the virus [25–27]. HCMV-specific T cells represent 10% of both the $CD4^+$ and $CD8^+$ memory compartments in the peripheral blood of CMV-seropositive individuals [28]. $CD8^+$ T cells release perforin and granzyme B to promote lysis of infected cells that present CMV peptides on MHC-I [29,30], while $CD4^+$ specific T cells present a typical Th1 cytokine secretion signature (IFN-γ and TNF-α) [31]. Immune repertoire interrogation using 13,687 spanning peptides to cover 213 predicted CMV-proteins [32] revealed that human T cells recognize at least 151 HCMV proteins. Among these, $CD4^+$ T cells recognize 125 proteins, while $CD8^+$ T cells recognize 107 proteins, and 81 proteins are recognized by both cell types. Although the HCMV-specific T cell response is very broad, the vast majority of the results points toward antigens that are highly conserved among different HCMV strains, such as the 65 kDa phosphoprotein (pp65) and the immediate early 1 (IE1) proteins, which are recognized by more than 50% of seropositive individuals [28]. $CD8^+$ T cells were proven to have a protective role in both HSCT and SOT recipients [33–35] and a function in preventing congenital HCMV infection [36]. However, one of the paradoxes of the cellular immunity against HCMV comes from the observation that HCMV does induce a very large T cell response, meanwhile the virus also possesses sophisticated and numerous immune evasion mechanisms [37]. Among those, the capacity of the virus to enter a latency state has been the subject of intense investigation. Indeed, while primary infection of immunocompetent individuals by HCMV is rarely the source of disease, the opposite is true for individuals with an immune system that is still immature (fetus) or compromised (HIV/AIDS and transplantations). Consequently, several studies sought to identify the antigens that are relevant for the latency phase. A vaccine able to boost the immune system against the latter would help clearing the latent reservoir of the virus. It is known that HCMV establishes latency in the myeloid cell lineage and viral genome has been detected in peripheral blood monocytes and in $CD34^+$ progenitors in the bone marrow [38–40]. The viral gene expression program in these cells is restricted and extremely different from the one established during lytic infections. HCMV latent transcriptome is an area of extensive research, and at present, the exact roles of many latency-associated genes remain unclear. Nevertheless, several studies identified a number of viral genes that are specifically associated with latency [41,42]. Notably, RNAs from the major IE region (UL122–123 CLTs) [43], Latency Unique Natural Antigen (LUNA) [44], UL138 [41], UL111a (encoding a viral IL-10 homologue (LAcmvIL-10)) [45], UL144 [46] and US28 [47] were identified [22]. Moreover, viral reactivation is also associated with the expression of the major immediate early proteins (IE72 and IE86) [48]. T-cell repertoire interrogation identified four viral proteins expressed during latency (LUNA, UL138, US28, and LAcmvIL-10). Interestingly, these proteins can be recognized by $CD4^+$ T cells and T-cell responses specific for all four proteins are detectable in healthy HCMV-positive donors [49]. Accordingly, future vaccine candidates should boost cellular immunity against some of these proteins representing key targets for viral clearance.

2.2. *Humoral Immune Response against HCMV*

Upon HCMV infection, a large quantity of the antibodies generated target the most abundant viral proteins. These include proteins from the tegument (i.e., pp65), the immediate early proteins (i.e., IE1), and envelope glycoproteins such as gB, gM/gN, and the gH/gL complexes (trimer and pentamer). Antibodies targeting antigens that are not exposed on the surface of the virion are unlikely to generate an efficient protection against the virus [10]. Nonetheless, antibodies targeting the envelope glycoproteins are able to neutralize viral infection in vitro and correlate with a decrease of viral transmission in primary infected pregnant women [50]. It is known that antibodies targeting the pentamer are the most potent neutralizers at least in vitro [51,52], while antibodies targeting gHgL and gB are a thousand times less potent [51]. This result is still not fully understood, since the gHgL and gB proteins form the core machinery for viral membrane fusion [53] and monoclonal antibodies (mAbs) targeting the fusion machinery of other herpesviruses, such as Epstein–Barr virus, are potent neutralizers [54]. Immune repertoire interrogation of HCMV seropositive donors allowed the identification of multiple mAbs targeting the pULs subunits. We recently demonstrated that these mAbs neutralize the virus by blocking the molecular recognition of the pentamer to its cellular host receptor Neuropilin 2 [55]. In contrast, mAbs targeting gH are supposed to prevent the activation of the fusion machinery [56]. These mAbs were assigned to only two antigenic regions of gH, indeed 3G16 and MSL-109 mAbs bind toward the C-terminus of gH, while the 13H11 mAb binds close to the gL interaction site [57].

Recently, two studies reported the results of the recombinant gB vaccine formulated in MF59 adjuvant, which demonstrated partial efficacy in reducing viraemia after SOT and preventing primary infection in women and adolescents [14,15]. Sera analysis from gB-vaccinated individuals allowed the characterization of at least five gB antigenic domains (AD-1 to AD-5). The AD-1 is a domain of 80 amino acids between amino acid 560 and 640 whereas AD-2 consists of two discontinuous binding sites: Site I, located between amino acids 68 and 77, is highly conserved among strains and is considered as a target of neutralizing responses, while Site II, located between amino acids 50 and 54, is less conserved. AD-3 is a linear epitope corresponding to amino acids 798–805 in the intraluminal region of gB. AD-4, like AD-2, is a discontinuous domain corresponding to amino acids 121–132 and 344–438. AD-5 matches to amino acids between 133 and 343 [58–60]. Interestingly, Baraniak et. al. demonstrated that vaccination only boosted AD-2 responses in the 50% of CMV+ individuals with a preexisting response and did not induce a new AD-2 response in those who lacked AD-2 antibodies following natural infection [15,61]. In parallel, Nelson et al. observed an increase of anti-gB IgG titer induced by the same vaccine in a cohort of CMV-post-partum women [14]. However, the authors also subsequently observed that 76% of the vaccine-induced IgG response recognized AD-3. Considering that AD-3 is located in the intraluminal part of the virus, antibodies against this region will be most probably non-protective [12].

The hypothesis that AD-3 is diverting the immune response away from antigenic sites that more likely induce protective antibody responses (AD-2), was recently proposed [62]. The next HCMV vaccines will have to contain multiple antigens that should induce a strong neutralizing antibody response protecting from primary infections and an efficient T-cell response to prevent viral reactivation and to clear the latent virus.

3. HCMV Antigens as Vaccine Candidates

HCMV is the largest virus infecting humans, with a genome containing a linear double-stranded DNA of about 230 kb, from which at least 170 open reading frames (ORFs) have been identified [63,64]. The virus contains over 30 structural proteins and encodes at least 20 membrane glycoproteins expressed on the virion envelope, which are involved in immune evasion, cell attachment, and viral entry. HCMV exhibits an extremely broad cellular tropism being able to infect different cell types ranging from epithelial, endothelial, fibroblasts, myeloid hematopoietic precursors, monocytes/macrophages to smooth muscle cells, stromal cells, neurons, astrocytes, hepatocytes and glial cells [65]. Identification of the host cellular receptors has been a subject of debate during the last decade. It is now accepted that the two main host cell receptors for HCMV involve the platelet-derived growth factor receptor α (PDGFRα) [66–68] and Neuropilin 2 (Nrp2) [55]. In addition, other cellular host factors were described as facilitators of viral entry such as the olfactory receptor family member OR14I1 [69], the adipocyte plasma membrane-associated protein (APMAP) [70], CD46 [71], and CD147 [72]. However, the biological relevance of this multitude of receptors remains to be understood. In contrast, the viral ligands responsible for the broad cellular tropism were clearly identified and correspond to two viral envelope complexes: the gHgLgO (trimer) and the gHgLpUL128pUL130pUL131A (pentamer) (Figure 1) [73]. The trimer is a heterocomplex, in which the heterodimer consisting of gH (UL75) and gL (UL115) is disulfide-linked to glycoprotein O (gO), a heavily N-glycosylated polypeptide encoded by UL74 [74–76]. The trimer complex binds PDGFRα and is required for entry in all cell types [77], representing an attractive target for vaccine design. However, the gO sequence heterogeneity and the large glycan shield present on this subunit are impairing the generation of potent neutralizing mAbs. Along with others, we speculate that these issues will probably slow down possible efforts to use the trimer as a vaccine candidate [78]. The pentamer complex is composed of the gHgL heterodimer bound to three additional glycoproteins encoded by pUL128, pUL130, and pUL131A. The pentamer complex is required for viral entry in epithelial, endothelial, and myeloid cells and binds Nrp2 [55,65,79]. It represents the main target of HCMV neutralizing antibodies, eliciting a protective response targeting the pULs subunits, which is several orders of magnitude more potent than any other response against HCMV glycoprotein [51,52,80]. However, anti-pULs mAbs are not able to block infection in all cell types, in contrast to mAbs directed against gH and gB subunits [81]. Indeed, membrane fusion and cell entry in all cell types is dictated by the core fusion machinery composed of gHgL and the glycoprotein B (gB) which are thus considered as primary targets for vaccine development [2]. gB is a class III viral fusion protein that forms homotrimers (Figure 1) and was initially reported to bind cell–surface proteins such as PDGFRα and EGFR. However, it is more likely that gB functions as a viral fusogen that is triggered when viral and host membranes are in close proximity [82]. In addition to the HCMV membrane glycoproteins, other viral antigens have been considered as potential vaccine targets. The phosphoprotein 65 (pp65) encoded by pUL83 and the immediate-early protein 1 (IE1) encoded by pUL123, both eliciting a robust T cell response, have undergone evaluation as subunit or vectored vaccines in human [83,84]. In conclusion, the aforementioned vaccine candidates failed to confer an appropriate protection from infection, viral reinfection or reactivation. We believe that the development of a protective vaccine should include antigens from the viral envelope to trigger the humoral response (mainly pentamer and newly designed gB) and antigens from the tegument or proteins that are specifically associated with latency (i.e., US28) to prompt the cellular response able to control viral reactivation.

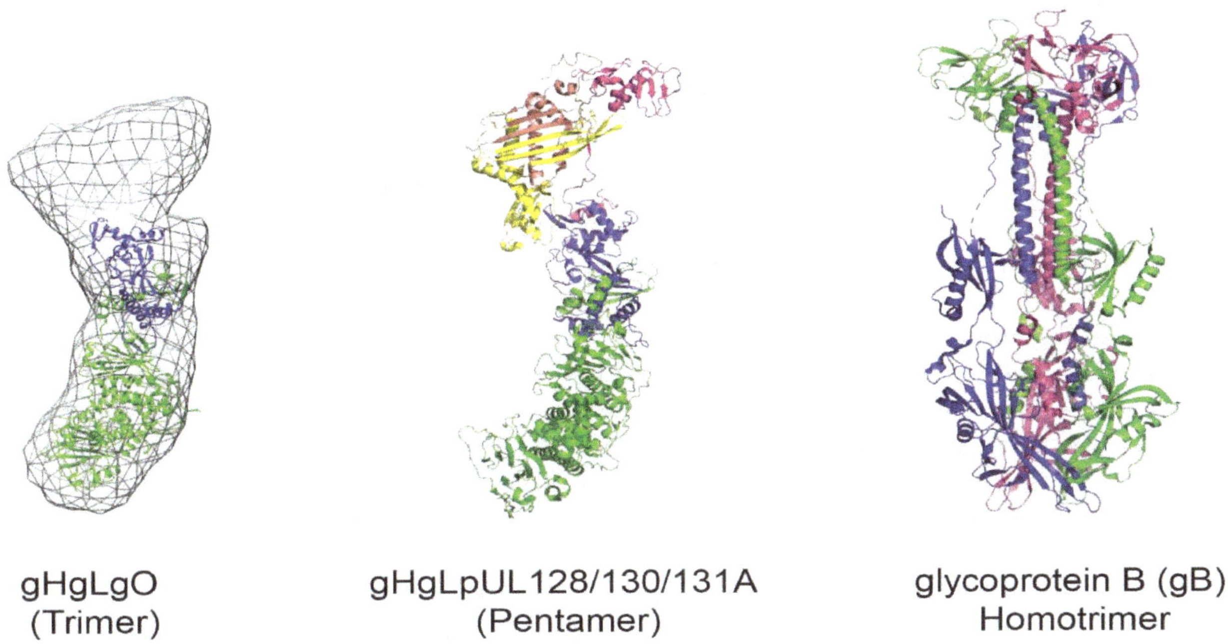

Figure 1. Structural representation of HCMV glycoproteins. Shown is the trimer, composed of the gHgL heterodimer and gO. Representation prepared with PDB: 5voc and EMD-3391. The pentamer is composed of the gHgL heterodimer and the three additional subunits pUL128, pUL130, and pUL131A. Representation prepared with PDB: 5voc. The gB homotrimer in its postfusion conformation is shown based on PDB: 5cxf. The figure was prepared using PyMOL software (The PyMOL Molecular Graphics System, Version 4.5 Schrödinger, LLC).

4. Virus-Like Particles and Nanoparticles for Antigen Display

Virus-like particles (VLPs) and nanoparticles (NPs) are protein structures that resemble wild type viruses but do not have a viral genome nor infectious ability, creating in principle safer vaccine candidates. Both VLPs and NPs are composed of self-assembling proteins displaying the epitope of interest at a high density on their surface. Antigen presentation as a repetitive array is known to drive stronger humoral immune responses when compared to the single soluble antigen [85]. This effect is thought to derive from some key properties of the VLPs/NPs presentation such as the increased antigen density that creates avidity leading to a stronger B cell activation through antigen-driven cross-linking of B cell receptors (BCRs) [86]. Moreover, VLPs/NPs are also supposed to enhance antigen uptake by antigen presenting cells (APCs) which subsequently support the adaptive arms of the immune system [87]. Finally, VLPs/NPs have also been proven, in some cases, to generate an epitope-focusing effect in which antigenic sites promoting the generation of potent neutralizing mAbs were preferentially targeted [88,89]. Over the last decades, several platforms for VLPs/NPs design have been generated, including the usage of viral core proteins, covalent links of individual folded proteins through site-specific ligations and de novo protein nanostructure formation via non-covalent intramolecular and intermolecular interactions. VLPs/NPs are currently recognized as one of the most promising and extensively studied molecular carriers for new vaccine development. Here we will present the current VLP HCMV vaccines in development and provide some examples that can be relevant for novel vaccine design.

4.1. Developed HCMV VLP Vaccine

Enveloped virus-like particles (eVLPs) are VLP structures wrapped with a lipid envelope obtained by transfection of the Moloney murine leukemia virus (MLV) gag protein in human or hamster cell lines (i.e., HEK or CHO cells). The MLV gag expression induces burgeoning of particles from membranes of transfected cells. Variation Biotechnologies Incorporated (VBI) laboratories generated an eVLP vaccine expressing an HCMV gB full-length or a chimeric gB protein, where the extracellular domain (ECD) of gB is membrane-anchored using the transmembrane and cytoplasmic domains of the vesicular stomatitis virus (VSV) G protein [90]. The chimeric gB-VSV-G protein is thought to maintain gB in a prefusion conformation. Both vaccines were used to immunize mice and induce a neutralizing antibody response 10-fold higher compared to their soluble recombinant protein counterpart [90]. The vaccine was entered in phase I clinical studies enrolling HCMV-seronegative individuals for evaluation of safety and immunogenicity in early 2016 [91]. An additional eVLP vaccine candidate, targeting both the gB and pp65 antigens, has also been manufactured by VBI. However, we believe that a combination of gB, pentamer, and pp65 or US28 would be more appealing. Finally, another eVLP HCMV vaccine candidate was developed by Redvax GmbH, a Swiss biopharmaceutical company. Unlike VBI, that used mammalian cells, they used the rePAX baculovirus co-expression technology minimizing the purification issues due to the relative large size of VLPs for the efficient generation of a VLP vaccine candidate containing HCMV pp65 and gB [92]. Redvax GmbH was later acquired by Pfizer and the vaccine was able to elicit high-titer neutralizing antibodies and good T cell responses after immunization. Nonetheless, no protection was demonstrated from viremia upon challenge.

4.2. Hepatitis B Core Antigen Nanoparticle

The core protein of the hepatitis B virus (HBc) self-assembles into highly immunogenic virus-like structures with icosahedral symmetry. The hepatitis B core nanoparticle (HBc) is assembled from dimers of 183 or 185 amino acids and occurs in two size classes with a T = 3 or T = 4 symmetry. Depending on the symmetry, HBc is formed by 90 or 120 dimeric subunits with a respective diameter of 24 or 31 nm [93]. The antigen of interest needs to be inserted between alpha helices 3 and 4 of the major immune-dominant region (MIR) domain (amino acids 78–82) (Figure 2A) of the HBc protein. This insertion allows the antigen to be exposed on spike structures at the surface of the assembled nanoparticle. HBc protomers first dimerize and then multimerize (Figure 2B,C). Several developments led to the success of this platform, such as splitting of the HBc protein between the α3 and α4 helices or fusing two monomers together using a flexible glycine serine linker that allowed the introduction of larger protein domains [94,95]. However, one limitation of this technology is the need for both the N- and C-termini of the inserted antigen to fit with the geometry of the core acceptor site, a requirement that is not always successfully met by natively folded proteins.

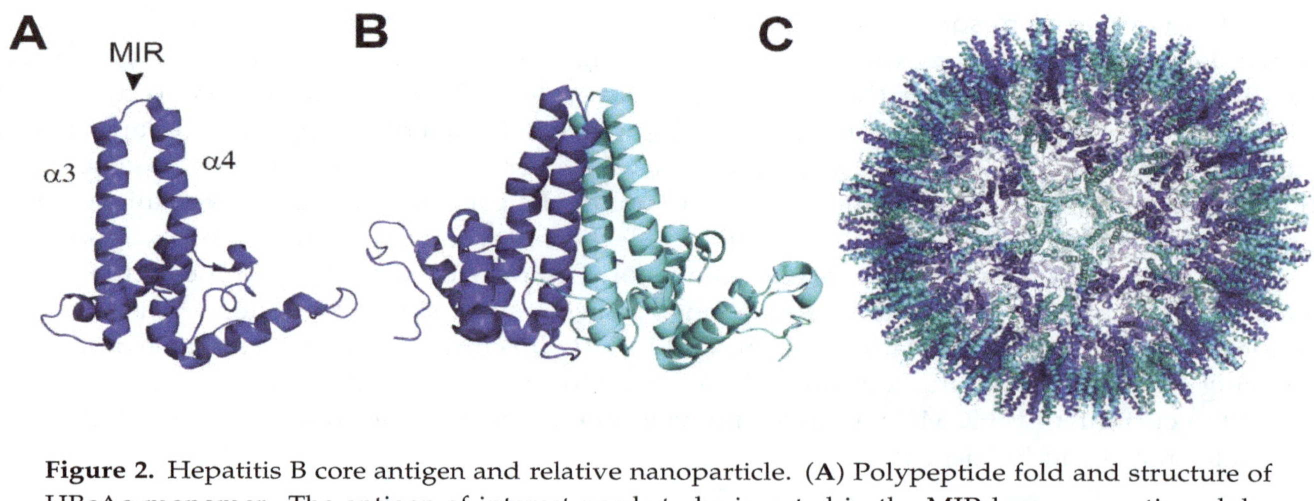

Figure 2. Hepatitis B core antigen and relative nanoparticle. (**A**) Polypeptide fold and structure of HBcAg monomer. The antigen of interest needs to be inserted in the MIR loop connecting alpha helices 3 and 4. (**B**) Two HBcAg monomers spontaneously interact to form a dimer, which acts as an intermediate in the nanoparticle formation. (**C**) Assembled nanoparticle containing either 90 or 120 dimers. The figure was prepared with PDB: 6htx using Pymol software (The PyMOL Molecular Graphics System, Version 4.5 Schrödinger, LLC).

In summary, the HBc is a powerful platform to generate nanoparticles and it is particularly useful in the case of small antigens. Indeed, it is unlikely that complex envelope glycoproteins such as gB or the gHgL complexes could be correctly displayed on HBc particles. Nevertheless, HBc could be very efficient to generate strong T cell responses [96]. For example, the viral-encoded G protein-coupled receptor US28 was recently shown to aid in the establishment and the maintenance of viral latency. US28 modulates host–cell proteins to suppress viral processes associated with lytic replication and thereby represent an important target promoting latent infection [97]. HBc particles displaying US28 peptides recognized by T cells could provide an important advancement to boost the existing immune responses necessary to control reactivation of latently infected individuals [98].

4.3. Ferritin-Based Nanoparticle

Ferritin is an intracellular globular protein that stores iron and releases it in a controlled fashion [99]. The protein is expressed in many tissues, mainly as a cytosolic protein, but it can be also found at low concentration in the serum where it functions as an iron carrier [100]. Ferritin is a four-helix bundle protein consisting of two couples of anti-parallel α-helices connected by a long loop and a short C-terminal α-helix (Figure 3A). The monomer can dimerize and further self-assemble to form a nanocage of 24 protein subunits, which has an internal and external diameter of 8 and 12 nm, respectively [101]. Ferritin nanoparticle (ferritin-NP) presents the advantage of being resistant to thermal and chemical stress [102]. Moreover, antigen display is achieved through genetic fusion at the N-terminus of each ferritin protomer. Ferritin-NP self-arranges as an octahedron composed of eight trimeric units (Figure 3B), each with a 3-fold symmetry axis that allows the correct presentation of trimeric antigens at the nanoparticle surface (Figure 3C).

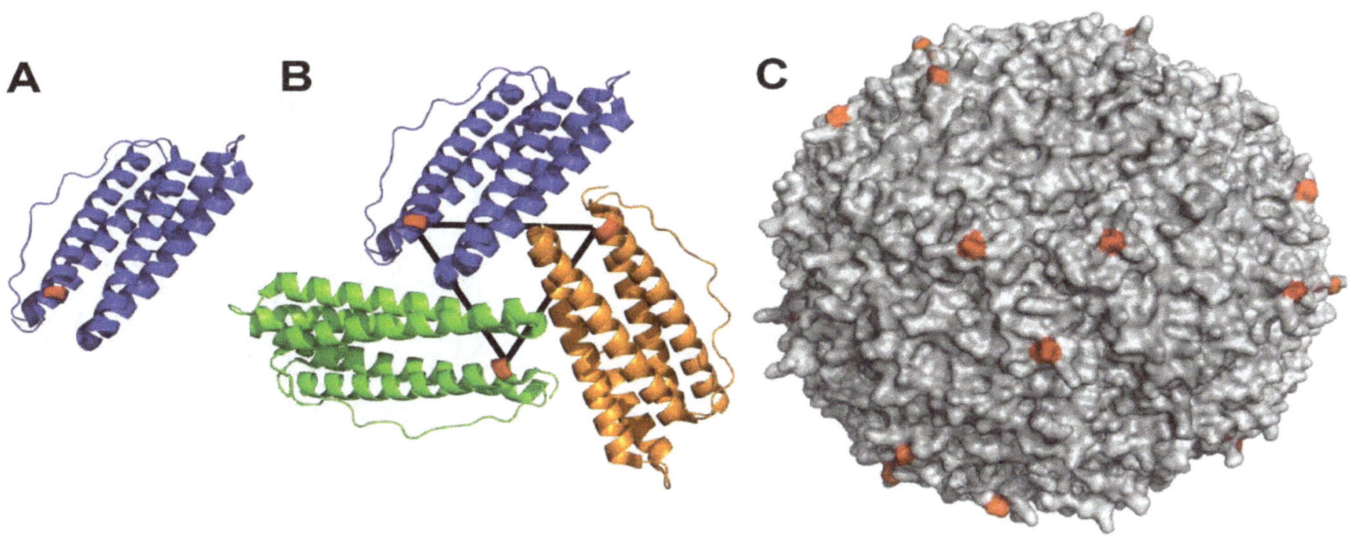

Figure 3. Structure of ferritin nanoparticle. (**A**) The antigen of interest is fused to the N-terminus of the ferritin polypeptide (shown in red). (**B**) Ferritin assembles to form symmetry units with threefold axes. (**C**) Fully assembled nanoparticle with surface-exposed N-termini colored in red. The figure was prepared using PDB: 3bve using PyMOL software (The PyMOL Molecular Graphics System, Version 4.5 Schrödinger, LLC).

A recent development and one of the major advantages of this carrier is the possibility to generate multivalent displays of different antigenic proteins. For example, ferritin-NP was first used to present HIV-1 and influenza antigens on the same particle [103]. Furthermore, Kanekiyo and coworkers at the Vaccine Research Center in the United States. further developed and exploited the ferritin-NP system using a ferritin hybrid protein [89] to generate a universal vaccine against influenza. The team co-displayed the receptor binding domain (RBD) of the last 90 years H1N1 influenza viruses [104] and showed that immunization with this mosaic RBD-NP elicited a broad antibody response covering all the known H1N1 strains. Multiple displays on ferritin-NP have opened up new possibilities for novel vaccines against different pathogens or against different antigens of a given pathogen.

In the case of HCMV, we can speculate that a mosaic ferritin-NP displaying both pentamer and gB ECDs should generate a potent humoral immune reaction. The antibodies generated targeting the gHgL and gB subunits will block infection of connective tissues and stroma (containing fibroblasts). On the other hand, antibodies directed against the pUL subunits will block infection of epithelial tissues.

4.4. Qβ Nanoparticle

The bacteriophage Qβ is a member of the *Leviviridae* family, forming 30 nm icosahedral nanoparticles of 180 copies from the 14 kDa coat protein [105]. The coat protein monomer (Figure 4A) forms Qβ dimers (Figure 4B) that further assemble into pentamers and hexamers by disulfide and hydrogen bond interactions to form a Qβ nanoparticle under physiological conditions (Figure 4C). This nanoparticle is highly stable and is used to display ligands and proteins on its exterior surface [106,107]. Co-expression of Qβ proteins displaying different antigens of interest or engineered Qβ proteins displaying functionalized groups for subsequent direct antigen conjugation can be easily produced in bacterial cells. Of note, the genetic fusion occurs at the C-terminus of the protein, a property that might impair the correct folding of some antigens of interest. Genes encoding the viral Qβ protein have been also successfully expressed in yeast cells but the possibility to generate a Qβ nanoparticle in prokaryotic hosts, maintaining therefore a low production cost, will be of great interest for the generation of a personalized T cell vaccine targeting the proteins associated to latency. Regarding mammalian cell expression, there is currently no evidence that the system is also compatible with it, which is a prerequisite for the production of most of the HCMV glycoprotein antigens.

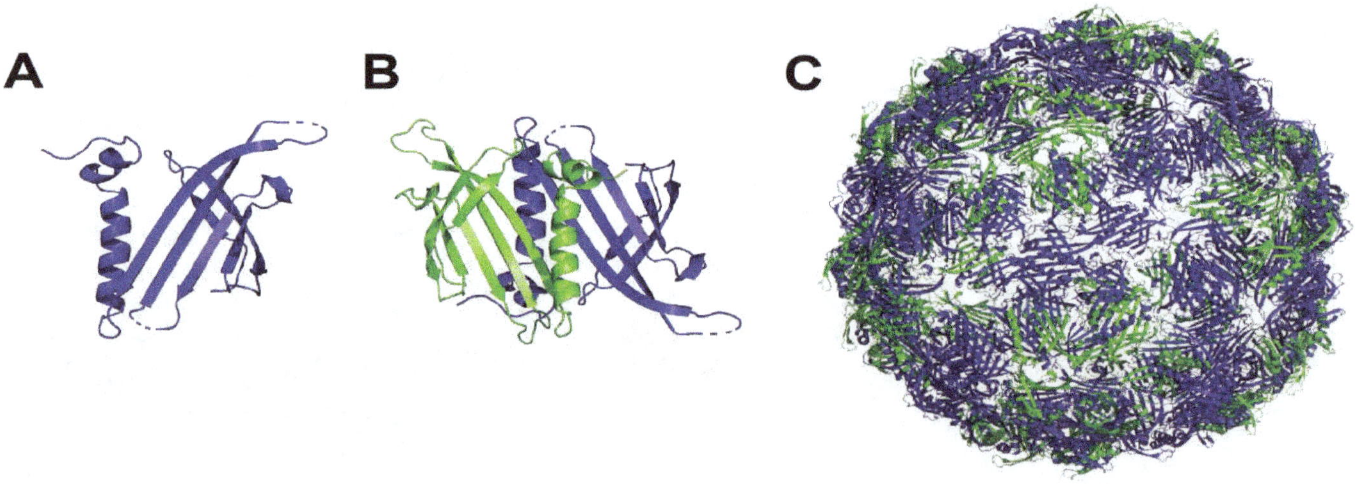

Figure 4. Structure and assembly of Qβ nanoparticle. Qβ protein is depicted as a monomer (**A**) and noncovalent dimer (**B**). (**C**) The fully self-assembled Qβ nanoparticle consists of 20 hexamers and 12 pentamers. The figure was prepared using 1qbe PDB structure and PyMOL software (The PyMOL Molecular Graphics System, Version 4.5 Schrödinger, LLC).

4.5. De Novo Design-Based Nanoparticle

Structure-based design of nanoparticle immunogens has been limited by the restricted number of scaffolds available and the fact that their physico-chemical properties are fixed (i.e., ferritin, encapsulins). Moreover, most of the self-assembling scaffolds spontaneously do so upon expression in the transfected host cell, a property that might lead to poor production yield. These constraints have pushed the exploration of new structural and functional geometries (i.e., icosahedron, dodecahedron) in the nanoparticle immunogen design field. Recent computational methods for designing novel self-assembling proteins with atomic-level accuracy offer the possibility to design self-assembling proteins with customized structures, offering new opportunities for structure-based vaccine design [108–110]. For instance, the HIV gp41 ectodomain trimer was displayed onto the I3–01 particle [108,111]. The gp41 antigen exposed on NPs, stimulated mAb-expressing B cells more effectively than the soluble trimers [111]. Two additional publications highlighted the potential of this de novo self-assembling nanoparticle for antigen display. The I5350 nanoparticle (Figure 5) was used to generate an enhanced vaccine against the respiratory syncytial virus (RSV). Self-assembling protein nanoparticles displaying 20 copies of the stabilized version of the RSV fusion glycoprotein trimer (DS-Cav1) induced a neutralizing antibody response ~10-fold higher than soluble trimeric DS-Cav1 [112]. In the second case, native-like HIV-1 envelope trimer antigens were displayed in a multivalent fashion on the I5350 nanoparticle scaffold and immunization studies revealed a more effective priming compared to the soluble SOSIP trimers [113]. SOSIP corresponds to a stabilized trimer with mutations that cross-link the cleaved gp120 and gp41. In contrast, the natural HIV trimer is comprised of three copies of a non-covalently linked gp120/gp41 heterodimer arising from cleavage of the viral gp160 precursor protein. It can be speculated that de novo design-based nanoparticles will have an increasing impact on next generation vaccines since they are customizable at will, supported by a multitude of expression platforms and able to generate multivalent display as well as encapsulation of small proteins or compounds [114,115].

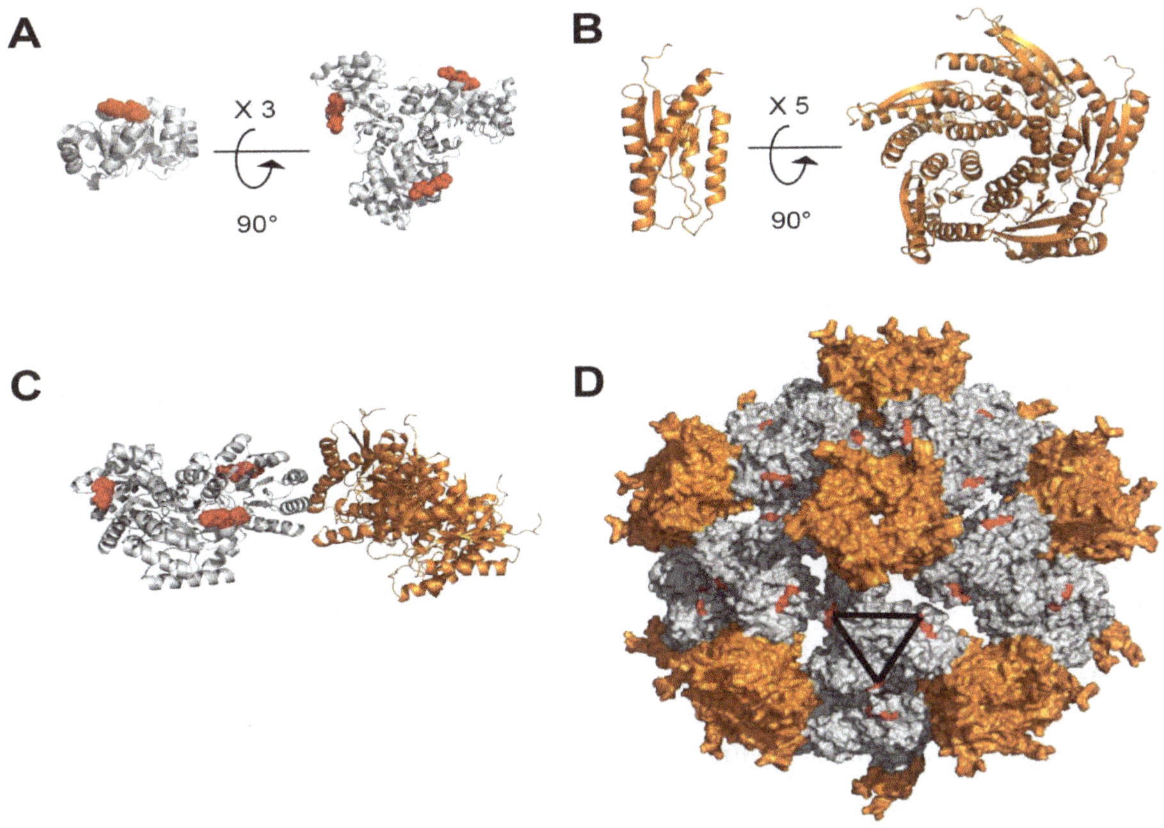

Figure 5. Self-assembly of the I5350 nanoparticle. (**A**) Polypeptide I53–50A.1NT1; shown in red is the N-terminus projecting outward, where antigens can be displayed. I53–50A.1NT1 naturally trimerizes forming a 3-fold symmetry axis. (**B**) The I53–50B.4PT1 protein (orange) assembles into a pentamer. (**C**) I53–50A.1NT1 trimer and I53–50B.4PT1 pentamer self-assemble as a nanoparticle. (**D**) Assembled nanoparticle formed by 20 trimers and 12 pentamers, the N-termini of I53–50A.1NT1 is shown in red, and the black triangle represents the 3-fold symmetry axis of each pair of trimers. The figure was prepared using PyMOL software (The PyMOL Molecular Graphics System, Version 4.5 Schrödinger, LLC).

Ideally, I5350 particles should present on their surface the pentamer and gB to generate a humoral response against the gH, gL, pULs, and gB molecules. Moreover, as I5350 nanoparticles are hollow, the in vitro assembly step with I53–50B.4PT1 could be performed in the presence of T-cell stimulating peptides (i.e., pp65, IE1 and US28) that would be encapsulated inside the particles. The resulting vaccine candidates should in this way stimulate both arms of the immune system, offering a maximal protection.

4.6. SpyCatcher and SpyTag for Nanoparticle Formation

The SpyTag/SpyCatcher system (referred as Spy-System) is based on the internal isopeptide bond of the CnaB2 domain of FbaB protein from *Streptococcus pyogenes*. An internal isopeptide bond forms spontaneously in this domain between the reactive amine of lysine K31 and the side chain carboxyl of aspartate D117. This reaction is catalyzed by the spatially adjacent glutamate E77. The resulting isopeptide bond confers high stability to the CnaB2 domain. The CnaB2 domain is cleaved into two subcomponents, the large and incomplete immunoglobulin-like domain, named SpyCatcher, composed of 138 amino acids, and the short beta strand, named SpyTag, composed of 13 amino acids [116]. While the SpyCatcher contains the reactive lysine (K31) and catalytic glutamate (E77), the SpyTag includes the reactive aspartate (D117). The two components can still recognize each other with high affinity and the isopeptide is formed within minutes. Despite the fact that this system is not able to generate nanoparticles on its own, the two components of the Spy-System can be genetically fused to a number of viral or designed self-assembling proteins leading to the generation of a stable nanoparticle displaying a large variety of antigens. Moreover, the Spy-System offers a great flexibility since components can be inserted at the N- or C-termini of the target proteins. Its simplicity is of particular interest to quickly screen if a nanoparticle formulation will be of benefit for vaccine design, before generating genetic fusion on the nanoparticle of interest. The first nanoparticle assembly with Spy-System was performed by genetically fusing the SpyCatcher to the N-terminus of the viral coat protein (CP3) of the RNA bacteriophage AP205 [117]. AP205 VLPs have been then further investigated as vaccine candidates against a number of targets, including malaria and cancer [117–119].

5. Conclusions and Future Directions

We described a large variety of systems to generate both VLPs and NPs. Self-assembling scaffolds have been used to present complex glycoprotein antigens and for vaccination studies against influenza [104], HIV [113,120–123], Epstein–Barr virus [89], and RSV [112]. In all cases, antigen immunogenicity was increased by multivalent presentation and in some cases, an epitope focusing effect could be observed. The rise of computational design to generate novel self-assembling proteins has now paved the way for new possibilities to display antigens without limitation in term of quantity or oligomeric state of the antigen. HCMV is still the principal viral cause of congenital malformations. About one quarter of infants infected by HCMV in utero will develop severe sequelae including microcephaly, sensorineural hearing and vision loss, or cognitive delay [1,6]. The recent identification of key HCMV antigenic targets for both humoral and cellular immune responses and the capacity to display and encapsulate proteins or nucleic acids (RNAs) on VLPs/NPs is likely to generate improved vaccine candidates able to redirect the immune response against specific targets.

Author Contributions: M.P. and L.P. conceptualized and wrote the review. All authors have read and agreed to the published version of the manuscript.

Acknowledgments: The authors acknowledge Mathilde Foglierini and Jessica Marcandalli for critical reading and helpful comments on the manuscript.

References

1. Kenneson, A.; Cannon, M.J. Review and meta-analysis of the epidemiology of congenital cytomegalovirus (CMV) infection. *Rev. Med. Virol.* **2007**, *17*, 253–276. [CrossRef] [PubMed]
2. Plotkin, S.A.; Boppana, S.B. Vaccination against the human cytomegalovirus. *Vaccine* **2018**, *37*, 7437–7442. [CrossRef] [PubMed]

3. Britt, W. Manifestations of human cytomegalovirus infection: Proposed mechanisms of acute and chronic disease. *Curr. Top. Microbiol. Immunol.* **2008**, *325*, 417–470. [CrossRef] [PubMed]
4. Gerna, G.; Zavattoni, M.; Baldanti, F.; Furione, M.; Chezzi, L.; Revello, M.G.; Percivalle, E. Circulating cytomegalic endothelial cells are associated with high human cytomegalovirus (HCMV) load in AIDS patients with late-stage disseminated HCMV disease. *J. Med. Virol.* **1998**, *55*, 64–74. [CrossRef]
5. Lilleri, D.; Gerna, G. Strategies to control human cytomegalovirus infection in adult hematopoietic stem cell transplant recipients. *Immunotherapy* **2016**, *8*, 1135–1149. [CrossRef] [PubMed]
6. Boppana, S.B.; Britt, W.J. Antiviral antibody responses and intrauterine transmission after primary maternal cytomegalovirus infection. *J. Infect. Dis.* **1995**, *171*, 1115–1121. [CrossRef]
7. Spinillo, A.; Gerna, G. Hyperimmune globulin to prevent congenital CMV infection. *N. Engl. J. Med.* **2014**, *370*, 2544–2545. [CrossRef]
8. James, S.H.; Kimberlin, D.W. Advances in the prevention and treatment of congenital cytomegalovirus infection. *Curr. Opin. Pediatrics* **2016**, *28*, 81–85. [CrossRef]
9. Marsico, C.; Kimberlin, D.W. Congenital Cytomegalovirus infection: Advances and challenges in diagnosis, prevention and treatment. *Ital. J. Pediatrics* **2017**, *43*, 38. [CrossRef]
10. Gomes, A.C.; Griffiths, P.D.; Reeves, M.B. The Humoral Immune Response Against the gB Vaccine: Lessons Learnt from Protection in Solid Organ Transplantation. *Vaccines* **2019**, *7*, 67. [CrossRef]
11. Schleiss, M.R. Recombinant cytomegalovirus glycoprotein B vaccine: Rethinking the immunological basis of protection. *Proc. Natl. Acad. Sci. USA* **2018**, *115*, 6110–6112. [CrossRef] [PubMed]
12. Nelson, C.S.; Herold, B.C.; Permar, S.R. A new era in cytomegalovirus vaccinology: Considerations for rational design of next-generation vaccines to prevent congenital cytomegalovirus infection. *Npj Vaccines* **2018**, *3*, 38. [CrossRef] [PubMed]
13. Foglierini, M.; Marcandalli, J.; Perez, L. HCMV Envelope Glycoprotein Diversity Demystified. *Front. Microbiol.* **2019**, *10*, 1005. [CrossRef]
14. Nelson, C.S.; Huffman, T.; Jenks, J.A.; Cisneros de la Rosa, E.; Xie, G.; Vandergrift, N.; Pass, R.F.; Pollara, J.; Permar, S.R. HCMV glycoprotein B subunit vaccine efficacy mediated by nonneutralizing antibody effector functions. *Proc. Natl. Acad. Sci. USA* **2018**, *115*, 6267–6272. [CrossRef]
15. Baraniak, I.; Kropff, B.; Ambrose, L.; McIntosh, M.; McLean, G.R.; Pichon, S.; Atkinson, C.; Milne, R.S.B.; Mach, M.; Griffiths, P.D.; et al. Protection from cytomegalovirus viremia following glycoprotein B vaccination is not dependent on neutralizing antibodies. *Proc. Natl. Acad. Sci. USA* **2018**, *115*, 6273–6278. [CrossRef] [PubMed]
16. Baraniak, I.; Gomes, A.C.; Sodi, I.; Langstone, T.; Rothwell, E.; Atkinson, C.; Pichon, S.; Piras-Douce, F.; Griffiths, P.D.; Reeves, M.B. Seronegative patients vaccinated with cytomegalovirus gB-MF59 vaccine have evidence of neutralising antibody responses against gB early post-transplantation. *EBioMedicine* **2019**, *50*, 45–54. [CrossRef] [PubMed]
17. Gerna, G.; Lilleri, D.; Fornara, C.; Bruno, F.; Gabanti, E.; Cane, I.; Furione, M.; Revello, M.G. Differential kinetics of human cytomegalovirus load and antibody responses in primary infection of the immunocompetent and immunocompromised host. *J. Gen. Virol.* **2015**, *96*, 360–369. [CrossRef]
18. Smith, C.J.; Quinn, M.; Snyder, C.M. CMV-Specific CD8 T Cell Differentiation and Localization: Implications for Adoptive Therapies. *Front. Immunol.* **2016**, *7*, 352. [CrossRef]
19. Bialas, K.M.; Westreich, D.; Cisneros de la Rosa, E.; Nelson, C.S.; Kauvar, L.M.; Fu, T.M.; Permar, S.R. Maternal Antibody Responses and Nonprimary Congenital Cytomegalovirus Infection of HIV-1-Exposed Infants. *J. Infect. Dis.* **2016**, *214*, 1916–1923. [CrossRef]
20. Itell, H.L.; Nelson, C.S.; Martinez, D.R.; Permar, S.R. Maternal immune correlates of protection against placental transmission of cytomegalovirus. *Placenta* **2017**, *60* (Suppl. 1), S73–S79. [CrossRef]
21. Stern, L.; Withers, B.; Avdic, S.; Gottlieb, D.; Abendroth, A.; Blyth, E.; Slobedman, B. Human Cytomegalovirus Latency and Reactivation in Allogeneic Hematopoietic Stem Cell Transplant Recipients. *Front. Microbiol.* **2019**, *10*, 1186. [CrossRef] [PubMed]
22. Collins-McMillen, D.; Buehler, J.; Peppenelli, M.; Goodrum, F. Molecular Determinants and the Regulation of Human Cytomegalovirus Latency and Reactivation. *Viruses* **2018**, *10*, 444. [CrossRef] [PubMed]
23. Krishna, B.A.; Wills, M.R.; Sinclair, J.H. Advances in the treatment of cytomegalovirus. *Br. Med. Bull.* **2019**, *131*, 5–17. [CrossRef] [PubMed]

24. Wilkinson, G.W.; Tomasec, P.; Stanton, R.J.; Armstrong, M.; Prod'homme, V.; Aicheler, R.; McSharry, B.P.; Rickards, C.R.; Cochrane, D.; Llewellyn-Lacey, S.; et al. Modulation of natural killer cells by human cytomegalovirus. *J. Clin. Virol.* **2008**, *41*, 206–212. [CrossRef]
25. Rist, M.; Cooper, L.; Elkington, R.; Walker, S.; Fazou, C.; Tellam, J.; Crough, T.; Khanna, R. Ex vivo expansion of human cytomegalovirus-specific cytotoxic T cells by recombinant polyepitope: Implications for HCMV immunotherapy. *Eur. J. Immunol.* **2005**, *35*, 996–1007. [CrossRef]
26. Rohrlich, P.S.; Cardinaud, S.; Lule, J.; Montero-Julian, F.A.; Prodhomme, V.; Firat, H.; Davignon, J.L.; Perret, E.; Monseaux, S.; Necker, A.; et al. Use of a lentiviral vector encoding a HCMV-chimeric IE1-pp65 protein for epitope identification in HLA-Transgenic mice and for ex vivo stimulation and expansion of CD8(+) cytotoxic T cells from human peripheral blood cells. *Hum. Immunol.* **2004**, *65*, 514–522. [CrossRef]
27. Boppana, S.B.; Britt, W.J. Recognition of human cytomegalovirus gene products by HCMV-specific cytotoxic T cells. *Virology* **1996**, *222*, 293–296. [CrossRef]
28. Sylwester, A.W.; Mitchell, B.L.; Edgar, J.B.; Taormina, C.; Pelte, C.; Ruchti, F.; Sleath, P.R.; Grabstein, K.H.; Hosken, N.A.; Kern, F.; et al. Broadly targeted human cytomegalovirus-specific CD4+ and CD8+ T cells dominate the memory compartments of exposed subjects. *J. Exp. Med.* **2005**, *202*, 673–685. [CrossRef]
29. Hertoghs, K.M.; Moerland, P.D.; van Stijn, A.; Remmerswaal, E.B.; Yong, S.L.; van de Berg, P.J.; van Ham, S.M.; Baas, F.; ten Berge, I.J.; van Lier, R.A. Molecular profiling of cytomegalovirus-induced human CD8+ T cell differentiation. *J. Clin. Invest.* **2010**, *120*, 4077–4090. [CrossRef]
30. Gillespie, G.M.; Wills, M.R.; Appay, V.; O'Callaghan, C.; Murphy, M.; Smith, N.; Sissons, P.; Rowland-Jones, S.; Bell, J.I.; Moss, P.A. Functional heterogeneity and high frequencies of cytomegalovirus-specific CD8(+) T lymphocytes in healthy seropositive donors. *J. Virol.* **2000**, *74*, 8140–8150. [CrossRef]
31. van Leeuwen, E.M.; Remmerswaal, E.B.; Vossen, M.T.; Rowshani, A.T.; Wertheim-van Dillen, P.M.; van Lier, R.A.; ten Berge, I.J. Emergence of a CD4+CD28- granzyme B+, cytomegalovirus-specific T cell subset after recovery of primary cytomegalovirus infection. *J. Immunol.* **2004**, *173*, 1834–1841. [CrossRef]
32. Kern, F.; Faulhaber, N.; Frommel, C.; Khatamzas, E.; Prosch, S.; Schonemann, C.; Kretzschmar, I.; Volkmer-Engert, R.; Volk, H.D.; Reinke, P. Analysis of CD8 T cell reactivity to cytomegalovirus using protein-spanning pools of overlapping pentadecapeptides. *Eur. J. Immunol.* **2000**, *30*, 1676–1682. [CrossRef]
33. Lilleri, D.; Zelini, P.; Fornara, C.; Zavaglio, F.; Rampino, T.; Perez, L.; Gabanti, E.; Gerna, G. Human cytomegalovirus (HCMV)-specific T cell but not neutralizing or IgG binding antibody responses to glycoprotein complexes gB, gHgLgO, and pUL128L correlate with protection against high HCMV viral load reactivation in solid-organ transplant recipients. *J. Med. Virol.* **2018**, *90*, 1620–1628. [CrossRef] [PubMed]
34. Reusser, P.; Gambertoglio, J.G.; Lilleby, K.; Meyers, J.D. Phase I-II trial of foscarnet for prevention of cytomegalovirus infection in autologous and allogeneic marrow transplant recipients. *J. Infect. Dis.* **1992**, *166*, 473–479. [CrossRef] [PubMed]
35. Greenberg, P.D.; Reusser, P.; Goodrich, J.M.; Riddell, S.R. Development of a treatment regimen for human cytomegalovirus (CMV) infection in bone marrow transplantation recipients by adoptive transfer of donor-derived CMV-specific T cell clones expanded in vitro. *Ann. N. Y. Acad. Sci.* **1991**, *636*, 184–195. [CrossRef] [PubMed]
36. Fornara, C.; Cassaniti, I.; Zavattoni, M.; Furione, M.; Adzasehoun, K.M.G.; De Silvestri, A.; Comolli, G.; Baldanti, F. Human Cytomegalovirus-Specific Memory CD4+ T-Cell Response and Its Correlation With Virus Transmission to the Fetus in Pregnant Women With Primary Infection. *Clin. Infect. Dis.* **2017**, *65*, 1659–1665. [CrossRef]
37. Reddehase, M.J. Antigens and immunoevasins: Opponents in cytomegalovirus immune surveillance. *Nat. Rev. Immunol.* **2002**, *2*, 831–844. [CrossRef]
38. Taylor-Wiedeman, J.; Sissons, J.G.; Borysiewicz, L.K.; Sinclair, J.H. Monocytes are a major site of persistence of human cytomegalovirus in peripheral blood mononuclear cells. *J. Gen. Virol.* **1991**, *72 Pt 9*, 2059–2064. [CrossRef]
39. Mendelson, M.; Monard, S.; Sissons, P.; Sinclair, J. Detection of endogenous human cytomegalovirus in CD34+ bone marrow progenitors. *J. Gen. Virol.* **1996**, *77 Pt 12*, 3099–3102. [CrossRef]
40. Hargett, D.; Shenk, T.E. Experimental human cytomegalovirus latency in CD14+ monocytes. *Proc. Natl Acad. Sci. USA* **2010**, *107*, 20039–20044. [CrossRef]
41. Goodrum, F.; Reeves, M.; Sinclair, J.; High, K.; Shenk, T. Human cytomegalovirus sequences expressed in latently infected individuals promote a latent infection in vitro. *Blood* **2007**, *110*, 937–945. [CrossRef] [PubMed]

42. Reeves, M.B.; Sinclair, J.H. Analysis of latent viral gene expression in natural and experimental latency models of human cytomegalovirus and its correlation with histone modifications at a latent promoter. *J. Gen. Virol.* **2010**, *91*, 599–604. [CrossRef] [PubMed]
43. Kondo, K.; Kaneshima, H.; Mocarski, E.S. Human cytomegalovirus latent infection of granulocyte-macrophage progenitors. *Proc. Natl Acad. Sci. USA* **1994**, *91*, 11879–11883. [CrossRef] [PubMed]
44. Bego, M.; Maciejewski, J.; Khaiboullina, S.; Pari, G.; St Jeor, S. Characterization of an antisense transcript spanning the UL81-82 locus of human cytomegalovirus. *J. Virol.* **2005**, *79*, 11022–11034. [CrossRef]
45. Avdic, S.; Cao, J.Z.; Cheung, A.K.; Abendroth, A.; Slobedman, B. Viral interleukin-10 expressed by human cytomegalovirus during the latent phase of infection modulates latently infected myeloid cell differentiation. *J. Virol.* **2011**, *85*, 7465–7471. [CrossRef]
46. Poole, E.; Walther, A.; Raven, K.; Benedict, C.A.; Mason, G.M.; Sinclair, J. The myeloid transcription factor GATA-2 regulates the viral UL144 gene during human cytomegalovirus latency in an isolate-specific manner. *J. Virol.* **2013**, *87*, 4261–4271. [CrossRef]
47. Beisser, P.S.; Laurent, L.; Virelizier, J.L.; Michelson, S. Human cytomegalovirus chemokine receptor gene US28 is transcribed in latently infected THP-1 monocytes. *J. Virol.* **2001**, *75*, 5949–5957. [CrossRef]
48. Gatherer, D.; Seirafian, S.; Cunningham, C.; Holton, M.; Dargan, D.J.; Baluchova, K.; Hector, R.D.; Galbraith, J.; Herzyk, P.; Wilkinson, G.W.; et al. High-resolution human cytomegalovirus transcriptome. *Proc. Natl. Acad. Sci. USA* **2011**, *108*, 19755–19760. [CrossRef]
49. Mason, G.M.; Jackson, S.; Okecha, G.; Poole, E.; Sissons, J.G.; Sinclair, J.; Wills, M.R. Human cytomegalovirus latency-associated proteins elicit immune-suppressive IL-10 producing CD4(+) T cells. *PLoS Pathog.* **2013**, *9*, e1003635. [CrossRef]
50. Lilleri, D.; Kabanova, A.; Revello, M.G.; Percivalle, E.; Sarasini, A.; Genini, E.; Sallusto, F.; Lanzavecchia, A.; Corti, D.; Gerna, G. Fetal human cytomegalovirus transmission correlates with delayed maternal antibodies to gH/gL/pUL128-130-131 complex during primary infection. *PLoS ONE* **2013**, *8*, e59863. [CrossRef]
51. Kabanova, A.; Perez, L.; Lilleri, D.; Marcandalli, J.; Agatic, G.; Becattini, S.; Preite, S.; Fuschillo, D.; Percivalle, E.; Sallusto, F.; et al. Antibody-driven design of a human cytomegalovirus gHgLpUL128L subunit vaccine that selectively elicits potent neutralizing antibodies. *Proc. Natl. Acad. Sci. USA* **2014**, *111*, 17965–17970. [CrossRef] [PubMed]
52. Macagno, A.; Bernasconi, N.L.; Vanzetta, F.; Dander, E.; Sarasini, A.; Revello, M.G.; Gerna, G.; Sallusto, F.; Lanzavecchia, A. Isolation of human monoclonal antibodies that potently neutralize human cytomegalovirus infection by targeting different epitopes on the gH/gL/UL128-131A complex. *J. Virol.* **2010**, *84*, 1005–1013. [CrossRef] [PubMed]
53. Vanarsdall, A.L.; Howard, P.W.; Wisner, T.W.; Johnson, D.C. Human Cytomegalovirus gH/gL Forms a Stable Complex with the Fusion Protein gB in Virions. *PLoS Pathog.* **2016**, *12*, e1005564. [CrossRef] [PubMed]
54. Bu, W.; Joyce, M.G.; Nguyen, H.; Banh, D.V.; Aguilar, F.; Tariq, Z.; Yap, M.L.; Tsujimura, Y.; Gillespie, R.A.; Tsybovsky, Y.; et al. Immunization with Components of the Viral Fusion Apparatus Elicits Antibodies That Neutralize Epstein-Barr Virus in B Cells and Epithelial Cells. *Immunity* **2019**. [CrossRef] [PubMed]
55. Martinez-Martin, N.; Marcandalli, J.; Huang, C.S.; Arthur, C.P.; Perotti, M.; Foglierini, M.; Ho, H.; Dosey, A.M.; Shriver, S.; Payandeh, J.; et al. An Unbiased Screen for Human Cytomegalovirus Identifies Neuropilin-2 as a Central Viral Receptor. *Cell* **2018**, *174*, 1158–1171.e1119. [CrossRef]
56. Malito, E.; Chandramouli, S.; Carfi, A. From recognition to execution-the HCMV Pentamer from receptor binding to fusion triggering. *Curr. Opin. Virol.* **2018**, *31*, 43–51. [CrossRef]
57. Ciferri, C.; Chandramouli, S.; Leitner, A.; Donnarumma, D.; Cianfrocco, M.A.; Gerrein, R.; Friedrich, K.; Aggarwal, Y.; Palladino, G.; Aebersold, R.; et al. Antigenic Characterization of the HCMV gH/gL/gO and Pentamer Cell Entry Complexes Reveals Binding Sites for Potently Neutralizing Human Antibodies. *PLoS Pathog.* **2015**, *11*, e1005230. [CrossRef]
58. Wiegers, A.K.; Sticht, H.; Winkler, T.H.; Britt, W.J.; Mach, M. Identification of a neutralizing epitope within antigenic domain 5 of glycoprotein B of human cytomegalovirus. *J. Virol.* **2015**, *89*, 361–372. [CrossRef]
59. Spindler, N.; Diestel, U.; Stump, J.D.; Wiegers, A.K.; Winkler, T.H.; Sticht, H.; Mach, M.; Muller, Y.A. Structural basis for the recognition of human cytomegalovirus glycoprotein B by a neutralizing human antibody. *PLoS Pathog.* **2014**, *10*, e1004377. [CrossRef]

60. Potzsch, S.; Spindler, N.; Wiegers, A.K.; Fisch, T.; Rucker, P.; Sticht, H.; Grieb, N.; Baroti, T.; Weisel, F.; Stamminger, T.; et al. B cell repertoire analysis identifies new antigenic domains on glycoprotein B of human cytomegalovirus which are target of neutralizing antibodies. *PLoS Pathog.* **2011**, *7*, e1002172. [CrossRef]
61. Baraniak, I.; Kropff, B.; McLean, G.R.; Pichon, S.; Piras-Douce, F.; Milne, R.S.B.; Smith, C.; Mach, M.; Griffiths, P.D.; Reeves, M.B. Epitope-Specific Humoral Responses to Human Cytomegalovirus Glycoprotein-B Vaccine With MF59: Anti-AD2 Levels Correlate With Protection From Viremia. *J. Infect. Dis.* **2018**, *217*, 1907–1917. [CrossRef] [PubMed]
62. Baraniak, I.; Kern, F.; Holenya, P.; Griffiths, P.; Reeves, M. Original Antigenic Sin Shapes the Immunological Repertoire Evoked by Human Cytomegalovirus Glycoprotein B/MF59 Vaccine in Seropositive Recipients. *J. Infect. Dis.* **2019**, *220*, 228–232. [CrossRef] [PubMed]
63. Varnum, S.M.; Streblow, D.N.; Monroe, M.E.; Smith, P.; Auberry, K.J.; Pasa-Tolic, L.; Wang, D.; Camp, D.G., 2nd; Rodland, K.; Wiley, S.; et al. Identification of proteins in human cytomegalovirus (HCMV) particles: The HCMV proteome. *J. Virol.* **2004**, *78*, 10960–10966. [CrossRef] [PubMed]
64. Stern-Ginossar, N.; Weisburd, B.; Michalski, A.; Le, V.T.; Hein, M.Y.; Huang, S.X.; Ma, M.; Shen, B.; Qian, S.B.; Hengel, H.; et al. Decoding human cytomegalovirus. *Science* **2012**, *338*, 1088–1093. [CrossRef] [PubMed]
65. Nguyen, C.C.; Kamil, J.P. Pathogen at the Gates: Human Cytomegalovirus Entry and Cell Tropism. *Viruses* **2018**, *10*, 704. [CrossRef] [PubMed]
66. Wu, K.; Oberstein, A.; Wang, W.; Shenk, T. Role of PDGF receptor-alpha during human cytomegalovirus entry into fibroblasts. *Proc. Natl. Acad. Sci. USA* **2018**, *115*, E9889–E9898. [CrossRef] [PubMed]
67. Wu, Y.; Prager, A.; Boos, S.; Resch, M.; Brizic, I.; Mach, M.; Wildner, S.; Scrivano, L.; Adler, B. Human cytomegalovirus glycoprotein complex gH/gL/gO uses PDGFR-alpha as a key for entry. *PLoS Pathog.* **2017**, *13*, e1006281. [CrossRef]
68. Kabanova, A.; Marcandalli, J.; Zhou, T.; Bianchi, S.; Baxa, U.; Tsybovsky, Y.; Lilleri, D.; Silacci-Fregni, C.; Foglierini, M.; Fernandez-Rodriguez, B.M.; et al. Platelet-derived growth factor-alpha receptor is the cellular receptor for human cytomegalovirus gHgLgO trimer. *Nat. Microbiol.* **2016**, *1*, 16082. [CrossRef]
69. E, X.; Meraner, P.; Lu, P.; Perreira, J.M.; Aker, A.M.; McDougall, W.M.; Zhuge, R.; Chan, G.C.; Gerstein, R.M.; Caposio, P.; et al. OR14I1 is a receptor for the human cytomegalovirus pentameric complex and defines viral epithelial cell tropism. *Proc. Natl. Acad. Sci. USA* **2019**, *116*, 7043–7052. [CrossRef]
70. Ye, X.; Gui, X.; Freed, D.C.; Ku, Z.; Li, L.; Chen, Y.; Xiong, W.; Fan, X.; Su, H.; He, X.; et al. Identification of adipocyte plasma membrane-associated protein as a novel modulator of human cytomegalovirus infection. *PLoS Pathog.* **2019**, *15*, e1007914. [CrossRef]
71. Stein, K.R.; Gardner, T.J.; Hernandez, R.E.; Kraus, T.A.; Duty, J.A.; Ubarretxena-Belandia, I.; Moran, T.M.; Tortorella, D. CD46 facilitates entry and dissemination of human cytomegalovirus. *Nat. Commun.* **2019**, *10*, 2699. [CrossRef] [PubMed]
72. Vanarsdall, A.L.; Pritchard, S.R.; Wisner, T.W.; Liu, J.; Jardetzky, T.S.; Johnson, D.C. CD147 Promotes Entry of Pentamer-Expressing Human Cytomegalovirus into Epithelial and Endothelial Cells. *MBio* **2018**, *9*. [CrossRef] [PubMed]
73. Wang, D.; Shenk, T. Human cytomegalovirus virion protein complex required for epithelial and endothelial cell tropism. *Proc. Natl. Acad. Sci. USA* **2005**, *102*, 18153–18158. [CrossRef] [PubMed]
74. Huber, M.T.; Compton, T. The human cytomegalovirus UL74 gene encodes the third component of the glycoprotein H-glycoprotein L-containing envelope complex. *J. Virol.* **1998**, *72*, 8191–8197.
75. Wille, P.T.; Knoche, A.J.; Nelson, J.A.; Jarvis, M.A.; Johnson, D.C. A human cytomegalovirus gO-null mutant fails to incorporate gH/gL into the virion envelope and is unable to enter fibroblasts and epithelial and endothelial cells. *J. Virol.* **2010**, *84*, 2585–2596. [CrossRef]
76. Ciferri, C.; Chandramouli, S.; Donnarumma, D.; Nikitin, P.A.; Cianfrocco, M.A.; Gerrein, R.; Feire, A.L.; Barnett, S.W.; Lilja, A.E.; Rappuoli, R.; et al. Structural and biochemical studies of HCMV gH/gL/gO and Pentamer reveal mutually exclusive cell entry complexes. *Proc. Natl. Acad. Sci. USA* **2015**, *112*, 1767–1772. [CrossRef]
77. Zhou, M.; Lanchy, J.M.; Ryckman, B.J. Human Cytomegalovirus gH/gL/gO Promotes the Fusion Step of Entry into All Cell Types, whereas gH/gL/UL128-131 Broadens Virus Tropism through a Distinct Mechanism. *J. Virol.* **2015**, *89*, 8999–9009. [CrossRef]
78. Bagdonaite, I.; Norden, R.; Joshi, H.J.; King, S.L.; Vakhrushev, S.Y.; Olofsson, S.; Wandall, H.H. Global Mapping of O-Glycosylation of Varicella Zoster Virus, Human Cytomegalovirus, and Epstein-Barr Virus. *J. Biol. Chem.* **2016**, *291*, 12014–12028. [CrossRef]

79. Nogalski, M.T.; Chan, G.C.; Stevenson, E.V.; Collins-McMillen, D.K.; Yurochko, A.D. The HCMV gH/gL/UL128-131 complex triggers the specific cellular activation required for efficient viral internalization into target monocytes. *PLoS Pathog.* **2013**, *9*, e1003463. [CrossRef]
80. Fouts, A.E.; Chan, P.; Stephan, J.P.; Vandlen, R.; Feierbach, B. Antibodies against the gH/gL/UL128/UL130/UL131 complex comprise the majority of the anti-cytomegalovirus (anti-CMV) neutralizing antibody response in CMV hyperimmune globulin. *J. Virol.* **2012**, *86*, 7444–7447. [CrossRef]
81. Zydek, M.; Petitt, M.; Fang-Hoover, J.; Adler, B.; Kauvar, L.M.; Pereira, L.; Tabata, T. HCMV infection of human trophoblast progenitor cells of the placenta is neutralized by a human monoclonal antibody to glycoprotein B and not by antibodies to the pentamer complex. *Viruses* **2014**, *6*, 1346–1364. [CrossRef] [PubMed]
82. Wille, P.T.; Wisner, T.W.; Ryckman, B.; Johnson, D.C. Human cytomegalovirus (HCMV) glycoprotein gB promotes virus entry in trans acting as the viral fusion protein rather than as a receptor-binding protein. *MBio* **2013**, *4*, e00332-13. [CrossRef] [PubMed]
83. Selinsky, C.; Luke, C.; Wloch, M.; Geall, A.; Hermanson, G.; Kaslow, D.; Evans, T. A DNA-based vaccine for the prevention of human cytomegalovirus-associated diseases. *Hum. Vaccin.* **2005**, *1*, 16–23. [CrossRef] [PubMed]
84. Yue, Y.; Kaur, A.; Zhou, S.S.; Barry, P.A. Characterization and immunological analysis of the rhesus cytomegalovirus homologue (Rh112) of the human cytomegalovirus UL83 lower matrix phosphoprotein (pp65). *J. Gen. Virol.* **2006**, *87*, 777–787. [CrossRef] [PubMed]
85. Bachmann, M.F.; Jennings, G.T. Vaccine delivery: A matter of size, geometry, kinetics and molecular patterns. *Nat. Reviews. Immunol.* **2010**, *10*, 787–796. [CrossRef]
86. Lopez-Sagaseta, J.; Malito, E.; Rappuoli, R.; Bottomley, M.J. Self-assembling protein nanoparticles in the design of vaccines. *Comput Struct Biotechnol J.* **2016**, *14*, 58–68. [CrossRef]
87. Manolova, V.; Flace, A.; Bauer, M.; Schwarz, K.; Saudan, P.; Bachmann, M.F. Nanoparticles target distinct dendritic cell populations according to their size. *Eur. J. Immunol.* **2008**, *38*, 1404–1413. [CrossRef]
88. Duan, H.; Chen, X.; Boyington, J.C.; Cheng, C.; Zhang, Y.; Jafari, A.J.; Stephens, T.; Tsybovsky, Y.; Kalyuzhniy, O.; Zhao, P.; et al. Glycan Masking Focuses Immune Responses to the HIV-1 CD4-Binding Site and Enhances Elicitation of VRC01-Class Precursor Antibodies. *Immunity* **2018**, *49*, 301–311.e305. [CrossRef]
89. Kanekiyo, M.; Bu, W.; Joyce, M.G.; Meng, G.; Whittle, J.R.; Baxa, U.; Yamamoto, T.; Narpala, S.; Todd, J.P.; Rao, S.S.; et al. Rational Design of an Epstein-Barr Virus Vaccine Targeting the Receptor-Binding Site. *Cell* **2015**, *162*, 1090–1100. [CrossRef]
90. Kirchmeier, M.; Fluckiger, A.C.; Soare, C.; Bozic, J.; Ontsouka, B.; Ahmed, T.; Diress, A.; Pereira, L.; Schodel, F.; Plotkin, S.; et al. Enveloped virus-like particle expression of human cytomegalovirus glycoprotein B antigen induces antibodies with potent and broad neutralizing activity. *Clin. Vaccine Immunol. Cvi.* **2014**, *21*, 174–180. [CrossRef]
91. Cui, X.; Snapper, C.M. Development of novel vaccines against human cytomegalovirus. *Hum. Vaccines Immunother.* **2019**, *15*, 2673–2683. [CrossRef] [PubMed]
92. Vicente, T.; Burri, S.; Wellnitz, S.; Walsh, K.; Rothe, S.; Liderfelt, J. Fully aseptic single-use cross flow filtration system for clarification and concentration of cytomegalovirus-like particles. *Eng. Life Sci.* **2014**, *14*, 318–326. [CrossRef]
93. Crowther, R.A.; Kiselev, N.A.; Bottcher, B.; Berriman, J.A.; Borisova, G.P.; Ose, V.; Pumpens, P. Three-dimensional structure of hepatitis B virus core particles determined by electron cryomicroscopy. *Cell* **1994**, *77*, 943–950. [CrossRef]
94. Roseman, A.M.; Berriman, J.A.; Wynne, S.A.; Butler, P.J.; Crowther, R.A. A structural model for maturation of the hepatitis B virus core. *Proc. Natl. Acad. Sci. USA* **2005**, *102*, 15821–15826. [CrossRef] [PubMed]
95. Walker, A.; Skamel, C.; Vorreiter, J.; Nassal, M. Internal core protein cleavage leaves the hepatitis B virus capsid intact and enhances its capacity for surface display of heterologous whole chain proteins. *J. Biol. Chem.* **2008**, *283*, 33508–33515. [CrossRef] [PubMed]
96. Schwarz, K.; Meijerink, E.; Speiser, D.E.; Tissot, A.C.; Cielens, I.; Renhof, R.; Dishlers, A.; Pumpens, P.; Bachmann, M.F. Efficient homologous prime-boost strategies for T cell vaccination based on virus-like particles. *Eur. J. Immunol.* **2005**, *35*, 816–821. [CrossRef]
97. Krishna, B.A.; Humby, M.S.; Miller, W.E.; O'Connor, C.M. Human cytomegalovirus G protein-coupled receptor US28 promotes latency by attenuating c-fos. *Proc. Natl. Acad. Sci. USA* **2019**, *116*, 1755–1764. [CrossRef]

98. Krishna, B.A.; Miller, W.E.; O'Connor, C.M. US28: HCMV's Swiss Army Knife. *Viruses* **2018**, *10*, 445. [CrossRef]
99. Watt, G.D.; Jacobs, D.; Frankel, R.B. Redox reactivity of bacterial and mammalian ferritin: Is reductant entry into the ferritin interior a necessary step for iron release? *Proc. Natl. Acad. Sci. USA* **1988**, *85*, 7457–7461. [CrossRef]
100. Theil, E.C. Ferritin: Structure, gene regulation, and cellular function in animals, plants, and microorganisms. *Annu. Rev. Biochem.* **1987**, *56*, 289–315. [CrossRef]
101. Cho, K.J.; Shin, H.J.; Lee, J.H.; Kim, K.J.; Park, S.S.; Lee, Y.; Lee, C.; Park, S.S.; Kim, K.H. The crystal structure of ferritin from Helicobacter pylori reveals unusual conformational changes for iron uptake. *J. Mol. Biol.* **2009**, *390*, 83–98. [CrossRef] [PubMed]
102. Pulsipher, K.W.; Villegas, J.A.; Roose, B.W.; Hicks, T.L.; Yoon, J.; Saven, J.G.; Dmochowski, I.J. Thermophilic Ferritin 24mer Assembly and Nanoparticle Encapsulation Modulated by Interdimer Electrostatic Repulsion. *Biochemistry* **2017**, *56*, 3596–3606. [CrossRef] [PubMed]
103. Georgiev, I.S.; Joyce, M.G.; Chen, R.E.; Leung, K.; McKee, K.; Druz, A.; Van Galen, J.G.; Kanekiyo, M.; Tsybovsky, Y.; Yang, E.S.; et al. Two-Component Ferritin Nanoparticles for Multimerization of Diverse Trimeric Antigens. *Acs. Infect. Dis.* **2018**, *4*, 788–796. [CrossRef] [PubMed]
104. Kanekiyo, M.; Joyce, M.G.; Gillespie, R.A.; Gallagher, J.R.; Andrews, S.F.; Yassine, H.M.; Wheatley, A.K.; Fisher, B.E.; Ambrozak, D.R.; Creanga, A.; et al. Mosaic nanoparticle display of diverse influenza virus hemagglutinins elicits broad B cell responses. *Nat. Immunol.* **2019**, *20*, 362–372. [CrossRef] [PubMed]
105. Golmohammadi, R.; Fridborg, K.; Bundule, M.; Valegard, K.; Liljas, L. The crystal structure of bacteriophage Q beta at 3.5 A resolution. *Structure* **1996**, *4*, 543–554. [CrossRef]
106. Cornuz, J.; Zwahlen, S.; Jungi, W.F.; Osterwalder, J.; Klingler, K.; van Melle, G.; Bangala, Y.; Guessous, I.; Muller, P.; Willers, J.; et al. A vaccine against nicotine for smoking cessation: A randomized controlled trial. *PLoS ONE* **2008**, *3*, e2547. [CrossRef]
107. Vasiljeva, I.; Kozlovska, T.; Cielens, I.; Strelnikova, A.; Kazaks, A.; Ose, V.; Pumpens, P. Mosaic Qbeta coats as a new presentation model. *Febs. Lett.* **1998**, *431*, 7–11. [CrossRef]
108. Hsia, Y.; Bale, J.B.; Gonen, S.; Shi, D.; Sheffler, W.; Fong, K.K.; Nattermann, U.; Xu, C.; Huang, P.S.; Ravichandran, R.; et al. Corrigendum: Design of a hyperstable 60-subunit protein icosahedron. *Nature* **2016**, *540*, 150. [CrossRef]
109. King, N.P.; Bale, J.B.; Sheffler, W.; McNamara, D.E.; Gonen, S.; Gonen, T.; Yeates, T.O.; Baker, D. Accurate design of co-assembling multi-component protein nanomaterials. *Nature* **2014**, *510*, 103–108. [CrossRef]
110. Bale, J.B.; Gonen, S.; Liu, Y.; Sheffler, W.; Ellis, D.; Thomas, C.; Cascio, D.; Yeates, T.O.; Gonen, T.; King, N.P.; et al. Accurate design of megadalton-scale two-component icosahedral protein complexes. *Science* **2016**, *353*, 389–394. [CrossRef]
111. He, L.; Kumar, S.; Allen, J.D.; Huang, D.; Lin, X.; Mann, C.J.; Saye-Francisco, K.L.; Copps, J.; Sarkar, A.; Blizard, G.S.; et al. HIV-1 vaccine design through minimizing envelope metastability. *Sci. Adv.* **2018**, *4*, eaau6769. [CrossRef]
112. Marcandalli, J.; Fiala, B.; Ols, S.; Perotti, M.; de van der Schueren, W.; Snijder, J.; Hodge, E.; Benhaim, M.; Ravichandran, R.; Carter, L.; et al. Induction of Potent Neutralizing Antibody Responses by a Designed Protein Nanoparticle Vaccine for Respiratory Syncytial Virus. *Cell* **2019**, *176*, 1420–1431.e1417. [CrossRef] [PubMed]
113. Brouwer, P.J.M.; Antanasijevic, A.; Berndsen, Z.; Yasmeen, A.; Fiala, B.; Bijl, T.P.L.; Bontjer, I.; Bale, J.B.; Sheffler, W.; Allen, J.D.; et al. Enhancing and shaping the immunogenicity of native-like HIV-1 envelope trimers with a two-component protein nanoparticle. *Nat. Commun.* **2019**, *10*, 4272. [CrossRef] [PubMed]
114. Boyken, S.E.; Benhaim, M.A.; Busch, F.; Jia, M.; Bick, M.J.; Choi, H.; Klima, J.C.; Chen, Z.; Walkey, C.; Mileant, A.; et al. De novo design of tunable, pH-driven conformational changes. *Science* **2019**, *364*, 658–664. [CrossRef] [PubMed]
115. Votteler, J.; Ogohara, C.; Yi, S.; Hsia, Y.; Nattermann, U.; Belnap, D.M.; King, N.P.; Sundquist, W.I. Designed proteins induce the formation of nanocage-containing extracellular vesicles. *Nature* **2016**, *540*, 292–295. [CrossRef]
116. Zakeri, B.; Fierer, J.O.; Celik, E.; Chittock, E.C.; Schwarz-Linek, U.; Moy, V.T.; Howarth, M. Peptide tag forming a rapid covalent bond to a protein, through engineering a bacterial adhesin. *Proc. Natl. Acad. Sci. USA* **2012**, *109*, E690–E697. [CrossRef]

117. Brune, K.D.; Leneghan, D.B.; Brian, I.J.; Ishizuka, A.S.; Bachmann, M.F.; Draper, S.J.; Biswas, S.; Howarth, M. Plug-and-Display: Decoration of Virus-Like Particles via isopeptide bonds for modular immunization. *Sci. Rep.* **2016**, *6*, 19234. [CrossRef]
118. Palladini, A.; Thrane, S.; Janitzek, C.M.; Pihl, J.; Clemmensen, S.B.; de Jongh, W.A.; Clausen, T.M.; Nicoletti, G.; Landuzzi, L.; Penichet, M.L.; et al. Virus-like particle display of HER2 induces potent anti-cancer responses. *Oncoimmunology* **2018**, *7*, e1408749. [CrossRef]
119. Thrane, S.; Janitzek, C.M.; Matondo, S.; Resende, M.; Gustavsson, T.; de Jongh, W.A.; Clemmensen, S.; Roeffen, W.; van de Vegte-Bolmer, M.; van Gemert, G.J.; et al. Bacterial superglue enables easy development of efficient virus-like particle based vaccines. *J. Nanobiotechnology* **2016**, *14*, 30. [CrossRef]
120. Abbott, R.K.; Lee, J.H.; Menis, S.; Skog, P.; Rossi, M.; Ota, T.; Kulp, D.W.; Bhullar, D.; Kalyuzhniy, O.; Havenar-Daughton, C.; et al. Precursor Frequency and Affinity Determine B Cell Competitive Fitness in Germinal Centers, Tested with Germline-Targeting HIV Vaccine Immunogens. *Immunity* **2018**, *48*, 133–146.e6. [CrossRef]
121. He, L.; de Val, N.; Morris, C.D.; Vora, N.; Thinnes, T.C.; Kong, L.; Azadnia, P.; Sok, D.; Zhou, B.; Burton, D.R.; et al. Presenting native-like trimeric HIV-1 antigens with self-assembling nanoparticles. *Nat. Commun.* **2016**, *7*, 12041. [CrossRef] [PubMed]
122. McGuire, A.T.; Gray, M.D.; Dosenovic, P.; Gitlin, A.D.; Freund, N.T.; Petersen, J.; Correnti, C.; Johnsen, W.; Kegel, R.; Stuart, A.B.; et al. Specifically modified Env immunogens activate B-cell precursors of broadly neutralizing HIV-1 antibodies in transgenic mice. *Nat. Commun.* **2016**, *7*, 10618. [CrossRef] [PubMed]
123. Sliepen, K.; Ozorowski, G.; Burger, J.A.; van Montfort, T.; Stunnenberg, M.; LaBranche, C.; Montefiori, D.C.; Moore, J.P.; Ward, A.B.; Sanders, R.W. Presenting native-like HIV-1 envelope trimers on ferritin nanoparticles improves their immunogenicity. *Retrovirology* **2015**, *12*, 82. [CrossRef] [PubMed]

5

Virus-Like Particle-Mediated Vaccination against Interleukin-13 May Harbour General Anti-Allergic Potential beyond Atopic Dermatitis

John Foerster * and Aleksandra Molęda *

Department of Molecular and Clinical Medicine, University of Dundee, Medical School, Ninewells Hospital, Jacquie Woods Centre, Ninewells Drive, Dundee DD1 9SY, UK

* Correspondence: j.foerster@dundee.ac.uk (J.F.); a.moleda@dundee.ac.uk (A.M.)

Abstract: Virus-like particle (VLP)-based anti-infective prophylactic vaccination has been established in clinical use. Although validated in proof-of-concept clinical trials in humans, no VLP-based therapeutic vaccination against self-proteins to modulate chronic disease has yet been licensed. The present review summarises recent scientific advances, identifying interleukin-13 as an excellent candidate to validate the concept of anti-cytokine vaccination. Based on numerous clinical studies, long-term elimination of IL-13 is not expected to trigger target-related serious adverse effects and is likely to be safer than combined targeting of IL-4/IL-13. Furthermore, recently published results from large-scale trials confirm that elimination of IL-13 is highly effective in atopic dermatitis, an exceedingly common condition, as well as eosinophilic esophagitis. The distinctly different mode of action of a polyclonal vaccine response is discussed in detail, suggesting that anti-IL-13 vaccination has the potential of outperforming monoclonal antibody-based approaches. Finally, recent data have identified a subset of follicular T helper cells dependent on IL-13 which selectively trigger massive IgE accumulation in response to anaphylactoid allergens. Thus, prophylactic IL-13 vaccination may have broad application in a number of allergic conditions.

Keywords: VLP; IL-13; interleukin-13; vaccine; Tfh cells

---

1. Introduction: Why Develop an Anti-IL-13 Vaccine?

In an age dominated by an avalanche of monoclonal antibodies (MAb) hitting the market for a dizzying variety of conditions, one may ask why replacing this obvious successful model with a vaccine strategy is sensible at all. The answer to this question is four-fold. Two of these are generic and would apply to many vaccines replacing a MAb treatment. First, it will be much more accessible to patients (economics). Second, it will have much broader applications thanks to the qualitatively different nature of a polyclonal vs. a monoclonal immune response (see below for details). The third reason is more limited to IL-13: it has an excellent safety profile as a target compared to almost all other cytokines, with the exception of IL-17. Fourth, and finally, very recent data suggest that targeting IL-13 with a VLP vaccine may have very broad anti-allergic potential, possibly leading to amelioration of allergies and being able to achieve synergistic effects with other anti-allergic treatments. The present review will discuss these four themes in turn, not aiming to be exhaustive, but rather with the intent to stimulate further efforts to tackle many open questions. By implication, therefore, this review does not intend to deliver a broader review of the signalling, structure, or immunobiology of IL-13 which have been reviewed excellently recently elsewhere [1–3].

2. Virus-Like Particles as a Construct for IL-13 Therapeutic Vaccine

Virus-like particle (VLP) vaccines are nanostructures generated by self-assembly of structural proteins resembling the native version in their morphology and composition but lack the genomic material of infectious capacity [4,5]. VLPs can be acquired from a variety of expression systems and platforms including bacteriophages (MS2, PP7 and AP205 [6–8]), yeast (*Hansenula polymorpha* and *Saccharomyces cerevisiae* [9,10]), bacteria (*Escherichia coli* [8]), mammalian cell lines (Vero, 293T and BHK cell lines [11–13]), plant cell culture (cowpea mosaic virus, cucumber mosaic virus, tobacco mosaic virus, and bean yellow dwarf virus [14–16]) and insect cell lines (Baculovirus and Sf9 cell line [12,17]) [18]. Vaccine development faces a clear challenge: production of sufficient amounts of quality antibodies to target the desired antigen. VLPs provide an excellent vaccine delivery platform due to their composition: their small size (usually 20–200 nm), geometry and flexibility during development [4]. Their size allows easy passage and drainage through the lymph to reach all areas such as secondary lymphoid organs resulting in profound effects in targeting follicular B cells [4,19–21]. Furthermore, CD8+ and plasmacytoid subsets of dendritic cells (DCs) can cross-present small-sized antigens such as VLPs and active B cells and T cells in the lymph nodes to induce cytotoxic effects [20,22,23]. Repetitive multivalent surface arrangement allows cross-linking of B cell receptors, perfect for inducing great amounts and long-lasting antibodies [20,24]. VLPs also act as a template for further engineering, where additional epitopes, proteins and nucleic acids are easily incorporated alongside vaccine targets that can significantly increase immunity such as Toll-like receptor (Tlr) ligands [20,25]. These characteristics can thus provide solutions for vaccine delivery challenges and are readily modified for a vast variety of constructs to boost immune responses in many individuals.

3. The Health Economics of IL-13-Targetable Diseases

In terms of economics, it is obvious that health care systems globally are under huge strain; personal bankruptcies due to health care expenditure in the US alone tell the story: a 2019 study in the American Journal of Public Health found that two-thirds of personal bankruptcies are filed due to medical bills, equating to more than half a million of affected people despite the Affordable Care Act [26]. While health care cost in other economies may not be quite as exorbitant, that fact is offset by the simple unavailability of many high-quality medicines to patients who cannot afford private health care. Given current demographic trends toward increased old age-related morbidity, including the dementia 'epidemic', as well as globally increased longevity, the search for truly affordable health care solutions represents a distinct priority.

The clinical indications amenable to anti-IL-13 vaccination based on documented action of anti-IL-13 MAbs to date include atopic dermatitis, subgroups of asthma, and eosinophilic esophagitis. However, the list of other potential indications is much longer and has been discussed in detail [27]. Crucially, in the context of competitive resource allocation vis-à-vis conditions such as dementia, cancer, and emerging infectious diseases, it is clear that per-case expenditure available by health care providers will not be able to satisfy the profit margins required to offset large-scale manufacture of monoclonal antibodies. Hence, vaccine approaches, which also avoid the need for laboratory monitoring infrastructure, will become eminently competitive in the near future.

4. Monoclonal Antibodies vs. Polyclonal Vaccine Responses

The rate of recent marketing approvals of MAbs and sometimes decoy receptors suggests that they are highly effective in ameliorating disease. However, a closer look prompts the question: do they reach full therapeutic potential? Specifically, it is becoming increasingly evident that the serum concentrations required for monoclonal antibodies to be effective are rather extreme. A striking example for this is the group of monoclonals targeting the p19 subunit of IL-23, currently licensed for psoriasis: guselkumab, risankizumab, and tildrakizumab. While the molecular mode of action is identical between all three antibodies, even the comparatively high affinity of tildrakizumab to its cytokine target (300 pM) is evidently suboptimal based on its inferior clinical activity compared to the competitor MAb, which feature Kd values in the vicinity of a staggering 2 pM (Table 1). Notably, the relatively low efficacy of tildrakizumab exists despite a much higher relative affinity of this MAb for the cytokine compared to the receptor (Table 1).

Table 1. Association of IL-23-targeting monoclonal antibody (MAb) affinity with clinical efficacy.

	Target MAb Affinity	Clinical Efficacy [1]	Fold-Increase Vs. Receptor Binding [2]	Ref
Guselkumab	2 pM	91%	3000-fold	[28,29]
Risankizumab	2 pM	91%	3000-fold	[30,31]
Tildrakizumab	300 pM	61%	20-fold	[32]

[1] Response of psoriasis severity, measured as the so-called PASI75 index, indicating 75% improvement from baseline, measured at twelve weeks after treatment start, in each study cited. [2] Compared to the 6 nM reported affinity of IL-23 to receptor [33].

For MAbs targeting the IL-4/13 system, this overall scenario appears similar. MAbs and their respective molecular targets are graphically summarised in Figure 1. Structural and signalling details have been summarised in detail recently elsewhere [2]. As detailed in Table 2, the picture emerging from an integrated review of clinical success (or failure) of related MAbs is that affinities of Kd values of approximately 60 pM or higher appear to correlate with clinical activity, justifying clinical development all the way through phase III trials. The failure of pascolinumab is mechanistically of interest, as this MAb harbours high affinity. By implication, its lack of satisfactory activity in clinical trials would clearly suggest that isolated IL-4 inhibition, with intact IL-13 signalling, is insufficient to achieve useful suppression of pro-inflammatory signalling.

Table 2. Ligand affinities and affinities relative to ligand–receptor binding of various cytokine-binding clinically used MAbs.

Mab/Blocker	Net Target [1]	Affinity (pM)	Tested in [2]	Effective in	Fold Affinity Vs. Receptor [3]	Ref
Group 1: IL-13-only blockers						
Lebrikizumab	IL-13Ra1	<10	Asthma, AD	AD, Asthma [4]	3.5	[35,36]
Anrukinzumab	IL-13Ra1	385	UC, Asthma	—	0.1	[37]
RPC4046	IL-13Ra1/Ra2	50	EoE	EoE	0.7	[38,39]
Tralokinumab	IL-13Ra1/Ra2	58	Asthma, AD	AD	0.8	[40]
Group 2: IL-4-selective and IL4/IL-13 combined blockers						
Pascolizumab	IL-4Ra	60	Asthma	—	1.4	[41]
Dupilumab	IL-4Ra, IL-13Ra1	9	Asthma, AD	Asthma, AD	10	[42]
Pitrankinra	IL-4Ra, IL-13Ra1	100 [5]	Asthma	—	1	[43]
Altrakincept	IL-4Ra, IL-13Ra1	1000	Asthma	—	0.1	[44,45]
AMG317	IL-4Ra, IL-13Ra1	180	Asthma	—	0.8	[46]

[1] Signal-transducing receptor pathway inactivated by monoclonal antibody. The actual targets of each IL-13- and IL-4-inhibiting MAb are shown in Figure 1. [2] Disease abbreviations: UC—ulcerative colitis, EoE—eosinophilic esophagitis, and Pso—psoriasis. [3] Target–receptor affinities are complex, involving sequential ternary complex formation of more than one receptor subunit. The data shown depict the ratio between MAb/cytokine affinity and cytokine/receptor affinity, respectively, for IL-13 -> IL-13Ra1/IL-4Ra (30–40 pM, for group 1), and for IL-4 -> IL-4Ra (100 pM, group two), as detailed in [47]. The highest affinity target/receptor binding reported was chosen as most relevant to gauge the competitive strength of drug circulating in serum. [4] In the high-biomarker patient subgroup. [5] Assuming retained affinity for the dual mutation differentiating pitankinra from native IL-4.

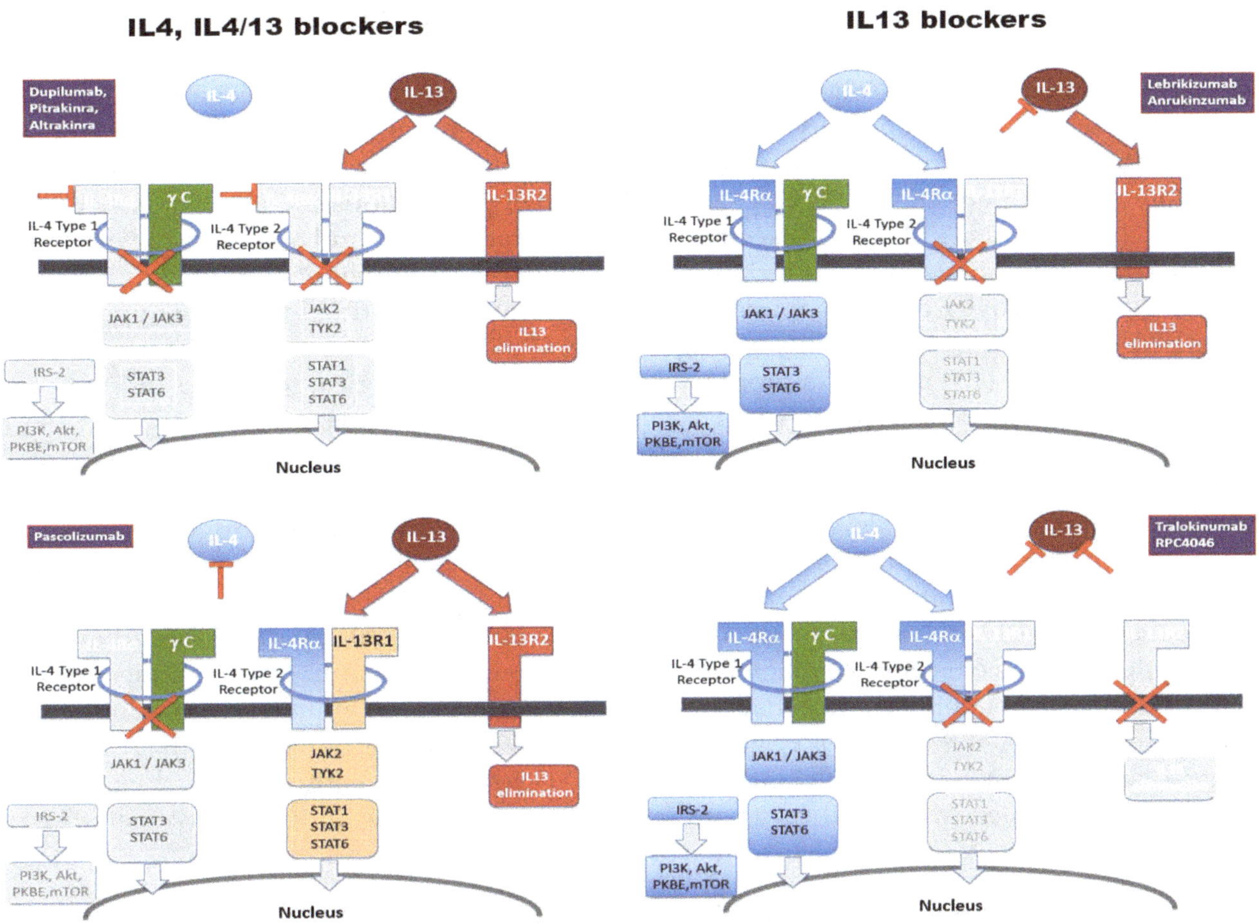

Figure 1. Molecular targets of monoclonal antibodies clinically evaluated to inhibit IL4/IL-13 signalling to date. For a list of antibodies and references, see Table 1. Colour codes used are blue for signalling transduced through IL-4, but not IL-13, beige for either IL-4 or IL-13 (through the IL-4Ra/IL-13Ra1 receptor dimer), and red for IL-13, but not IL-4. IL-13Ra2, also depicted in red, acts primarily as a cellular disposal facility for IL-13 [34]. For details on structure and signalling, see 2.

The apparent requirement for ultra-high cytokine affinity of MAbs is all the more noteworthy, as trough serum concentrations are usually above 5 g/mL. By contrast, serum concentrations reported for IL-13 range from below 1 pg/mL, regardless of whether in healthy probands or symptomatic asthma patients [48], to between 0.16 and 0.24 ng/mL in diverse populations and patient groups [49]. Even if concentrations in target tissues (lung or skin) may be significantly higher than in serum, it is remarkable that molar excess of several orders of magnitude of MAb to cytokine still can prove clinically insufficient.

By contrast, polyclonal responses act by combining various affinities of different antibody species. The quantity of B cell clones, as well as resulting affinities, can vary widely. Thus, a bivalent VLP-based vaccine against norovirus consisting of Gll.1 and Gll.4 sequence strains was found to produce an oligoclonal response, with < 3 antibodies accounting for 58–86% of epitope-specific clones [14]. This study utilised the VEE replicon vector to transfect ORF2 genes of norovirus for production of viral protein 1, a capsid protein that can self-assembly into a VLP when introduced into BHK-21 cells. By contrast, a recent in-depth analysis showed that influenza virus vaccination in humans triggered 36 ± 12 (mean ± SD, range 16–49) B cell lineages expanding >50-fold and, collectively, accounting for 22 ± 12% of each subject's antibody repertoire during peak response [50]. In another influenza vaccine study, vaccination elicited between 40 and 147 clonotypes where the top 6% most abundant clonotypes accounted for > 60% of the entire repertoire [51]. In terms of affinity, Kd values between 2.5 pM and 160 nM were found [51]. A large-scale analysis of influenza vaccination in healthy controls and SLE patients elicited antibody affinities between 1 and 100 nM [52]. A single-protein vaccination of HIV-Env produced final affinity-matured Ig affinities to the antigen between approximately 3 and 10 nM in Rhesus monkeys [53]. Collectively, these data strongly suggest that vaccine-triggered natural effector antibodies show significantly less single-clone affinity compared to the engineered MAbs detailed in Table 1 but bear the potential of significant cooperative action. Although no detailed studies are available on therapeutic VLP vaccines, these likely trigger responses comparable to anti-virus vaccines. Accordingly, the VLP-based vaccines targeting interleukin-1 and angiotensin both met their pharmacodynamic endpoints in clinical trials [54,55]. Likewise, a number of VLP-based vaccines have been shown to be effective in other mammalian species, including treating insect bite hypersensitivity in horses [56]. Here, IL-5 was chemically conjugated to a VLP from cucumber mosaic virus engineered with the tetanus toxoid (TT) epitope, a property to enhance immunological responses of T helper cells and memory B cells [56]. This characteristic was also employed in vaccine constructs against psoriasis, cat allergy and Alzheimer's disease [57]. Designing a VLP vaccine that contains the TT epitope alongside the target antigen can be a useful tool in ensuring enhanced immune protection across majority of immunised individuals, especially those that are aging [57]. Similarly, for influenza vaccines, polyclonal approaches may outperform monoclonal targeting based on broader antigen coverage [58].

Apart from the affinity and polyclonality of a vaccine response, a third fundamental difference between MAbs and polyclonal responses is that MAbs are of a singular—mostly IgG1—isotype, which is efficient in engaging effector functions such as antibody-dependent cytotoxity (ADCC), antibody-dependent cellular phagocytosis (ADCP), or pro-inflammatory cytokine activation, mediated by Fc binding of a variety of Fc gamma receptors (FcγRs). It is noteworthy that dupilumab is of the IgG4 isotype, which is less efficient in engaging FcγRs [59]. By contrast, polyclonal responses produce a mix of isotypes, which will vary between vaccine recipients in addition to cooperative action between various species targeting the cytokine at different epitopes.

5. The Inhibition of Anaphylactic TfH Cells: A Novel Role for IL-13 Neutralisation

Very recently, the paradigm in IL-4/IL-13 immune function in the germinal centre reaction was that IL-4 is central to germinal centre-based affinity maturation, as well as isotype switching toward IgE of B-cells, but not IL-13, through follicular T-helper (TfH) 2 cells characterised by IL-4 secretion (reviewed in [60]). However, a very recent landmark study identified a new Tfh subset characterised by IL-13 secretion which is responsible for the generation of IgE^{high} B cells in response to stimulation with allergens [61] (Figure 2). Crucially, TfH13 cells were not only identified in the newly created hyper-IgE-harbouring mouse model, but also detectable and increased in humans with peanut allergy. Importantly, TfH13 cells did not drive IgE^{high} B cell and peripheral IgE production in response to parasitic (helminth) infection but only in response to anaphylactoid allergen challenge (also reviewed in [62]). Moreover, T cell-specific ablation of IL-13 was found to profoundly suppress IgE synthesis. These data suggest that elimination of IL-13 function may lead to suppression of anaphylactic reaction to a wide range of allergens.

As detailed above, the response to such therapeutic intervention may profoundly differ between anti-IL-13 MAb administration and anti-IL-13 vaccination, in particular since the latter is expected to induce IL-13-targeted memory clones (both B and T cells), which could modulate the germinal centre reaction by cytokine secretion and which would not feature in MAb-mediated IL-13 suppression. In addition, it is intriguing that TfH1 cells, which would mediate class switching in response to a VLP-type vaccine, would be instrumentalised in this way to suppress the activity of TfH13 cells. In fact, this concept appears to already have been validated for TfH2 cells, since blocking of IL-4 caused a profound block in Th2-class switch and improved antibody responses to oxycodone and diptheria-pertussis-tetanus vaccination [64]. Clinically, it is very possible that the routinely observed major drop in serum IgE levels in patients treated with dupilumab is in part mediated by suppression of TfH2 cells. It would therefore be of interest to compare the performance of monoclonal- vs. vaccine-mediated IL-13 inhibition in the novel DOCK8-/- mouse model established in the above cited study. Moreover, given the different mode of action of a polyclonal response, combined with the novel anti-TfH13 mode of action, it is entirely possible that VLP vaccine-based IL-13 targeting will perform different to MAb-based treatment in allergic asthma.

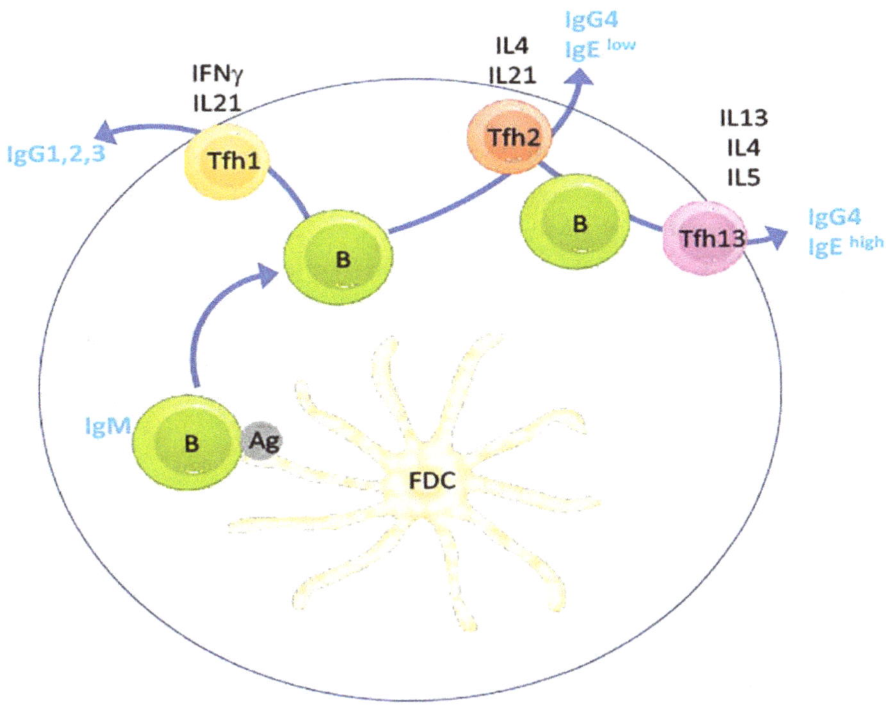

Figure 2. Function of IL-13-dependent TfH cells in IgE production in response to allergens. Simplified schematic showing the light zone of a peripheral lymphoid germinal centre (GC) where a naïve IgM-positive B cell survives apoptosis after antigen (Ag) encounter presented by a follicular dendritic cell (FDC). Prior and additional interaction with Th cells are not shown. Depending on the type of antigen, the B cell may then receive stimulation by TfH1 cells, resulting in class switching to Ig-isoforms, as indicated. Further, sequential stimulation by TfH2 cells may cause secondary class switching to IgG4 or IgE^{low} phenotypes. Finally, the newly identified IL-13-dependent TfH13 cells, may cause tertiary switching to IgE^{high} in the context of allergen stimulation. The schematic is based on figures in [61,63].

6. Safety of Anti-IL-13 Vaccination

In light of the above-detailed roles of IL-13 and IL-4, it is both highly significant and reassuring that a large double-blind controlled study on almost 180 patients did not find any effect of tetanus vaccine-induced specific IgG formation after twelve weeks of dupilumab treatment [65]. Furthermore, emerging post-marketing surveillance data of patients on dupilumab confirms an approximately 10% incidence of conjunctivitis. In one recent real-world review of 54 patients, 2 patients had to discontinue due to, or for reasons related to, conjunctivitis symptoms [66]. Since this drug-specific side effect had already been recognised during pre-marketing phase II–III studies and continues to be non-reported in any anti-IL-13 treated cohort, it is highly likely that conjunctivitis will not be associated with long-term IL-13 elimination. Furthermore, a growing array of meta-analyses, and systematic reviews of anti-IL-13 MAb-treated patients fail to uncover target-related limiting adverse events in large patient groups [27,67–69].

7. Conclusions

Utilising VLPs as vaccine constructs provides flexibility and many prospects in design that can significantly enhance protection and immunogenicity. IL-13 represents an excellent proof-of-concept target to validate anti-cytokine vaccination as a therapeutic strategy in humans based on validated vaccine targets, an excellent target safety profile, and broad vaccine applicability. Treating IL-13-related immunological disorders with a therapeutic vaccine will offer a new avenue in medical intervention.

Author Contributions: J.F. and A.M. wrote and edited the manuscript. All authors have read and agreed to the published version of the manuscript.

Acknowledgments: The authors would like to acknowledge the support of Jean-Christophe Bourdon in the co-supervision of AM research.

References

1. Bao, K.; Reinhardt, R.L. The differential expression of IL-4 and IL-13 and its impact on type-2 immunity. *Cytokine* **2015**, *75*, 25–37. [CrossRef] [PubMed]
2. Junttila, I. Tuning the Cytokine Responses: An Update on Interleukin (IL)-4 and IL-13 Receptor Complexes. *Front. Immunol.* **2018**, *9*, 888. [CrossRef] [PubMed]
3. LaPorte, S.L.; Juo, Z.S.; Vaclavikova, J.; Colf, L.A.; Qi, X.; Heller, N.M.; Keegan, A.D.; Garcia, K.C. Molecular and structural basis of cytokine receptor pleiotropy in the interleukin-4/13 system. *Cell* **2008**, *132*, 259–272. [CrossRef] [PubMed]
4. Cimica, V.; Galarza, J.M. Adjuvant formulations for virus-like particle (VLP) based vaccines. *Clin. Immunol.* **2017**, *183*, 99–108. [CrossRef] [PubMed]
5. Fuenmayor, J.; Gòdia, F.; Cervera, L. Production of virus-like particles for vaccines. *N. Biotechnol.* **2017**, *39*, 174–180. [CrossRef]
6. Lino, C.A.; Caldeira, J.C.; Peabody, D.S. Display of single-chain variable fragments on bacteriophage MS2 virus-like particles. *J. Nanobiotechnol.* **2017**, *15*, 13. [CrossRef]
7. Tumban, E.; Peabody, J.; Peabody, D.S.; Chackerian, B. A Pan-HPV Vaccine Based on Bacteriophage PP7 VLPs Displaying Broadly Cross-Neutralizing Epitopes from the HPV Minor Capsid Protein, L2. *PLoS ONE* **2011**, *6*, e23310. [CrossRef]
8. Janitzek, C.M.; Matondo, S.; Thrane, S.; Nielsen, M.; Kavishe, R.; Mwakalinga, S.B.; Theander, T.; Salanti, A.; Sander, A.F. Bacterial superglue generates a full-length circumsporozoite protein virus-like particle vaccine capable of inducing high and durable antibody responses. *Malar. J.* **2016**, *15*, 545. [CrossRef]
9. Wetzel, D.; Rolf, T.; Suckow, M.; Kranz, A.; Barbian, A.; Chan, J.A.; Leitsch, J.; Weniger, M.; Jenzelewski, V.; Kouskousis, B.; et al. Establishment of a yeast-based VLP platform for antigen presentation. *Microb. Cell Factories* **2018**, *17*, 17. [CrossRef]
10. Kim, H.J.; Kim, H.-J. Yeast as an expression system for producing virus-like particles: What factors do we need to consider? *Lett. Appl. Microbiol.* **2017**, *64*, 111–123. [CrossRef]
11. Huang, X.; Wang, X.; Zhang, J.; Xia, N.; Zhao, Q. Escherichia coli-derived virus-like particles in vaccine development. *NPJ Vaccines* **2017**, *2*, 3. [CrossRef] [PubMed]
12. Wu, C.-Y.; Yeh, Y.-C.; Yang, Y.-C.; Chou, C.; Liu, M.-T.; Wu, H.-S.; Chan, J.-T.; Hsiao, P.-W. Mammalian Expression of Virus-Like Particles for Advanced Mimicry of Authentic Influenza Virus. *PLoS ONE* **2010**, *5*, e9784. [CrossRef]
13. Arevalo, M.T.; Wong, T.M.; Ross, T.M. Expression and Purification of Virus-like Particles for Vaccination. *J. Vis. Exp.* **2016**, *112*, e54041. [CrossRef] [PubMed]
14. Lindesmith, L.C.; McDaniel, J.R.; Changela, A.; Verardi, R.; Kerr, S.A.; Costantini, V.; Brewer-Jensen, P.D.; Mallory, M.L.; Voss, W.N.; Boutz, D.R.; et al. Sera Antibody Repertoire Analyses Reveal Mechanisms of Broad and Pandemic Strain Neutralizing Responses after Human Norovirus Vaccination. *Immunity* **2019**, *50*, 1530–1541. [CrossRef] [PubMed]
15. Sainsbury, F.; Saxena, P.; Aljabali, A.A.; Saunders, K.; Evans, D.; Lomonossoff, G.P. *Genetic Engineering and Characterization of Cowpea Mosaic Virus Empty Virus-Like Particles*; Humana Press: Totowa, NJ, USA, 2014; pp. 139–153.
16. Storni, F.; Zeltins, A.; Balke, I.; Heath, M.D.; Kramer, M.F.; Skinner, M.A.; Zha, L.; Roesti, E.; Engeroff, P.; Muri, L.; et al. Vaccine against peanut allergy based on engineered virus-like particles displaying single major peanut allergens. *J. Allergy Clin. Immunol.* **2019**, *145*, 1240–1253. [CrossRef]

17. Larkin, E.J.; Brown, A.D.; Culver, J.N. Fabrication of Tobacco Mosaic Virus-Like Nanorods for Peptide Display. In *Methods in Molecular Biology (Clifton, N.J.)*; Humana Press: Totowa, NJ, USA, 2018; Volume 1776, pp. 51–60.
18. Abdoli, A.; Soleimanjahi, H.; Fotouhi, F.; Teimoori, A.; Pour Beiranvand, S.; Kianmehr, Z. Human Papillomavirus Type16- L1 VLP Production in Insect Cells. *Iran. J. Basic Med. Sci.* **2013**, *16*, 891–895.
19. Jennings, G.T.; Bachmann, M.F. Immunodrugs: Therapeutic VLP-Based Vaccines for Chronic Diseases. *Annu. Rev. Pharmacol. Toxicol.* **2008**, *49*, 303–326. [CrossRef]
20. Mohsen, M.O.; Zha, L.; Cabral-Miranda, G.; Bachmann, M.F. Major findings and recent advances in virus–like particle (VLP)-based vaccines. *Semin. Immunol.* **2017**, *34*, 123–132. [CrossRef]
21. Bachmann, M.F.; Jennings, G.T. Vaccine delivery: A matter of size, geometry, kinetics and molecular patterns. *Nat. Rev. Immunol.* **2010**, *10*, 787–796. [CrossRef]
22. Bachmann, M.; Rohrer, U.; Kündig, T.; Burki, K.; Hengartner, H.; Zinkernagel, R. The influence of antigen organization on B cell responsiveness. *Science* **1993**, *262*, 1448–1451. [CrossRef]
23. Phan, T.G.; Grigorova, I.; Okada, T.; Cyster, J.G. Subcapsular encounter and complement-dependent transport of immune complexes by lymph node B cells. *Nat. Immunol.* **2007**, *8*, 992–1000. [CrossRef] [PubMed]
24. Keller, S.A.; Bauer, M.; Manolova, V.; Muntwiler, S.; Saudan, P.; Bachmann, M.F. Cutting Edge: Limited Specialization of Dendritic Cell Subsets for MHC Class II-Associated Presentation of Viral Particles. *J. Immunol.* **2010**, *184*, 26–29. [CrossRef] [PubMed]
25. Bachmann, M.F.; El-Turabi, A.; Fettelschoss-Gabriel, A.; Vogel, M. The Prospects of an Active Vaccine Against Asthma Targeting IL-5. *Front. Microbiol.* **2018**, *9*, 2522. [CrossRef] [PubMed]
26. Himmelstein, D.U.; Lawless, R.M.; Thorne, D.; Foohey, P.; Woolhandler, S. Medical Bankruptcy: Still Common Despite the Affordable Care Act. *Am. J. Public Health* **2019**, *109*, 431–433. [CrossRef] [PubMed]
27. Foerster, J.; Molęda, A. Feasibility Analysis of Interleukin-13 as a Target for a Therapeutic Vaccine. *Vaccines (Basel)* **2019**, *7*, 20. [CrossRef] [PubMed]
28. FDA Application Review Guselkumab. Available online: https://www.accessdata.fda.gov/drugsatfda_docs/nda/2017/761061Orig1s000MultidisciplineR.pdf. (accessed on 1 March 2020).
29. Blauvelt, A.; Papp, K.; Griffiths, C.E.M.; Randazzo, B.; Wasfi, Y.; Shen, Y.-K.; Li, S.; Kimball, A. Efficacy and safety of guselkumab, an anti-interleukin-23 monoclonal antibody, compared with adalimumab for the continuous treatment of patients with moderate to severe psoriasis: Results from the phase III, double-blinded, placebo- and active comparator–controlled VOYAGE 1 trial. *J. Am. Acad. Dermatol.* **2017**, *76*, 405–417.
30. Singh, S.; Kroe-Barrett, R.R.; Canada, K.A.; Zhu, X.; Sepulveda, E.; Wu, H.; He, Y.; Raymond, E.L.; Ahlberg, J.; Frego, L.E.; et al. Selective targeting of the IL23 pathway: Generation and characterization of a novel high-affinity humanized anti-IL23A antibody. *MAbs* **2015**, *7*, 778–791. [CrossRef]
31. Gordon, K.B.; Strober, B.; Lebwohl, M.; Augustin, M.; Blauvelt, A.; Poulin, Y.; Papp, K.; Sofen, H.; Puig, L.; Foley, P.; et al. Efficacy and safety of risankizumab in moderate-to-severe plaque psoriasis (UltIMMa-1 and UltIMMa-2): Results from two double-blind, randomised, placebo-controlled and ustekinumab-controlled phase 3 trials. *Lancet* **2018**, *392*, 650–661. [CrossRef]
32. Reich, K.; Papp, K.; Blauvelt, A.; Tyring, S.K.; Sinclair, R.; Thaçi, D.; Nograles, K.; Mehta, A.; Cichanowitz, N.; Li, Q.; et al. Tildrakizumab versus placebo or etanercept for chronic plaque psoriasis (reSURFACE 1 and reSURFACE 2): Results from two randomised controlled, phase 3 trials. *Lancet* **2017**, *390*, 276–288. [CrossRef]
33. Bloch, Y.; Bouchareychas, L.; Merceron, R.; Składanowska, K.; Van den Bossche, L.; Detry, S.; Govindarajan, S.; Elewaut, D.; Haerynck, F.; Dullaers, M.; et al. Structural Activation of Pro-inflammatory Human Cytokine IL-23 by Cognate IL-23 Receptor Enables Recruitment of the Shared Receptor IL-12Rbeta1. *Immunity* **2018**, *48*, 45–58. [CrossRef]
34. Kasaian, M.T.; Raible, D.; Marquette, K.; Cook, T.A.; Zhou, S.; Tan, X.-Y.; Tchistiakova, L. IL-13 Antibodies Influence IL-13 Clearance in Humans by Modulating Scavenger Activity of IL-13Ralpha2. *J. Immunol.* **2011**, *187*, 561–569. [CrossRef] [PubMed]
35. Liu, Y.; Zhang, S.; Chen, R.; Wei, J.; Guan, G.; Zhou, M.; Dong, N.; Cao, Y. Meta-analysis of randomized controlled trials for the efficacy and safety of anti-interleukin-13 therapy with lebrikizumab in patients with uncontrolled asthma. *Allergy Asthma Proc.* **2018**, *39*, 332–337. [CrossRef]

36. Hanania, N.A.; Korenblat, P.; Chapman, K.; Bateman, E.D.; Kopecky, P.; Paggiaro, P.; Yokoyama, A.; Olsson, J.; Gray, S.; Holweg, C.T.J.; et al. Efficacy and safety of lebrikizumab in patients with uncontrolled asthma (LAVOLTA I and LAVOLTA II): Replicate, phase 3, randomised, double-blind, placebo-controlled trials. *Lancet Respir. Med.* **2016**, *4*, 781–796. [CrossRef]
37. Tiwari, A.; Kasaian, M.; Heatherington, A.C.; Jones, H.M.; Hua, F. A mechanistic PK/PD model for two anti-IL13 antibodies explains the difference in total IL-13 accumulation observed in clinical studies. *MAbs* **2016**, *8*, 983–990. [CrossRef] [PubMed]
38. Tripp, C.S.; Cuff, C.; Campbell, A.L.; Hendrickson, B.A.; Voss, J.; Melim, T.; Wu, C.; Cherniack, A.D.; Kim, K. RPC4046, A Novel Anti-interleukin-13 Antibody, Blocks IL-13 Binding to IL-13 alpha1 and alpha2 Receptors: A Randomized, Double-Blind, Placebo-Controlled, Dose-Escalation First-in-Human Study. *Adv. Ther.* **2017**, *34*, 1364–1381. [CrossRef] [PubMed]
39. Hirano, I.; Collins, M.H.; Dayan, Y.A.; Evans, L.; Gupta, S.; Schoepfer, A.M.; Straumann, A.; Safroneeva, E.; Grimm, M.; Smith, H.; et al. RPC4046, a Monoclonal Antibody Against IL13, Reduces Histologic and Endoscopic Activity in Patients With Eosinophilic Esophagitis. *Gastroenterology* **2019**, *156*, 592–603. [CrossRef]
40. Popovic, B.; Breed, J.; Rees, D.; Gardener, M.; Vinall, L.; Kemp, B.; Spooner, J.; Keen, J.; Minter, R.; Uddin, F.; et al. Structural Characterisation Reveals Mechanism of IL-13-Neutralising Monoclonal Antibody Tralokinumab as Inhibition of Binding to IL-13Ralpha1 and IL-13Ralpha2. *J. Mol. Biol.* **2017**, *429*, 208–219. [CrossRef]
41. Hart, T.K.; Blackburn, M.N.; Brigham-Burke, M.; DeDe, K.; Al-Mahdi, N.; Zia-Amirhosseini, P.; Cook, R.M. Preclinical efficacy and safety of pascolizumab (SB 240683): A humanized anti-interleukin-4 antibody with therapeutic potential in asthma. *Clin. Exp. Immunol.* **2002**, *130*, 93–100. [CrossRef]
42. Kim, J.-E.; Jung, K.; Kim, J.-A.; Kim, S.-H.; Park, H.-S.; Kim, Y.S. Engineering of anti-human interleukin-4 receptor alpha antibodies with potent antagonistic activity. *Sci. Rep.* **2019**, *9*, 7772. [CrossRef]
43. Getz, E.B.; Fisher, D.M.; Fuller, R. Human Pharmacokinetics/Pharmacodynamics of an Interleukin-4 and Interleukin-13 Dual Antagonist in Asthma. *J. Clin. Pharmacol.* **2009**, *49*, 1025–1036. [CrossRef]
44. Maliszewski, C.R.; Sato, T.A.; Bos, T.V.; Waugh, S.; Dower, S.K.; Slack, J.; Beckmann, M.P.; Grabstein, K.H. Cytokine receptors and B cell functions. I. Recombinant soluble receptors specifically inhibit IL-1- and IL-4-induced B cell activities in vitro. *J. Immunol.* **1990**, *144*, 3028–3033. [PubMed]
45. Borish, L.C.; Nelson, H.S.; Lanz, M.J.; Claussen, L.; Whitmore, J.B.; Agosti, J.M.; Garrison, L. Interleukin-4 receptor in moderate atopic asthma. A phase I/II randomized, placebo-controlled trial. *Am. J. Respir. Crit. Care Med.* **1999**, *160*, 1816–1823. [CrossRef] [PubMed]
46. Corren, J.; Busse, W.; Meltzer, E.O.; Mansfield, L.; Bensch, G.; Fahrenholz, J.; Wenzel, S.E.; Chon, Y.; Dunn, M.; Weng, H.H.; et al. A randomized, controlled, phase 2 study of AMG 317, an IL-4Ralpha antagonist, in patients with asthma. *Am. J. Respir. Crit. Care Med.* **2010**, *181*, 788–796. [CrossRef] [PubMed]
47. Kraich, M.; Klein, M.; Patiño, E.; Harrer, H.; Nickel, J.; Sebald, W.; Mueller, T.D. A modular interface of IL-4 allows for scalable affinity without affecting specificity for the IL-4 receptor. *BMC Biol.* **2006**, *4*, 13. [CrossRef] [PubMed]
48. Ledger, K.S.; Agee, S.J.; Kasaian, M.T.; Forlow, S.B.; Durn, B.L.; Minyard, J.; Lu, Q.A.; Todd, J.; Vesterqvist, O.; Burczynski, M.E. Analytical validation of a highly sensitive microparticle-based immunoassay for the quantitation of IL-13 in human serum using the Erenna®immunoassay system. *J. Immunol. Methods* **2009**, *350*, 161–170. [CrossRef]
49. Hua, F.; Ribbing, J.; Reinisch, W.; Cataldi, F.; Martin, S. A pharmacokinetic comparison of anrukinzumab, an anti- IL-13 monoclonal antibody, among healthy volunteers, asthma and ulcerative colitis patients. *Br. J. Clin. Pharmacol.* **2015**, *80*, 101–109. [CrossRef]
50. Horns, F.; Vollmers, C.; Dekker, C.L.; Quake, S.R. Signatures of selection in the human antibody repertoire: Selective sweeps, competing subclones, and neutral drift. *Proc. Natl. Acad. Sci. USA* **2019**, *116*, 1261–1266. [CrossRef]
51. Lee, J.; Boutz, D.R.; Chromikova, V.; Joyce, M.G.; Vollmers, C.; Leung, K.; Horton, A.P.; DeKosky, B.J.; Lee, C.-H.; Lavinder, J.J.; et al. Molecular-level analysis of the serum antibody repertoire in young adults before and after seasonal influenza vaccination. *Nat. Med.* **2016**, *22*, 1456–1464. [CrossRef]
52. Kaur, K.; Zheng, N.-Y.; Smith, K.; Huang, M.; Li, L.; Pauli, N.T.; Dunand, C.J.H.; Lee, J.-H.; Morrissey, M.; Wu, Y.; et al. High Affinity Antibodies against Influenza Characterize the Plasmablast Response in SLE Patients After Vaccination. *PLoS ONE* **2015**, *10*, e0125618. [CrossRef]

53. Wang, Y.; Sundling, C.; Wilson, R.; O'Dell, S.; Chen, Y.; Dai, K.; PhaD, G.E.; Zhu, J.; Xiao, Y.; Mascola, J.R.; et al. High-Resolution Longitudinal Study of HIV-1 Env Vaccine-Elicited B Cell Responses to the Virus Primary Receptor Binding Site Reveals Affinity Maturation and Clonal Persistence. *J. Immunol.* **2016**, *196*, 3729–3743. [CrossRef]
54. Cavelti-Weder, C.; Timper, K.; Seelig, E.; Keller, C.; Osranek, M.; Lässing, U.; Spohn, G.; Maurer, P.; Müller, P.; Jennings, G.T.; et al. Development of an Interleukin-1beta Vaccine in Patients with Type 2 Diabetes. *Mol. Ther.* **2016**, *24*, 1003–1012. [CrossRef]
55. Tissot, A.C.; Maurer, P.; Nussberger, J.; Sabat, R.; Pfister, T.; Ignatenko, S.; Volk, H.-D.; Stocker, H.; Müller, P.; Jennings, G.T.; et al. Effect of immunisation against angiotensin II with CYT006-AngQb on ambulatory blood pressure: A double-blind, randomised, placebo-controlled phase IIa study. *Lancet* **2008**, *371*, 821–827. [CrossRef]
56. Fettelschoss-Gabriel, A.; Fettelschoss, V.; Thoms, F.; Giese, C.; Daniel, M.; Olomski, F.; Kamarachev, J.; Birkmann, K.; Bühler, M.; Kummer, M.; et al. Treating insect-bite hypersensitivity in horses with active vaccination against IL-5. *J. Allergy Clin. Immunol.* **2018**, *142*, 1194–1205. [CrossRef]
57. Zeltins, A.; West, J.; Zabel, F.; El-Turabi, A.; Balke, I.; Haas, S.; Maudrich, M.; Storni, F.; Engeroff, P.; Jennings, G.T.; et al. Incorporation of tetanus-epitope into virus-like particles achieves vaccine responses even in older recipients in models of psoriasis, Alzheimer's and cat allergy. *NPJ Vaccines* **2017**, *2*, 30. [CrossRef]
58. Berry, C.M. Antibody immunoprophylaxis and immunotherapy for influenza virus infection: Utilization of monoclonal or polyclonal antibodies? *Hum. Vaccin. Immunother.* **2017**, *14*, 796–799. [CrossRef]
59. Wang, X.; Mathieu, M.; Brezski, R. IgG Fc engineering to modulate antibody effector functions. *Protein Cell* **2017**, *9*, 63–73. [CrossRef]
60. Sahoo, A.; Wali, S.; Nurieva, R. T helper 2 and T follicular helper cells: Regulation and function of interleukin-4. *Cytokine Growth Factor Rev.* **2016**, *30*, 29–37. [CrossRef]
61. Gowthaman, U.; Chen, J.S.; Zhang, B.; Flynn, W.F.; Lu, Y.; Song, W.; Joseph, J.; Gertie, J.A.; Xu, L.; Collet, M.A.; et al. Identification of a T follicular helper cell subset that drives anaphylactic IgE. *Science* **2019**, *365*, 6456. [CrossRef]
62. Gowthaman, U.; Chen, J.S.; Eisenbarth, S.C. Regulation of IgE by T follicular helper cells. *J. Leukoc. Biol.* **2020**, *107*, 409–418. [CrossRef]
63. Heesters, B.A.; Van Der Poel, C.E.; Das, A.; Carroll, M.C. Antigen Presentation to B Cells. *Trends Immunol.* **2016**, *37*, 844–854. [CrossRef]
64. Laudenbach, M.; Baruffaldi, F.; Robinson, C.; Carter, P.; Seelig, D.; Baehr, C.; Pravetoni, M. Blocking interleukin-4 enhances efficacy of vaccines for treatment of opioid abuse and prevention of opioid overdose. *Sci. Rep.* **2018**, *8*, 5508. [CrossRef] [PubMed]
65. Blauvelt, A.; Simpson, E.L.; Tyring, S.K.; Purcell, L.A.; Shumel, B.; Petro, C.D.; Akinlade, B.; Gadkari, A.; Eckert, L.; Graham, N.M.; et al. Dupilumab does not affect correlates of vaccine-induced immunity: A randomized, placebo-controlled trial in adults with moderate-to-severe atopic dermatitis. *J. Am. Acad. Dermatol.* **2019**, *80*, 158–167. [CrossRef] [PubMed]
66. Jo, C.E.; Georgakopoulos, J.R.; Ladda, M.; Ighani, A.; Mufti, A.; Drucker, A.M.; Piguet, V.; Yeung, J. Evaluation of long-term efficacy, safety, and reasons for discontinuation of dupilumab for moderate-to-severe atopic dermatitis in clinical practice: A retrospective cohort study. *J. Am. Acad. Dermatol.* **2020**, *82*. In Press. [CrossRef] [PubMed]
67. Luo, J.; Liu, D.; Liu, C.-T. The Efficacy and Safety of Antiinterleukin 13, a Monoclonal Antibody, in Adult Patients With Asthma: A Systematic Review and Meta-Analysis. *Medicine (Baltimore)* **2016**, *95*, e2556. [CrossRef] [PubMed]
68. Zhang, Y.; Cheng, J.; Li, Y.; He, R.; Pan, P.; Su, X.; Hu, C. The Safety and Efficacy of Anti–IL-13 Treatment with Tralokinumab (CAT-354) in Moderate to Severe Asthma: A Systematic Review and Meta-Analysis. *J. Allergy Clin. Immunol. Pr.* **2019**, *7*, 2661–2671. [CrossRef]
69. Carlsson, M.; Braddock, M.; Li, Y.; Wang, J.; Xu, W.; White, N.; Megally, A.; Hunter, G.; Colice, G. Evaluation of Antibody Properties and Clinically Relevant Immunogenicity, Anaphylaxis, and Hypersensitivity Reactions in Two Phase III Trials of Tralokinumab in Severe, Uncontrolled Asthma. *Drug Saf.* **2019**, *42*, 769–784. [CrossRef]

6

Differential Immune Transcriptome and Modulated Signalling Pathways in Rainbow Trout Infected with Viral Haemorrhagic Septicaemia Virus (VHSV) and Its Derivative Non-Virion (NV) Gene Deleted

Blanca Chinchilla [1], Paloma Encinas [2], Julio M. Coll [2] and Eduardo Gomez-Casado [2,*]

[1] Ocular Genomics Institute, Department of Ophthalmology, Massachusetts Eye and Ear Infirmary and Harvard Medical School, Boston, MA 02114, USA; Blanca_chinchillarodriguez@meei.harvard.edu

[2] Department of Biotechnology, National Agricultural and Food Research and Technology Institute (INIA), 28040 Madrid, Spain; paloma.encinas@inia.es (P.E.); juliocoll@inia.es (J.M.C.)

* Correspondence: casado@inia.es

Abstract: Viral haemorrhagic septicaemia virus (VHSV) is one of the worst viral threats to fish farming. Non-virion (NV) gene-deleted VHSV (dNV-VHSV) has been postulated as an attenuated virus, because the absence of the *NV* gene leads to lower induced pathogenicity. However, little is known about the immune responses driven by dNV-VHSV and the wild-type (wt)-VHSV in the context of infection. Here, we obtained the immune transcriptome profiling in trout infected with dNV-VHSV and wt-VHSV and the pathways involved in immune responses. As general results, dNV-VHSV upregulated more trout immune genes than wt-VHSV (65.6% vs 45.7%, respectively), whereas wt-VHSV maintained more non-regulated genes than dNV-VHSV (45.7% vs 14.6%, respectively). The modulated pathways analysis (Gene-Set Enrichment Analysis, GSEA) showed that, when compared to wt-VHSV infected trout, the dNV-VHSV infected trout upregulated signalling pathways (n = 19) such as RIG-I (retinoic acid-inducible gene-I) like receptor signalling, Toll-like receptor signalling, type II interferon signalling, and nuclear factor kappa B (NF-kappa B) signalling, among others. The results from individual genes and GSEA demonstrated that wt-VHSV impaired the activation at short stages of infection of pro-inflammatory, antiviral, proliferation, and apoptosis pathways, delaying innate humoral response and cellular crosstalk, whereas dNV-VHSV promoted the opposite effects. Therefore, these results might support future studies on using dNV-VHSV as a potential live vaccine.

Keywords: VHSV; non-virion (NV); transcriptome profiling; rainbow trout; immune pathways

1. Introduction

Viral haemorrhagic septicaemia virus (VHSV) belongs to the *Novirhabdovirus* genus, together with infectious haematopoietic necrosis virus (IHNV), snakehead rhabdovirus (SHRV), and hirame rhabdovirus (HIRV). They are all enveloped negative-stranded RNA viruses with a single RNA genome of ~11 Kb [1–3], which encodes five virion proteins (N, P, M, G, and L proteins) and the non-virion (NV) protein that gives the name to the *Novirhabdovirus* genus and differentiates it from other fish rhabdoviruses such as spring viremia carp virus (SVCV). VHSV has been isolated from more than 50 fish species from North America, Asia, and Europe, including 15 farmed [4] and free-living marine fish species [5] like trout, salmon, turbot, and eel, among others. Within a farm, the presence of VHSV infection, even if in only one individual fish, has to be notified to the Office International des Epizooties (OIE, Paris, France) and implies the sacrifice of all the farmed fish, thus leading to serious economic losses [6,7]. The *NV* gene was firstly characterised and named from IHNV genome studies [8]. Some years later, the *NV* gene from VHSV was further characterised by comparative genome studies [9]. Despite the presence of the *NV* gene in the four novirhabdovirus species mentioned above, their NV proteins showed very divergent inter-species sequences [10,11]. Initial studies regarding NV role showed that it was required for the highest efficient replication of IHNV in rainbow trout [12–14] and that of VHSV in olive flounder [13,15] and in *Epithelioma papulosum cyprinid* (EPC) cells [13]. However, NV was not essential for in vitro or in vivo SHRV production in warm-water flatfish [16,17]. Further, in vitro studies using the wild-type (wt) and NV knock-out IHNV or VHSV suggested that NV downregulated the host *ifn1/mx* transcriptional levels during in vitro infection in trout (RTG-2, Rainbow Trout Gonad-2) [18] or EPC cells [15], respectively. The higher levels of IFN-induced *mx* transcript in NV knock-out VHSV vs. wt-VHSV injected flounder found in these studies suggested that NV also interferes with IFN defences in vivo to favour VHSV replication [15]. The early anti-apoptotic role of NV during the first stages of VHSV infection has been also demonstrated [19]. Using recombinant NV protein (rNV) and a trout immune-targeted microarray, we have previously determined not only an anti-apoptotic role for NV, but also a plethora of novel expression changes (mainly downregulated) in genes associated with immune innate and adaptive response (i.e., interferons, MX, tumour necrosis factors, antigen presentation, interleukins) [6]. However, the effects driven by the injection of the rNV protein alone will probably differ from those induced by the NV in the course of VHSV infection. Recently, a microarray study in olive flounder liver infected with VHSV described differential gene expression and gene ontology classification of these genes [20], resulting in a global transcriptome profiling where only a few genes have been classified as immune-related. Gene expression has been also characterised with microarrays in olive flounder infected with a VHSV strain that produces high mortality in this species [21]. In addition, the protection of olive flounder against VHSV was previously assessed by immunization with the *NV* gene-knockout recombinant VHSV, which led to good protection against virulent VHSV [22]. However, the underlying mechanisms of olive flounder protection remain unknown. The aim of this work was to characterise the transcriptomic profiling of immune-related genes in trout infected with the wild-type VHSV (expressing NV) and dNV-VHSV (*NV* gene-deleted) in order to find targeted immune genes and signalling pathways implied in the course of a VHSV infection. This study will contribute to better understand how NV modulates gene expression and how the expression pattern changes in response to dNV-VHSV. The results will help tailoring future vaccines against viral haemorrhagic septicaemia virus and other novirhabdoviruses.

1.1. Viral Haemorrhagic Septicaemia Viruses (VHSV)

Wild type VHSV-23.75 (wt-VHSV) isolated from brown trout [23] (GenBank accession number FN665788) and its derivative *NV* gene-deleted (dNV-VHSV), obtained as previously described [13], were used to infect rainbow trout (*Oncorhynchus mykiss*) by intraperitoneal injection. Both wt- and dNV-VHSV viruses were kindly provided by Dr. Michel Brémont (INRA, France), and further propagated in EPC cells at 14 °C and titrated by the plaque-forming assay (pfu) as previously described [14].

1.2. Virus Dosages and Injection of Fingerling Rainbow Trout

Fingerling rainbow trout (*Oncorhynchus mykiss*) of 6–12 g (approximately 10 cm in length), free of IPNV (Infectious Pancreatic Necrosis Virus) and VHSV antibodies, were obtained from a local fish farm (Los Molinos, Madrid). They were maintained at 14 °C in a 200 L aquarium with tap-dechlorinated carbon-filtered water provided with biological filters and fed with a commercial fish diet. After two weeks of acclimation, fish were separated into seven groups of six trout per group. Due to the non-virion (NV) expression by wt-VHSV, a different replication rate of wt-VHSV and dNV-VHSV in the EPC cell line was established [13], and since the maximum NV expression by wt-VHSV is reached at 48 hpi (hours post-infection), we aimed at establishing the equivalent infectious dosage yielding comparable transcriptomic profile for each virus at 48 hpi. For that, we injected trout intraperitoneally with 100 μL of wt-VHSV (10^4, 10^5 or 35×10^6 pfu), dNV-VHSV (10^4, 10^5 or 35×10^6 pfu) or phosphate-buffered saline (PBS). Each group of injected trout was then released into a 50-L aquarium and maintained at 14 °C. Two days after injection, trout were sacrificed, head kidney and spleen (whole organs) were pooled, and immediately immersed in RNAlater (Ambion, Austin, USA) at 4 °C overnight, before being frozen at −70 °C until further analysis.

1.3. RNA Extraction and cDNA Synthesis

The pooled head kidney and spleen (whole organs) from each individual trout were homogenized using the Tissue Lyser Cell Disruptor (Qiagen Iberia, S.L., Madrid, Spain) for 10 min at 50 Hz with 3 mm glass beads in an RTL buffer (Qiagen Iberia, S.L., Madrid, Spain). RNA was then extracted from the homogenates by using the RNAeasyPlus kit (Qiagen Iberia, S.L., Madrid, Spain) and eluted in RNase-free water. RNA concentrations were estimated by Nanodrop and the presence of 18S and 28S rRNA bands was confirmed by denaturing RNA agarose electrophoresis (Sigma-Aldrich Quimica SA, Madrid, Spain). For qPCR experiments of the nucleoprotein (*N*) and non-virion (*NV*) genes, cDNA synthesis was carried out from RNA (1 μg) by using oligo-dT and PrimeScript^{TM} reverse transcriptase (RR037A TAKARA, Japan) according to the manufacturer's instructions. For microarray experiments, additional RNA quality controls (RNA integrity number, RIN) were performed by NIMGenetics (Madrid, Spain). For each experimental six-trout group, the four trout with best RNA quality (RIN > 7.0) were chosen for microarray hybridisation. cDNA was synthesized by using SuperScript III reverse transcriptase (Invitrogen) and oligo(dT) primer, labelled with Cy3 (GE Healthcare, Spain), and purified with Microcon YM30 (Merck Millipore, Spain).

1.4. Design of Oligo-Microarrays Enriched in Rainbow Trout Immune-Related Genes (Targeted Microarrays)

Oligo-microarrays were enriched in rainbow trout immune-related genes as previously described (immune-targeted microarrays) [6,24,25]. The final 8 × 15K microarray corresponds to Agilent's ID032303 (Gene Expression Omnibus GEO platform submission number GPL14155) and contains 1474 annotated immune-related probes (60-mer) per duplicate. In order to simplify the analysis of results, annotated probes were classified according to the following gene groups: VIG, VHSV-induced genes (number of probes, $n = 22$); IFN, interferons and their receptors ($n = 20$); MX, interferon-inducible proteins mx ($n = 3$); CO, complement components ($n = 6$); IL, interleukins and their receptors ($n = 19$); APM, antigen-presenting machinery genes ($n = 4$); TNFSF, tumour necrosis factor superfamily ($n = 16$); CD, cluster differentiation antigens ($n = 15$); CK, chemokines and their receptors ($n = 32$); CASP, caspases ($n = 3$); and TF, transcription factors ($n = 10$). The trout microarray used for these experiments was previously validated by real-time quantitative PCR (RTqPCR) [24,25]. The number of biological replicas was four. Four chips of eight samples per chip were used and hybridised simultaneously. This home-made rainbow trout oligo-microarray contains more immune-related genes than any other trout microarray available, since it includes all the immune-related genes from the Agilent's EST-derived rainbow trout oligo-microarray (ID16271) [6,24–26].

1.5. Hybridisation and Gene Expression Changes of Trout Transcripts to the Immune-Targeted Microarrays

The labelling of 2 μg of RNA (approximately 50 μg/mL) and hybridisation to the microarrays were performed by NIMGenetics (Madrid, Spain) complying with the Minimum Information about a Microarray Experiment (MIAME) standards [24].

Normalisations were performed by correcting the individual fluorescence in each microarray with the sum of all the fluorescent values according to the formula: fluorescence of each probe/sum of all the probe fluorescence signals per microarray. Raw and normalised data were deposited in GEO [27,28]. After normalisation, outlier values (defined by those fluorescence values above or below mean ± standard deviation per probe) were identified and eliminated from the calculations programmed in Origin Pro 8.6 (OriginLab Corporation, Northampton, MA, USA). Fold-change (FC) for each probe was calculated by the following formula: values of wt-VHSV or dNV-VHSV injected trout/mean of PBS injected trout ($n = 4$). Means and standard deviations of individual folds were calculated for each oligonucleotide probe by the following formula: fluorescent value/mean fluorescent value of the control ($n = 4$). Venn diagrams reflect the percentage of genes which FC value was upregulated, downregulated, and non-regulated for each comparison with these arbitrary criteria previously used [6]: (1) upregulated: FC $\geq$ 1.5; (2) downregulated: FC ≤ -1.5; and (3) non-regulated (basal) gene expression: $-1.5 <$ FC < 1.5. On the other hand, the heatmap figures reflect the FC for each gene comparison using an arbitrary criteria previously described [6]: (1) non-regulated (basal) gene expression: $-1.5 <$ FC $<$ 1.5 (black); (2) upregulated: $1.5 \leq$ FC < 2 (light red box), $2 \leq$ FC < 5 (red box), $5 \leq$ FC (dark red box); and (3) downregulated: $-1.5 \geq$ FC > -2 (light green box), $-2 \geq$ FC > -5 (green box), $-5 \geq$ FC (dark green box). Differentially expressed gene transcripts were considered significant when FC $\geq$ 1.5 or FC ≤ -1.5. Negative folds were calculated for those values below 0.66 applying the formula $-1/$FC. Therefore, FC = 0.66 corresponds to a –1.5 value; FC = 0.5 (more downregulated) corresponds to a –2 value; and FC = 0.2 (even more downregulated) corresponds to a –5 value.

1.6. *Quantitative Estimation of Transcripts by Real-Time Quantitative PCR (RTqPCR)*

To estimate the wt- or dNV-VHSV replication in rainbow trout head kidney and spleen, both *N* and *NV* transcript levels were estimated by RTqPCR amplification after intraperitoneal injection of the corresponding VHSV, as described in Section 1.2. RNA extraction and cDNA synthesis were carried out as described above. RTqPCR was carried out by mixing 100 ng of cDNA, 0.9 μM of forward primer, 0.9 μM of reverse primer, and Power SYBR Green PCR Master Mix (Life Technologies, Madrid, Spain). The thermal profile was 10 min at 95 °C, followed by 40 cycles of 95 °C for 15 s, and 60 °C for 1 min. For each experiment, the expression level of the analysed genes was calculated using the $2^{-\Delta\Delta Ct}$ relative quantitation method. The Ct for each viral gene was normalised to *β-actin* gene ($\Delta Ct^{gene} = Ct^{gene} - Ct^{\beta\text{-}actin}$), which was used as an internal control due to its low coefficient of variation (CV) among different virus dosages (CV $\leq$ 3% for 10^4 pfu/trout and 10^5 pfu/trout of wt- and dNV-VHSV; trout injected with 35×10^6 pfu of both viruses showed a CV close to 8%). Means and standard deviations were calculated for each experimental infection by intraperitoneal (ip) injection of either the wt- or dNV-VHSV in trout groups ($n = 6$) with 10^4, 10^5, or 35×10^6 pfu/trout. Primer sequences used were: *β-actin* (accession number AF550583.1) forward 5′CATCACCATCGGCAACGA and reverse 5′GATGTCCACGTCACACTTCAT; nucleoprotein (accession number AJ233396) forward 5′TCTCCGCTCGTCCTCCGTGAG and reverse 5′GTGAGCCCAGAGCCTCTTGTC; and non-virion (*NV*, accession number AJ233396) forward 5′TCAAGGTGACACAGGCAGTCA and reverse 5′CCAGTTCTCTCATGGGCATCAT. Calculated RTqPCR efficiency was 59% for *β-actin*, 45% for *N*, and 43% for *NV* genes. Efficiency was considered to correct the transcript levels obtained by RTqPCR assays.

1.7. *Calculations used for Gene Set Enrichment Analysis (GSEA)*

In order to explore the possible biological effects of simultaneous and small changes in several related genes, we screened the transcriptional data with the previously described 51 rainbow trout from the immune-related gene-set (GS) collection [25]. The trout GS collection was manually designed from the KEGG (K) and WIKI (W) trout orthologous human pathways (as accessed in 2013), using the trout genes contained in our home-designed microarray. The trout GS collection was then used for analysis by the Gene-Set Enrichment Analysis (GSEA) program [29–31]. Transcriptional data from the dNV-VHSV and wt-VHSV injected trout were analysed by GSEA to assign a normalised enrichment score (NES) for each GS of the collection in each of the three cases [25].

1.8. *Ethics Statement*

All the animal procedures used in this study were approved by the INIA (National Agricultural and Food Research and Technology Institute) ethical and biosecurity committee (authorization CEEA 2011/022) and performed following the National and European Commission guidelines and regulations on laboratory animals' care. Periodic examinations were performed several times a day during infections so as to euthanize fish with abnormal behaviour. To minimize animal suffering, fingerling rainbow trout were sacrificed by using a lethal dose of tricaine methanesulfonate (MS-222, 50 mg/mL, Sigma, Madrid, Spain).

2. Results and Discussion

2.1. dNV- and wt-VHSV Dosages used for Microarray Analysis

In this work, we have firstly defined the appropriate infectious dosage for wt-VHSV and dNV-VHSV in order to establish the comparative transcriptomic profiling between them. At 48 h post-infection, the RNA transcripts from head kidney and spleen were analysed by RTqPCR to estimate the corresponding viral replication loads based on *N* transcript levels (Figure 1). The trout injected with 10^4 pfu, 10^5 pfu, and 35×10^6 pfu of the wt-VHSV yielded the following *N* (±SD) values: 2.3 ± 1.1, 9.0 ± 4.1, and 348.8 ± 125, respectively (Figure 1). On the other hand, trout injected with 10^4 pfu, 10^5 pfu and 35×10^6 pfu of the dNV-VHSV yielded the following *N* (±SD) values: 0.6 ± 0.2, 1.1 ± 0.4, and 19.3 ± 7.6, respectively (Figure 1). Wild-type-VHSV/dNV-VHSV ratio for *N* transcripts yielded an approximately 18-fold higher replication rate for the wt-VHSV when both viruses were applied at a dose of 35×10^6 pfu/trout dose. However, this proportion was close to 1 when with the dose used was 10^5 pfu for wt-VHSV and 35×10^6 pfu for dNV-VHSV. For this reason, we considered it best to use the latter for the microarray study. Therefore, we compared the transcriptomic profile of trout injected with 10^5 pfu of wt-VHSV (NV presence) (data deposited on GEO GSE37330) and trout injected with a 350-fold more infectious dose (35×10^6 pfu) of dNV-VHSV (NV absence) (data deposited at GEO GSE43285).

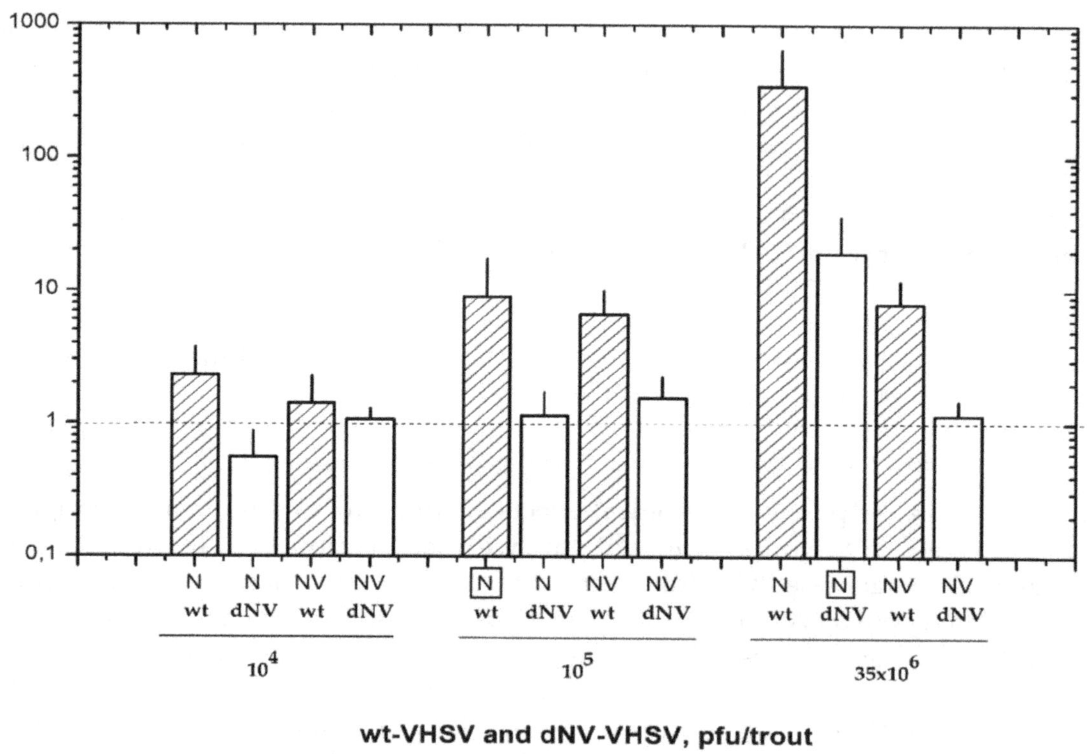

Figure 1. Nucleoprotein (*N*) and non-virion (*NV*) gene expression values (mean ± SD) obtained by RTqPCR of six trout injected with wild-type (wt)-VHSV (hatched bars) and *NV* gene-deleted (dNV)-VHSV (white bars). Animals were injected with three different dosages (10^4, 10^5, and 35×10^6 pfu/trout) of each virus and analysed 48 hpi. The results showed similar nucleoprotein (boxed N) transcript levels of wt-VHSV (10^5 pfu/trout) and dNV-VHSV (35×10^6 pfu/trout), indicating their similar replication levels. Horizontal dotted line corresponds to negative control. VHSV: viral haemorrhagic septicaemia virus.

2.2. *Overview of the Expression Profiles Obtained*

Normalised FC values of microarray datasets from wt-VHSV (10^5 pfu/trout) and dNV-VHSV ($35x10^6$ pfu/trout) were classified based on the groups defined for this study (see Section 1.5) and calculated the percentage of upregulated, downregulated and non-regulated genes. Figure 2A shows the upregulated genes between groups (wt-VHSV and dNV-VHSV) with fold changes (FC) ≥ 1.5 in Venn diagrams. The trout injected with dNV-VHSV showed the highest number of upregulated genes (65.6%), followed by those injected with wt-VHSV (45.7%). Probably, the upregulation increase in the dNV-VHSV injected trout was due to the absence of NV. In addition, dNV-VHSV and wt-VHSV shared 25.8% of the upregulated genes, which should be due to other viral proteins rather than NV.

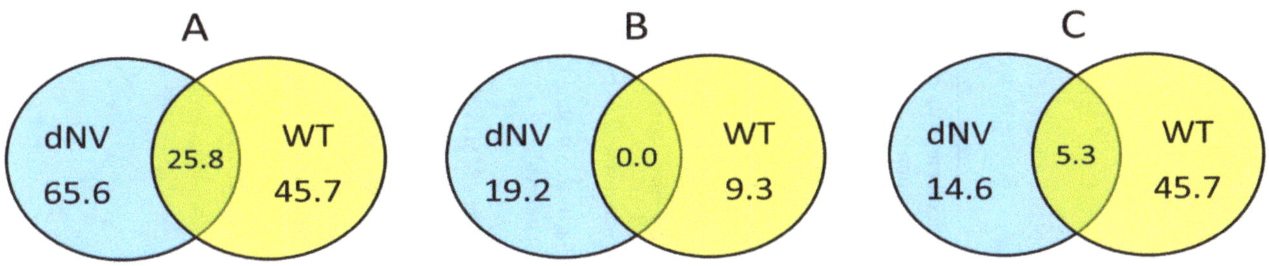

Figure 2. Venn diagrams showing the general transcriptomic relationships between trout injected with dNV-VHSV and wt-VHSV. Numbers indicate the percentage of upregulated (fold change, FC ≥ 1.5, (**A**), downregulated (FC ≤ −1.5, (**B**), and non-regulated (−1.5 < FC < 1.5, (**C**) genes, 48 h after injection with dNV-VHSV and wt-VHSV.

Figure 2B displays Venn diagrams with downregulated genes (FC ≤ −1.5), which indicate that fish infected with dNV-VHSV downregulated more genes than fish infected with wt-VHSV (19.2% vs 9.3%, respectively). On the other hand, dNV-VHSV and wt-VHSV do not have any downregulated genes in common.

When the non-regulated gene transcript levels with folds −1.5 < FC < 1.5 (Figure 2C) were analysed by Venn diagrams, the trout infected with wt-VHSV had the highest number of non-regulated genes (45.7%), followed by dNV-VHSV (14.6%). The Venn diagram also showed that 5.3% of non-regulated genes were shared by wt-VHSV and dNV-VHSV.

2.3. *dNV- and wt-VHSV Infection Effects on Trout Immune-Related Genes*

A detailed study of the transcriptomic changes driven by wt-VHSV and dNV-VHSV at 48 hpi was conducted. A heatmap was generated with the FC of the genes grouped in the categories described in methods. In addition, individual genes were also correlated with the pathways (KEGG database) [32] in which they participate (Table 1).

Table 1. Pathways related to modulated genes by WT-VHSV and dNV-VHSV. The pathways were obtained from the KEGG database [32]. See also Figures 3 and 4 for correlation with the genes.

(a) Antigen processing and presentation (b) Apoptosis (c) B-cell receptor signalling (d) Chemokine signalling (e) Complement and coagulation cascades	(q) Th1 and Th2 cell differentiation (r) Th17 cell differentiation (s) TLR (Toll-like receptor) signalling (t) TNF (Tumour necrosis factor) signalling (u) Cytokine-cytokine receptor interaction
(f) ErbB (Erb-B2 Receptor Tyrosine Kinase 2) signalling	(v) PI3-Akt (phosphatidylinositol 3-kinase and Protein kinase B) signalling (w) FoxO (Forkhead box O)signalling
(g) IL-17 signalling	(x) Natural killer cell-mediated cytotoxicity
(h) Jak–Stat signalling (Janus kinase-Signal transducer and activator of transcription)	(y) cAMP (Cyclic adenosine 3′,5′-monophosphate) signalling
(i) MAPK (Mitogen-Activated Protein Kinase) signalling (j) Necroptosis signalling (k) NF-kappa B signalling (Nuclear Factor kappa-light-chain-enhancer of activated B cells)	(z) AMPK (AMP-activated protein kinase) signalling (aa) Cell adhesion molecules (bb) Proteasome (cc) Wnt (wingless-type MMTV integration site family) signalling
(l) NOD-like (nucleotide-binding oligomerization domain-like) receptor signalling	(dd) General transcription factors (ee) Hematopoietic cell lineage (ff) TGFb (Transforming growth factor beta) signalling
(m) p53 signalling (n) Protein processing in endoplasmic reticulum (o) RIG-I-like receptor signalling (p) T-cell receptor signalling	(gg) mTOR (mammalian target of rapamycin) signalling

2.3.1. Cytosolic Sensors

Upon infection, viruses are recognised by host receptors and cytosolic sensors that activate mechanisms (signalling molecules) involved in diverse cellular processes such as the antiviral immune response. The cytosolic sensors studied belong to different gene groups and signalling pathways (Figures 3 and 4, and Table 1, RIG-I-like, and NOD-like signalling). Among the genes involved in these pathways, *tnf*, *ifna*, *irf7*, and *dhx58* and *mavs* (Figure 3, IFN and TNFSF) were upregulated by wt-VHSV and slightly more by dNV-VHSV. *Mavs*, another important cytosolic sensor, was upregulated by dNV-VHSV but non-regulated by wt-VHSV. This fact could be due to the NV expression by wt-VHSV and might indicate that *mavs* would be more functional for starting an appropriate immune response against dNV-VSHV as vaccine virus. Other important signalling molecules are *traf2* and *traf3* (Figure 3, TNFSF), and they are also upregulated by dNV-VHSV and non-regulated by wt-VHSV. These findings also support that dNV-VHSV activates better than wt-VHSV at these stages.

2.3.2. IFN System

We studied different genes belonging to the IFN system and IFN-related group of genes that belong to different signalling pathways (Figure 3, IFN pathways, $n = 14$). Regarding the IFN group of genes (IFN, $n = 20$), wt-VHSV induced the upregulation of the lowest number of genes (35%) compared to dNV-VHSV (85%) (Figure 3, IFN). This fact might be due to an inhibitory effect driven by NV after its expression from wt-VHSV. Among the downregulated and non-regulated (basal) genes, we found *iip30*, *ifng1*, *ifng2*, *iip1*, *iip2*, *ifp58*, *ifp35*, *mavs*, *ifn1*, *ifn2*, and *ifn5* (Figure 3, IFN). On the other hand, the expressions of *dhx58*, *hep*, *ifn3*, *ifna*, *irf1*, *irf7*, and *ifn4* were upregulated by wt-VHSV. Thus, some of them (i.e., *dhx58*, *hep*, *irf7*, *ifn3*) were even more upregulated by dNV-VHSV, probably due to the lack of the NV protein. The NV protein expressed by wt-VHSV induced the non-regulation of *mx2* and *mx3*, whereas *mx1* was slightly upregulated. The results also showed that all *mx* genes were upregulated by dNV-VHSV (Figure 3, MX). Mx proteins are implicated in the antiviral interferon-mediated response. In summary, in contrast to wt-VHSV, dNV-VHSV improved the antiviral immune response based on interferons (and related molecules), which would support its use as a potential live vaccine.

2.3.3. TNF Superfamily and Caspases

This gene group is comprised of molecules with diverse functionality that participate in several signalling pathways ($n = 20$, Figure 3 TNFSF, and Table 1). Most of the 16 TNF superfamily genes (*tnfsf*) studied here were upregulated (75%) by dNV-VHSV, whereas wt-VHSV induced a lower upregulation (50%) of these genes (Figure 3, TNFSF). The *tnfsf* genes upregulated by dNV-VHSV but downregulated or non-regulated by wt-VHSV were *balm*, *tnfd* (decoy), *tnfdr* (decoy receptor), *tnfr*, *tnfsf10*, *tnfsf13*, *tnfsf14*, and *tnfsf6* (Figure 3, TNFSF), which participate in several multipaths (Figure 3, TNFSF, Table 1). The *balm* gene is closely related to *tnfsf13b* (BAFF) and *tnfsf13* (APRIL) genes, and seems to be unique to teleost [33]. The *balm* gene has a constitutive expression in adult trout, mainly in the spleen, lymphocytes, posterior kidney, and anterior kidney and, therefore, *balm* has been assigned an immunological role [33]. The *tnfsf6* (FAS ligand, FASL) and *tnfsf13* (APRIL) genes modulate ligand-induced apoptosis [34]. In addition, *tnfsf10* (or TRAIL) is an inductor of apoptosis acting through *casp3* and *casp8*. Among the upregulated genes induced by wt- and dNV-VHSV injection were *tnfsf14* (stimulator of apoptosis), *tnf* (most important inducer of systemic inflammation), and *ltb1/ltb2* (involved in proliferation, differentiation, survival, and growth). Another member of TNFSF gene group is *tnfaip3* (A20 protein), which is upregulated in trout infected with wt-VHSV and downregulated in those infected with dNV-VHSV. Previous studies showed that A20 inhibited NF-kappa B and apoptosis [35,36] and our results support that dNV-VHSV would promote NF-kappa B signalling in order to set up a successful immune response.

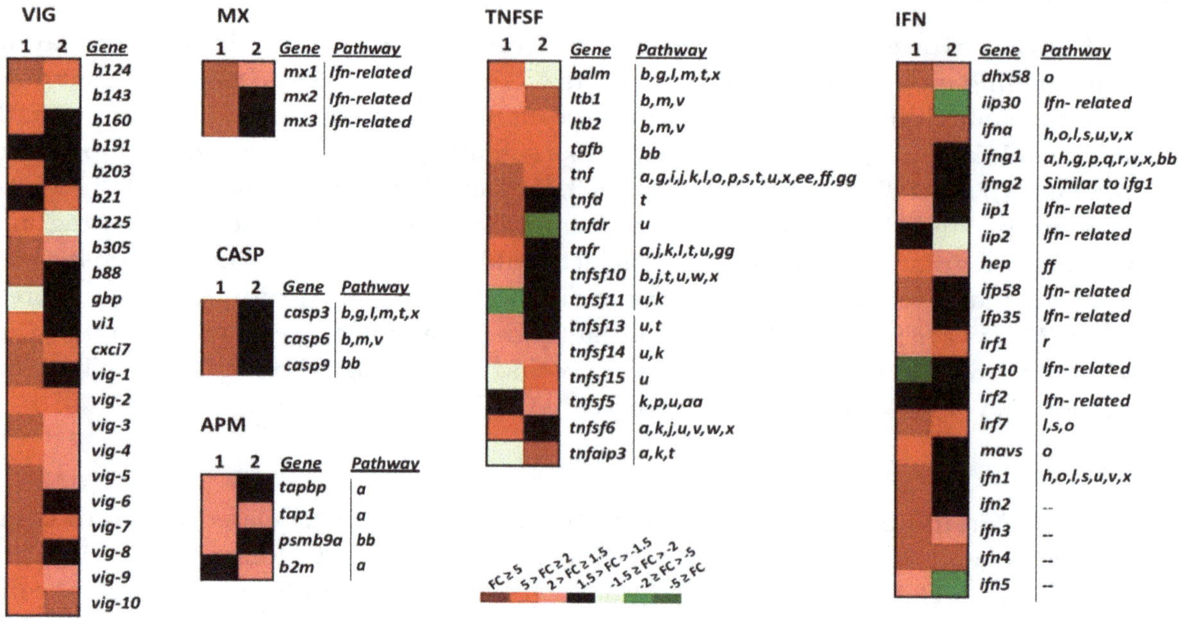

Figure 3. Heatmap showing the transcriptional expression fold changes (FCs) of the selected gene groups VHSV-induced (VIG), myxovirus resistance proteins (MX), caspases (CASP), tumour necrosis factor superfamily (TNFSF), interferon (IFN), and antigen-presenting machinery (APM) induced by dNV-VHSV and wt-VHSV in infected trout. *Gene* denotes names, and the *Pathway* column correlates with Table 1. –, unassigned pathway. Column 1, dNV-VHSV, each box corresponds to the average FC from four trout. Column 2, wt-VHSV, each box corresponds to the average FC from four trout. VIG group: b191 (c-lectin, AF483535), vig-1 (AF076620), vig-2 (AF290477), vig-3 (AF483529), vig-4 (AF483530), vig-5 (clone B17), vig-6 (clone B126), vig-7 (AF483527), vig-8 (clone B68), vig-9 (AF483533), vig-10 (AF483534), b203 (AF483538), b143 (AF483539), b225 (AF483540), b88 (AF483541), b160 (AF483545), b124 (AF483546), b305 (AF483542), cxci7 (VHSV induced protein 7 (vig7)), vi1 (VHSV induced protein 1), gbp (guanylate-binding protein GTPase, b21 (CD9, AF483544)). MX group: mx1 (myxovirus resistance 1), mx2 (myxovirus resistance 2), mx3 (myxovirus resistance 3). CASP group: casp3 (caspase 3), casp6 (caspase 6), casp9 (caspase 9). TNFSF group: balm (BAFF and APRIL-like molecule), ltb1 (lymphotoxin beta 1), ltb2 (lymphotoxin beta 2), tgfb (tumour growth factor beta), tnf (tumour necrosis factor alpha), tnfd (tumour necrosis factor decoy), tnfdr (tumour necrosis factor decoy receptor), tnfr (tumour necrosis factor receptor), tnfsf10 (tumour necrosis factor superfamily 10), tnfsf11 (tumour necrosis factor superfamily 11), tnfsf13 (tumour necrosis factor superfamily 13), tnfsf14 (tumour necrosis factor superfamily 14), tnfsf15 (tumour necrosis factor superfamily 15), tnfsf5 (tumour necrosis factor superfamily 5 (CD40)), tnfsf6 (tumour necrosis factor superfamily 6), tnfaip3 (tumour necrosis factor alpha-induced protein 3). IFN group: dhx58 (RIG-I-like receptor LGP2), iip30 (interferon gamma inducible protein 30), ifna (interferon alpha), ifng1 (interferon gamma 1), ifng2 (interferon gamma 2), iip1 (interferon inducible protein 1), iip2 (interferon inducible protein 2), hep (hepcidin), ifp58 (interferon-induced protein 58), ifp35 (interferon-induced protein 35), irf1 (interferon regulatory factor 1), irf10 (interferon regulatory factor 10), irf2 (interferon regulatory factor 2), irf7 (interferon regulatory factor 7), mavs (mitochondrial antiviral signalling protein), ifn1 (type 1 interferon 1), ifn2 (type 1 interferon 2), ifn3 (type 1 interferon 3), ifn4 (type 1 interferon 4), ifn5 (type 1 interferon 5). APM group: tapbp (tapasin (TAP binding protein)), tap1 (transporter associated with antigen processing 1), psmb9a (proteasome subunit type 9), b2m (beta-2 microglobulin).

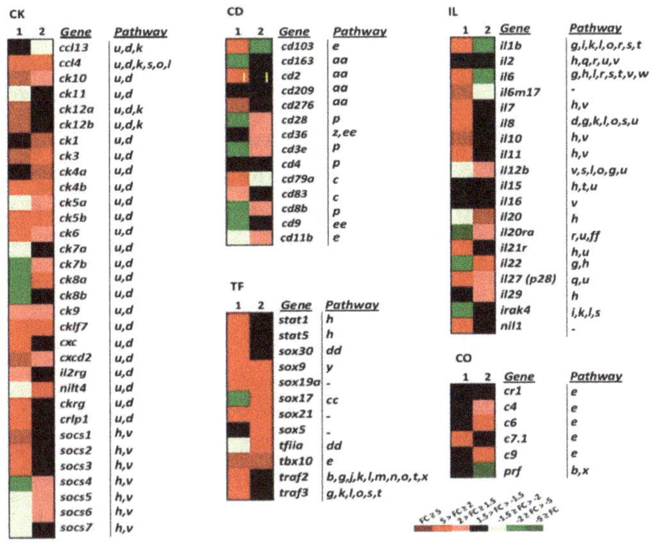

Figure 4. Heatmap showing the transcriptional expression fold changes (FCs) of the selected gene groups cytokines (CK), interleukins (IL), cluster of differentiation antigens (CD), complement (CO) and transcription factor (TF), induced by dNV-VHSV and wt-VHSV. *Gene* denotes names, and the *Pathway* column correlates with Table 1. –, unassigned pathway. Column 1, dNV-VHSV, each box corresponds to the average FC from four trout. Column2, wt-VHSV, each box corresponds to the average FC from four trout. CK group: ccl13 (cc-chemokine 13), ccl4 (cc-chemokine 4), ck10 (cc-chemokine 10), ck11 (cc-chemokine 11), ck12a (cc-chemokine 12a), ck12b (cc-chemokine 12b), ck1 (cc-chemokine 1), ck3 (cc-chemokine 3), ck4a (cc-chemokine 4a), ck4b (cc-chemokine 4b), ck5a (cc-chemokine 5a), ck5b (cc-chemokine 5b), ck6 (cc-chemokine 6), ck7a (cc-chemokine 7a), ck7b (cc-chemokine 7b), ck8a (cc-chemokine 8a), ck8b (cc-chemokine 8b), ck9 (cc-chemokine 9), cklf7 (chemokine-like factor superfamily member 7), cxc (α-chemokines), cxcd2 (cxc d2 chemokine), il2rg (il2 receptor gamma), nilt4 (novel immunoglobulin-like transcript 4 (FM200774.1)), ckrg (cytokine receptor gamma), crlp1 (chemokine receptor-like protein 1 (AJ620468.1)), socs1 (suppressor of cytokine signalling 1), socs2 (suppressor of cytokine signalling 2), socs3 (suppressor of cytokine signalling 3), socs4 (suppressor of cytokine signalling 4), socs5 (suppressor of cytokine signalling 5), socs6 (suppressor of cytokine signalling 6), socs7 (suppressor of cytokine signalling 7). IL group (r means receptor): il1b, il2, il6, il6m17, il7, il8, il10, il12b, il15, il16, il20, il20ra, il21r, il22, il27 (p28 subunit), il29, Irak4 (interleukin-1 receptor-associated kinase 4), nil1 (novel il-1 cytokine family member). CD group: cd103, cd163, cd2, cd209, cd276, cd28, cd36, cd3e (epsilon), cd4, d79a, cd83, cd8b (beta), cd9. CO group: cr1 (complement receptor type 1), c4 (complement component 4), c6 (complement component 6), c7.1 (complement component 7-1), c9 (complement component 9), prf (perforin). TF group: stat1 (signal transducer and activator of transcription 1), stat5 (signal transducer and activator of transcription 5), sox30 (SRY-related HMG box 30 gene family), sox9 (SRY-related HMG box 9 gene family), sox19a (SRY-related HMG box 19a gene family), sox17 (SRY-related HMG box 17 gene family), sox21 (SRY-related HMG box 21 gene family), sox5 (SRY-related HMG box 5 gene family), tfiia (transcription factor IIA), tbx10 (T-box 10 gene).

TNFs have a role as 'double-edged swords' in cellular proliferation, survival, differentiation or apoptosis. Ligands such as APRIL (*tnfsf13* gene), LIGHT (*tnfsf14* gene), RANKL (*tnfsf11* gene), LT-β (*ltb1*, *ltb2* genes), and CD40L (*tnfsf5* gene) bind to receptors with a TRAF-interacting motifs (TIM) domain, leading to the recruitment of TRAF molecules, and the activation of multiple signal transduction pathways such as NF-kappa B, Jun N-terminal kinase (JNK), p38, extracellular signal regulated kinase (ERK), and phosphoinositide-3 kinase (PI3K). On the other hand, ligands such as TNF-α (*tnf* gene), TRAIL (*tnfsf10* gene), FASL (*tnfsf6* gene), and decoy receptor have a dead domain (DD), which ultimately activates apoptosis through caspases. In summary, most of the *tnfsf* genes were upregulated by dNV-VHSV, giving rise to both activation signalling (NF-Kappa B, JNK, etc) and apoptosis signalling pathways.

Regarding the caspase group (Figure 3, CASP, and Table 1), the effector (*casp3, casp6*) and initiator (*casp9*) caspase genes were highly upregulated in the dNV-VHSV infected group while maintained at normal transcription levels in the wt-VHSV infected group. These results suggest that NV expressed by wt-VHSV impairs the upregulation and, consequently, the activation of apoptosis at 48 h post-infection (Figure 3, CASP). Moreover, the upregulation of the *casp* genes by dNV-VHSV promotes the activation of different pathways in which they participate, supporting an appropriate immune response developed by dNV-VHSV.

2.3.4. Antigen Presentation

Among the antigen presenting machinery (APM, n = 4) genes studied, TAPASIN (*tapbp*) and proteasome subunit (*psmb9a*) were non-regulated genes, whereas *tap1* and *b2m* were upregulated in wt-VHSV (Figure 3, APM). The APM genes belong to innate and adaptive immune responses. They act within the proteasome for peptide generation (*psmb9a*) and the transport of peptides (*tapbp, tap1*) into the endoplasmic reticulum. MHC (Major histocompatibility complex) class I molecules (together with *b2m*) bind these antigenic peptides to present them to CD8+ T-lymphocytes. Other genes belonging to TNFSF and IFN groups are also implicated in the antigen presentation signalling pathway (Figure 3). Overall, the results indicated that dNV-VHSV favoured the antigen processing and presentation in relation to wt-VHSV.

2.3.5. Cluster of Differentiation: B-Cell, T-Cell, and Cell-to-Cell Interactions

Cluster of differentiation genes (CD) conform a functional heterogeneous group of genes that have been involved in cell adhesion, B-cell receptor signalling, T-cell receptor signalling, complement and coagulation cascades, and hematopoietic markers (Figure 4 CD, and Table 1). In this study, 14 CD genes have been analysed. Downregulated and non-regulated CD genes (CD, n = 5 genes, Figure 4 CD) were found in the wt-VHSV dataset. The downregulated genes by wt-VHSV were *cd103* (a marker of dendritic cells) [37] and *cd79a* (associated with membrane-bound immunoglobulin in B-cells). On the other hand, the non-regulated genes in wt-VHSV were *cd2* (implicated in the adhesion T cell-APC through the *CD58* protein), *cd276* (participating in the regulation of the T-cell-mediated immune response), *cd83* (involved in the regulation of antigen presentation) [38], and *cd163* (exclusively expressed in monocytes and macrophages in humans), which was downregulated by dNV-VHSV. Some of the CD markers were found upregulated by dNV-VHSV (*cd103, cd2, cd276, cd279, cd83*) and others upregulated by wt-VHSV (*cd28, cd36, cd3e, cd83, cd11*). This fact might indicate that 48 hpi is a too short time to observe adaptive cellular responses against VHSV.

2.3.6. Cytokines: Chemokines and Interleukins

Among the chemoattractant cytokines or chemokines genes (CK, n = *32*), 53% were upregulated by wt-VHSV, whereas dNV-VHSV induced the upregulation by 50%. The chemokines showing downregulated or non-regulated fold changes by wt-VHSV were *ccl13, ck11, ck12a, ck12b, ck8b, cxc, ckrg, crlp1*, suppressor of cytokine 1 (*socs1*), *socs2, socs3*, and *socs7* (Figure 4, CK). In addition, dNV-VHSV induced the downregulation or non-regulation of the chemokines *ccl13* (basal), *ck1, ck4a, ck5a, ck7a, ck7b, ck8a, ck11, nilt4, socs4*, and *socs5*. Chemokines have different roles in the coordination of the immune response and may promote the activation or inhibition of different pathways (Figure 4 IL, Table 1), and for the most of them their function is unknown on the basis of viral infections.

Previous studies in rainbow trout have shown that recombinant CK1 has an attractant effect for blood leukocytes) [39]. In addition, CK6 is a chemoattractant for mature macrophages from the RTS11 rainbow trout monocyte-macrophage cell line and may also induce interleukin 8 (IL-8), inducible nitric oxide synthase (iNOS), and the CD-18 integrin in these cells, revealing additional immunomodulatory effects [40]. The capacity of trout recombinant CK12 to attract splenocytes has also been reported, establishing that IgM + B cells were one of the target cells recruited [41]. In the present study, CK1, CK6 and CK12 are upregulated by dNV-VHSV in relation to wt-VHSV. Regarding the interleukin genes group (IL, $n = 20$), the transcriptomic profile obtained after wt-VHSV injection was different from that of dNV-VHSV. Wild-type VHSV downregulated important pleiotropic pro- and anti-inflammatory interleukins such as *il1b*, *il6*, and its related *il6m17* (Figure 4, IL). On the contrary, interleukins *il1*, *il6*, *il6m7*, *il7*, *il8*, *il11*, *il21r*, *il27* and *nil1* were upregulated by dNV-VHSV. These interleukins have a key role in immune pathways (Figure 4 IL, Table 1) and their upregulation are required for an effective immune response followed vaccination, suggesting that dNV-VHSV could be an effective attenuated live vaccine.

2.3.7. General Transcription Factors

This group of genes (TF, $n = 10$ selected genes, Figure 4) are implicated in important cellular processes and pathways: Jak–Stat signalling (*stat1*, *stat5*), general transcription factors and regulatory elements (*sox* genes), and multipath genes previously mentioned (*traf2*, *traf3*). In the dNV-VHSV-injected trout, all the TF selected genes were upregulated except for *sox5* (non-regulated) and *tfiia* (downregulated). In wt-VHSV, all the genes studied were upregulated except for *traf2*, *traf3*, *sox30*, *stat5* and *stat1*, which were non-upregulated. These data reflected that Jak–Stat signalling pathway is upregulated by dNV-VHSV, which in turn promoted interferon responses leading to an improved antiviral stage.

2.3.8. Complement and VIG Genes

Among complement genes studied (CO, $n = 6$, Figure 4), the trout injected with dNV-VHSV maintained most of the genes non-regulated and only one was upregulated. It is interesting to note that C9 was upregulated by wt-VHSV, whereas perforin (*prf*) was downregulated by the same virus.

VHSV-induced genes (VIG, $n = 22$) were firstly identified by subtractive hybridisation performed in a previous work [42]. We found that NV from wt-VHSV inhibited the upregulation of 50% of all *vig* genes (*b143*, *b160*, *b191*, *b203*, *b225*, *b88*, *gbp*, *vi1*, *vig-1*, *vig-6*, *vig-8*) while these genes were upregulated in dNV-VHSV, except for *b191* and *gbp* (Figure 3, VIG). Viperin (*vig1*) is expressed by mitochondria and is an IFN-inducible protein that inhibits the replication of a variety of viruses [43]. In addition, *vig-2* [44], *vig-3*, *vig-4*, *vig5*, and probably *vig-6* are also induced by interferon [42]. On the other hand, *vig-7*, *vig-8*, *vig-9* have chemoattractant function, *vig-9* also has an apoptotic function, and *vig-10* is related to apoptosis and transcription repression [42].

The present study is the first one describing the trout transcriptomic profile driven by dNV-VHSV. There are scarce studies regarding whole gene effects upon VHSV infection in trout, the most relevant to our study is the characterization of the RNA microarray profile in olive flounder liver after VHSV infection by immersion [20]. Regarding the role of immune-related genes, we found that both wt-VHSV and dNV-VHSV induced an upregulation of hepcidin, (a regulator of the iron metabolism that is implicated in inflammatory processes) in trout similar to the results observed in VHSV infected olive flounder. However, the *irf2* gene was found non-regulated in the wt-VHSV injected trout, which differs from the upregulation found in olive flounder .The differences found between trout and olive flounder could be due to the expression profile of immune response genes in spleen/head kidney, which could be slightly different from those in liver.

Another recent study determined the miRNA expression profile after VHSV infection. Among the immunity-associated target genes of 63 differentially expressed miRNA after VHSV infection of olive flounder, the authors described IL (*il1b, il8, il10*), *mx*, interferon regulatory factors (*irf3, irf5, irf7*), TNF (*tnfsf*), and heat shock proteins (*hsp10, hsp60, hsp70, hsp90*) [45]. For instance, *mx* mRNA was regulated by one miRNA (pol-miR-1388-5p) only, for which the highest expression was at 0 hpi and the lowest at 72 hpi. At 48 hpi, the *mx* expression was not modulated by this miRNA. Our data in trout showed a non-regulation of *mx* at 48h after wt-VSHV injection, being coincident with those of miRNA in olive flounder. Maybe in the future, a correlation between miRNA and mRNA expression levels could be established in infected VHSV fish, as it has been done for some miRNAs in primary human osteoblasts from healthy individuals [46].

2.4. *Modulated Pathways in dNV- and wt-VHSV-Injected Trout using GSEA*

To define the impact of dNV-VHSV or wt-VHSV when targeting different pathways or gene sets (GS) in head kidney/spleen, we used the Gene-Set Enrichment Analysis (GSEA) program. Briefly, 51 trout GS collection previously defined [25] were used to obtain normalised enrichment scores (NES). The GS were then classified according to their NES values, as follows: (1) upregulation in dNV-VHSV in relation to wt-VHSV ($n = 19$), and (2) no regulation in dNV-VHSV in relation to wt-VHSV (Figure 5). Among the upregulated GS in dNV-VHSV in relation to wt-VHSV (Figure 5A), higher differences were found in those corresponding to "Protein processing in endoplasmic reticulum", "Regulation of autophagy", and "Autoimmune thyroid disease" (> 2 to 4-fold) (Figure 5A, red lines and symbols). Other GSs which showed lower improvement of upregulations with dNV-VHSV were those implicated in anti-viral interferon networks ("Toll-like receptor signalling pathway", "Toll-like receptor wikipathway", "Type II interferon signalling (IFNG)"), inflammation ("TNFa NF-kappa B signalling", "Cytokine inflammatory response pathway"), recognition of nucleic acids ("Cytosolic DNA sensing pathway", "RIG-I-like receptor signalling"), viral- and bacterial-caused diseases ("Hepatitis C", "Influenza A", "Measles", "Herpes simplex infection", "Epithelial cell *Helicobacter pylori*"), and others ("NF-kappa B signalling pathway", "T cell receptor signalling pathway", "Natural killer cell mediated cytotoxicity-K", "Interleukin 5"). The remaining GSs showed no differences between dNV-VHSV and wt-VHSV (Figure 5B). The "Type II IFN signalling (IFNG)" pathway was one of the top enriched GS found in VHSV survivor zebrafish [47], indicating that both species share similar mechanisms to fight VHSV. Other improved pathways in dNV-VHSV such as "Toll-like receptor signalling", "RIG-I-like receptor signalling", "Natural killer cell-mediated cytotoxicity", "Hepatitis C", and "Influenza A and Measles" were among the most targeted pathways in SVCV zebrafish infections [48]. Finally, "NF-kappa B signalling pathway", "Toll-like receptor wikipathway", "Natural killer cell mediated cytotoxicity", "RIG-I-like receptor signalling", "Autoimmune thyroid disease", "Influenza A", and "Herpes simplex infection" were also modulated in trout when injected with thyroid hormone analogues [25]. All the above-mentioned pathways participated in generating resistance to fish viral infections and underlined the importance that their upregulation by dNV-VHSV might have in case this defective virus is used as a potential attenuated live vaccine.

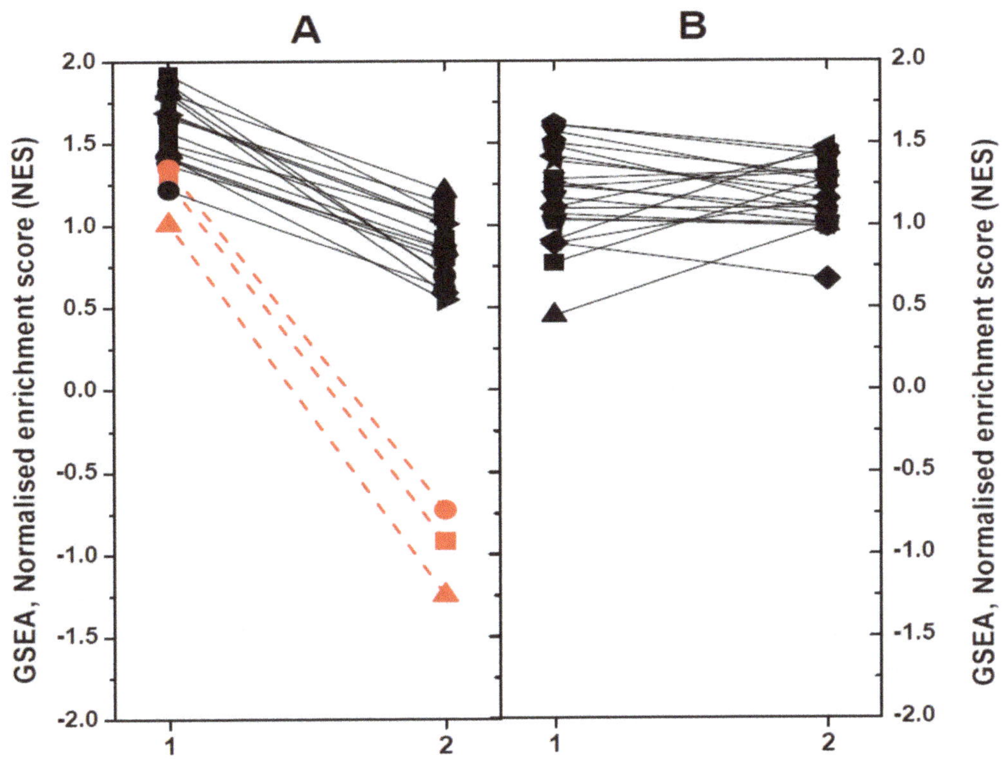

Figure 5. Comparison of significant normalised enrichment scores (NESs) of rainbow trout gene-sets (GSs) by Gene-Set Enrichment Analysis (GSEA). X axis: 1, dNV-VHSV. 2, wt-VHSV. Trout GSs were obtained from the KEGG (-K) and WIKI (-W) pathway databases as described before [25]. For comparative purposes, the NESs calculated by GSEA were represented in a diagram by linking the results obtained with lines. For better clarity, the results were not individually identified by GS. (**A**) GS which show upregulation in dNV-VHSV in relation to wt-VHSV: Toll-like receptor wikipathway-W, Hepatitis C-K, Toll-like receptor signalling pathway-W, RIG-I-like receptor signalling-K, Influenza A-K, Type II interferon signalling (IFNG)-W, Measles-K, NF-kappa B signalling pathway-K, TNFa NF-kappa B signalling-W, Herpes simplex infection-K, Epithelial cell *Helicobacter pylori*-K, T cell receptor signalling pathway-K, Cytosolic DNA sensing pathway-K, Natural killer cell mediated cytotoxicity-K, Interleukin 5-W, Cytokine inflammatory response pathway-W. The most upregulated pathways by dNV-VHSV in relation to wt-VHSV were: Red circle, Autoimmune thyroid disease-K; Red square, Regulation of autophagy-K; and Red triangle, Protein processing in endoplasmic reticulum-K. (**B**) GS which showed no regulation in relation to wt-VHSV: Interferon type I-W, Interferon alpha beta signalling-W, Apoptosis modulation by HSP70-W, B-cell receptor signalling pathway-W, EGFR1 signalling pathway-W, MAPK signalling pathway-K, Interleukin 6-W, Ubiquitin mediated proteolysis-K, TSH signalling pathway-W, Antigen processing and presentation-K, MAPK signalling pathway-W, Interleukin 2-W, HTLV-K, androgen receptor signalling-W, TP53 network signalling-W, AHR pathway-W, Interleukin 3-W, Hematopoietic cell lineages-K, T-cell receptor pathway-W, JAK–STAT signalling pathway-K, PI3K–AKT signalling pathway-K, FGF signalling pathway-W.

3. Conclusions

The results presented in this study support the hypothesis that dNV-VHSV can be considered an attenuated virus and a potential live vaccine, based on the fact that many critical host gene pathways are activated upon infection. On the contrary, NV expressed at first stages of infection by wt-VHSV modulates the expression levels of interferons, VIG, chemokines, CD, transcription factors, and other immune-related genes, leading to an immune unresponsiveness state that interferes with the early innate immune response. Importantly, this work opens new avenues for the use of NV-deleted novirhabdoviruses as a tool to study the regulation of immune pathways in other teleost fish.

Author Contributions: Experimental design, E.G.C. and J.M.C.; Methodology, B.C., P.E., J.M.C., and E.G.C.; Formal analysis, E.G.C.; Original draft preparation, B.C. and E.G.C; Writing—review and editing, B.C., P.E., and E.G.C.; Funding acquisition, J.M.C. and E.G.C. All authors have read and agreed to the published version of the manuscript.

Acknowledgments: Authors are in debt to Dr. Rosario Fernández-Godino for her helpful comments.

References

1. Nishizawa, T.; Iida, H.; Takano, R.; Isshiki, T.; Nakajima, K.; Muroga, K. Genetic relatedness among Japanese, American and European isolates of viral hemorrhagic septicemia virus (VHSV) based on partial G and P genes. *Dis. Aquat. Org.* **2002**, *48*, 143–148. [CrossRef] [PubMed]
2. Schutze, H.; Enzmann, P.J.; Kuchling, R.; Mundt, E.; Niemann, H.; Mettenleiter, T.C. Complete genomic sequence of the fish rhabdovirus infectious haematopoietic necrosis virus. *J. Gen. Virol.* **1995**, *76*, 2519–2527. [CrossRef] [PubMed]
3. Schutze, H.; Mundt, E.; Mettenleiter, T.C. Complete genomic sequence of viral hemorrhagic septicemia virus, a fish rhabdovirus. *Virus Genes* **1999**, *19*, 59–65. [CrossRef] [PubMed]
4. Skall, H.F.; Olesen, N.J.; Mellergaard, S. Viral haemorrhagic septicaemia virus in marine fish and its implications for fish farming - a review. *J. Fish Dis.* **2005**, *28*, 509–529. [CrossRef] [PubMed]
5. Brudeseth, B.E.; Evensen, O. Occurrence of viral haemorrhagic septicaemia virus (VHSV) in wild marine fish species in the coastal regions of Norway. *Dis. Aquat. Org.* **2002**, *52*, 21–28. [CrossRef] [PubMed]
6. Chinchilla, B.; Encinas, P.; Estepa, A.; Coll, J.M.; Gomez-Casado, E. Transcriptome analysis of rainbow trout in response to non-virion (NV) protein of viral haemorrhagic septicaemia virus (VHSV). *Appl. Microbiol. Biotechnol.* **2015**, *99*, 1827–1843. [CrossRef]
7. Wahli, T.; Bergmann, S.M. Viral haemorrhagic septicaemia (VHS): Detection, distribution and combat. *Cab. Rev: Persp. Agric. Vet. Sci. Nutr. Nat. Resour.* **2011**, *6*, 1–10. [CrossRef]
8. Kurath, G.; Leong, J.C. Characterization of infectious hematopoietic necrosis virus mRNA species reveals a nonvirion rhabdovirus protein. *J. Virol.* **1985**, *53*, 462–468. [CrossRef]
9. Schutze, H.; Enzmann, P.J.; Mundt, E.; Mettenleiter, T.C. Identification of the non-virion (NV) protein of fish rhabdoviruses viral haemorrhagic septicaemia virus and infectious haematopoietic necrosis virus. *J. Gen. Virol.* **1996**, *77*, 1259–1263. [CrossRef]
10. Einer-Jensen, K.; Ahrens, P.; Lorenzen, N. Parallel phylogenetic analyses using the N, G or Nv gene from a fixed group of VHSV isolates reveal the same overall genetic typing. *Dis. Aquat. Org.* **2005**, *67*, 39–45. [CrossRef]
11. Kurath, G.; Higman, K.H.; Björklund, H.V. Distribution and variation of NV genes in fish rhabdoviruses. *J. Gen. Virol.* **1997**, *78*, 113–117. [CrossRef] [PubMed]
12. Biacchesi, S.; Thoulouze, M.I.; Bearzotti, M.; Yu, Y.X.; Bremont, M. Recovery of NV knockout infectious hematopoietic necrosis virus expressing foreign genes. *J. Virol.* **2000**, *74*, 11247–11253. [CrossRef] [PubMed]
13. Biacchesi, S.; Lamoureux, A.; Merour, E.; Bernard, J.; Bremont, M. Limited interference at the early stage of infection between two recombinant novirhabdoviruses: Viral hemorrhagic septicemia virus and infectious hematopoietic necrosis virus. *J. Virol.* **2010**, *84*, 10038–10050. [CrossRef] [PubMed]
14. Thoulouze, M.I.; Bouguyon, E.; Carpentier, C.; Bremont, M. Essential role of the NV protein of Novirhabdovirus for pathogenicity in rainbow trout. *J. Virol.* **2004**, *78*, 4098–4107. [CrossRef] [PubMed]
15. Kim, M.S.; Kim, K.H. Effects of NV gene knock-out recombinant viral hemorrhagic septicemia virus (VHSV) on Mx gene expression in *Epithelioma papulosum cyprini* (EPC) cells and olive flounder (*Paralichthys olivaceus*). *Fish Shellfish Immunol.* **2012**, *32*, 459–463. [CrossRef]
16. Alonso, M.; Kim, C.H.; Johnson, M.C.; Pressley, M.; Leong, J.A. The NV gene of snakehead rhabdovirus (SHRV) is not required for pathogenesis, and a heterologous glycoprotein can be incorporated into the SHRV envelope. *J. Virol.* **2004**, *78*, 5875–5882. [CrossRef]
17. Johnson, M.C.; Simon, B.E.; Kim, C.H.; Leong, J.A. Production of recombinant snakehead rhabdovirus: The NV protein is not required for viral replication. *J. Virol.* **2000**, *74*, 2343–2350. [CrossRef]
18. Choi, M.K.; Moon, C.H.; Ko, M.S.; Lee, U.H.; Cho, W.J.; Cha, S.J.; Do, J.W.; Heo, G.J.; Jeong, S.G.; Hahm, Y.S.; et al. A nuclear localization of the infectious haematopoietic necrosis virus NV protein is necessary for optimal viral growth. *PLoS ONE* **2011**, *6*, e22362. [CrossRef]

19. Ammayappan, A.; Vakharia, V.N. Nonvirion protein of novirhabdovirus suppresses apoptosis at the early stage of virus infection. *J. Virol.* **2011**, *85*, 8393–8402. [CrossRef]
20. Cho, H.K.; Kim, J.; Moon, J.Y.; Nam, B.H.; Kim, Y.O.; Kim, W.J.; Park, J.Y.; An, C.M.; Cheong, J.; Kong, H.J. Microarray analysis of gene expression in olive flounder liver infected with viral haemorrhagic septicaemia virus (VHSV). *Fish Shellfish Immunol.* **2016**, *49*, 66–78. [CrossRef]
21. Hwang, J.Y.; Kwon, M.G.; Seo, J.S.; Do, J.W.; Park, M.A.; Jung, S.H.; Ahn, S.J. Differentially expressed genes after viral haemorrhagic septicaemia virus infection in olive flounder (Paralichthys olivaceus). *Vet. Microbiol.* **2016**, *193*, 72–82. [CrossRef] [PubMed]
22. Kim, M.S.; Kim, K.H. Protection of olive flounder, Paralichthys olivaceus, against viral hemorrhagic septicemia virus (VHSV) by immunization with NV gene-knockout recombinant VHSV. *Aquaculture* **2011**, *314*, 39–43. [CrossRef]
23. De Kinkelin, P.; LeBerre, M. Isolament d'un rhabdovirus pathogéne de la truite fario (*Salmo trutta L.*,1766). *C R Acad. Sci. Hebd. Seances Acad. Sci. D* **1977**, *284*, 101–104. (in French). [PubMed]
24. Ballesteros, N.A.; Saint-Jean, S.S.; Encinas, P.A.; Perez-Prieto, S.I.; Coll, J.M. Oral immunization of rainbow trout to infectious pancreatic necrosis virus (IPNV) induces different immune gene expression profiles in head kidney and pyloric ceca. *Fish Shellfish Immunol* **2012**, *33*, 174–185. [CrossRef]
25. Quesada-Garcia, A.; Encinas, P.; Valdehita, A.; Baumann, L.; Segner, H.; Coll, J.M.; Navas, J.M. Thyroid active agents T3 and PTU differentially affect immune gene transcripts in the head kidney of rainbow trout (*Oncorhynchus mykiss*). *Aquat. Toxicol.* **2016**, *174*, 159–168. [CrossRef]
26. Salem, M.; Kenney, P.B.; Rexroad, C.E.; Yao, J. Development of a 37 k high-density oligonucleotide microarray: A new tool for functional genome research in rainbow trout. *J. Fish Biol.* **2008**, *72*, 2187–2206. [CrossRef]
27. Gene Expression Omnibus. Available online: https://www.ncbi.nlm.nih.gov/geo/query/acc.cgi?acc=GSE37330 (accessed on 29 January 2020).
28. Gene Expression Omnibus. Available online: http://www.ncbi.nlm.nih.gov/geo/query/acc.cgi?acc=GSE37797 (accessed on 29 January 2020).
29. GSEA - Broad Institute. Available online: http://www.broad.mit.edu/GSEA (accessed on 29 January 2020).
30. Subramanian, A.; Tamayo, P.; Mootha, V.K.; Mukherjee, S.; Ebert, B.L.; Gillette, M.A.; Paulovich, A.; Pomeroy, S.L.; Golub, T.R.; Lander, E.S.; et al. Gene set enrichment analysis: A knowledge-based approach for interpreting genome-wide expression profiles. *Proc. Natl. Acad. Sci. USA* **2005**, *102*, 15545–15550. [CrossRef]
31. Subramanian, A.; Kuehn, H.; Gould, J.; Tamayo, P.; Mesirov, J.P. GSEA-P: A desktop application for Gene Set Enrichment Analysis. *Bioinformatics* **2007**, *23*, 3251–3253. [CrossRef]
32. KEGG: Kyoto Encyclopedia of Genes and Genomes. Available online: http://www.kegg.jp (accessed on 29 January 2020).
33. Glenney, G.W.; Wiens, G.D. Early diversification of the TNF superfamily in teleosts: Genomic characterization and expression analysis. *J. Immunol.* **2007**, *178*, 7955–7973. [CrossRef]
34. Roth, W.; Wagenknecht, B.; Klumpp, A.; Naumann, U.; Hahne, M.; Tschopp, J.; Weller, M. APRIL, a new member of the tumor necrosis factor family, modulates death ligand-induced apoptosis. *Cell Death Differ.* **2001**, *8*, 403–410. [CrossRef]
35. De Valck, D.; Jin, D.Y.; Heyninck, K.; Van de Craen, M.; Contreras, R.; Fiers, W.; Jeang, K.T.; Beyaert, R. The zinc finger protein A20 interacts with a novel anti-apoptotic protein which is cleaved by specific caspases. *Oncogene* **1999**, *18*, 4182–4190. [CrossRef] [PubMed]
36. Kelly, C.; Shields, M.D.; Elborn, J.S.; Schock, B.C. A20 regulation of nuclear factor-kappaB: Perspectives for inflammatory lung disease. *Am. J. Respir. Cell Mol. Biol.* **2011**, *44*, 743–748. [CrossRef] [PubMed]
37. Zelante, T.; Wong, A.Y.; Ping, T.J.; Chen, J.; Sumatoh, H.R.; Vigano, E.; Hong Bing, Y.; Lee, B.; Zolezzi, F.; Fric, J.; et al. CD103(+) Dendritic Cells Control Th17 Cell Function in the Lung. *Cell Rep.* **2015**, *12*, 1789–1801. [CrossRef] [PubMed]
38. Chapoval, A.I.; Ni, J.; Lau, J.S.; Wilcox, R.A.; Flies, D.B.; Liu, D.; Dong, H.; Sica, G.L.; Zhu, G.; Tamada, K.; et al. B7-H3: A costimulatory molecule for T cell activation and IFN-gamma production. *Nat. Immunol.* **2001**, *2*, 269–274. [CrossRef]
39. Dixon, B.; Shum, B.; Adams, E.J.; Magor, K.E.; Hedrick, R.P.; Muir, D.G.; Parham, P. CK-1, a putative chemokine of rainbow trout (*Oncorhynchus mykiss*). *Immunol. Rev.* **1998**, *166*, 341–348. [CrossRef]

40. Montero, J.; Coll, J.; Sevilla, N.; Cuesta, A.; Bols, N.C.; Tafalla, C. Interleukin 8 and CK-6 chemokines specifically attract rainbow trout (*Oncorhynchus mykiss*) RTS11 monocyte-macrophage cells and have variable effects on their immune functions. *Dev. Comp. Immunol.* **2008**, *32*, 1374–1384. [CrossRef]
41. Montero, J.; Ordas, M.C.; Alejo, A.; Gonzalez-Torres, L.; Sevilla, N.; Tafalla, C. CK12, a rainbow trout chemokine with lymphocyte chemo-attractant capacity associated to mucosal tissues. *Mol. Immunol.* **2011**, *48*, 1102–1113. [CrossRef]
42. O'Farrell, C.; Vaghefi, N.; Cantonnet, M.; Buteau, B.; Boudinot, P.; Benmansour, A. Survey of transcript expression in rainbow trout leukocytes reveals a major contribution of interferon-responsive genes in the early response to a rhabdovirus infection. *J. Virol.* **2002**, *76*, 8040–8049. [CrossRef]
43. Seo, J.; Yaneva, Y.R.; Cresswell, P. Viperin: A multifunctional, interferon-inducible protein that regulates virus replication. *Cell Host Microbe* **2011**, *10*, 534–539. [CrossRef]
44. Boudinot, P.; Salhi, S.; Blanco, M.; Benmansour, A. Viral haemorrhagic septicaemia virus induces vig-2, a new interferon-responsive gene in rainbow trout. *Fish Shellfish Immunol.* **2001**, *11*, 383–397. [CrossRef]
45. Najib, A.; Kim, M.S.; Choi, S.H.; Kang, Y.J.; Kim, K.H. Changes in microRNAs expression profile of olive flounder (*Paralichthys olivaceus*) in response to viral hemorrhagic septicemia virus (VHSV) infection. *Fish Shellfish Immunol.* **2016**, *51*, 384–391. [CrossRef] [PubMed]
46. Laxman, N.; Rubin, C.J.; Mallmin, H.; Nilsson, O.; Pastinen, T.; Grundberg, E.; Kindmark, A. Global miRNA expression and correlation with mRNA levels in primary human bone cells. *Rna* **2015**, *21*, 1433–1443. [CrossRef] [PubMed]
47. Estepa, A.; Coll, J. Innate Multigene Family Memories Are Implicated in the Viral-Survivor Zebrafish Phenotype. *PLoS ONE* **2015**, *10*, e0135483. [CrossRef] [PubMed]
48. Encinas, P.; Garcia-Valtanen, P.; Chinchilla, B.; Gomez-Casado, E.; Estepa, A.; Coll, J. Identification of multipath genes differentially expressed in pathway-targeted microarrays in zebrafish infected and surviving spring viremia carp virus (SVCV) suggest preventive drug candidates. *PLoS ONE* **2013**, *8*, e73553. [CrossRef] [PubMed]

7

Hepatitis B Virus (HBV) Subviral Particles as Protective Vaccines and Vaccine Platforms

Joan Kha-Tu Ho [1], Beena Jeevan-Raj [1] and Hans-Jürgen Netter [1,2,*]

1 Victorian Infectious Diseases Reference Laboratory (VIDRL), Melbourne Health, The Peter Doherty Institute, Melbourne, Victoria 3000, Australia; Joan.Ho@mh.org.au (J.K.-T.H.); Beena.JeevanRaj@mh.org.au (B.J.-R.)

2 Royal Melbourne Institute of Technology (RMIT) University, School of Science, Melbourne, Victoria 3001, Australia

* Correspondence: Hans.Netter@mh.org.au

Abstract: Hepatitis B remains one of the major global health problems more than 40 years after the identification of human hepatitis B virus (HBV) as the causative agent. A critical turning point in combating this virus was the development of a preventative vaccine composed of the HBV surface (envelope) protein (HBsAg) to reduce the risk of new infections. The isolation of HBsAg sub-viral particles (SVPs) from the blood of asymptomatic HBV carriers as antigens for the first-generation vaccines, followed by the development of recombinant HBsAg SVPs produced in yeast as the antigenic components of the second-generation vaccines, represent landmark advancements in biotechnology and medicine. The ability of the HBsAg SVPs to accept and present foreign antigenic sequences provides the basis of a chimeric particulate delivery platform, and resulted in the development of a vaccine against malaria (RTS,S/AS01, Mosquirix^{TM}), and various preclinical vaccine candidates to overcome infectious diseases for which there are no effective vaccines. Biomedical modifications of the HBsAg subunits allowed the identification of strategies to enhance the HBsAg SVP immunogenicity to build potent vaccines for preventative and possibly therapeutic applications. The review provides an overview of the formation and assembly of the HBsAg SVPs and highlights the utilization of the particles in key effective vaccines.

Keywords: hepatitis B virus; surface (envelope) antigen; sub-viral particle; virus-like particle

1. Introduction

Hepatitis B is globally one of the most common infectious diseases in humans, which is associated with significant morbidity and mortality. Approximately 2 billion people worldwide have been infected with hepatitis B virus (HBV) and approximately 257 million people live with chronic HBV infections. An estimated 887,000 persons died in 2015 from acute or chronic consequences of hepatitis B [1–4]. The ability of the HBV structural proteins, including the hepatitis B surface (envelope) proteins (HBsAg) to assemble into non-infectious sub-viral particles (SVPs), allows the generation of highly organized particles displaying neutralizing epitopes that promote protective immune responses against the parent virus. The approval of the recombinant hepatitis B vaccine Recombivax HB (Merck Sharp and Dohme) in 1986, based on HBsAg SVPs and produced in the yeast *Saccharomyces cerevisiae,* was the first developed vaccine using recombinant DNA technology. The recombinant vaccine, together with the recombinant products, human insulin (licensed 1982), human growth hormone (licensed 1985), and alpha interferon (licensed 1986), demonstrated the capability of biotechnological approaches to generate innovative medicines [1]. The ability to accept foreign antigenic sequences into the SVP structure can provide the basis for the development of delivery platforms for targeted medically relevant sequences, as in the case of the RTS,S/AS01 (Mosquirix™) vaccine against malaria. The antigenic components of Mosquirix™ are chimeric SVPs containing HBsAg proteins fused to a *Plasmodium falciparum*-specific circumsporozoite (CS) polypeptide [5–7]. The design and generation of chimeric SVPs holds enormous potential in the treatment of infectious diseases, for which there are no effective vaccines [8–10].

2. Hepatitis B Virus, Classification, and Gene Products

HBV is a hepatocyte-tropic virus and is assigned to the family of hepatitis DNA viruses, *Hepadnaviridae* [11–13]. HBV is divided into 10 main genotypes, A–J, which differ by more than 8% at the nucleotide level [14,15]. The HBV genome has a size of approximately 3.2 kilobases (kb), and is represented by a relaxed circular, partially double-stranded DNA (rcDNA), which is delivered to the nucleus of the host cell and converted into a covalently closed circular DNA (cccDNA) molecule [12]. The cccDNA represents a non-integrated stable episome and forms the template for all viral RNA transcripts. In the absence of an origin of replication site required for DNA-dependent DNA amplification, one of the viral transcripts, the pre-genomic RNA (pgRNA), serves as the template for replication to generate rcDNA via reverse transcription [12]. HBV contains four open reading frames (C, P, S, and X) and encodes seven proteins (polymerase, X protein, HBcAg, HBeAg, HBsAgL, HBsAgM, and HBsAgS). The polymerase is essential for several steps in the replication pathway through its reverse transcriptase, RNaseH, and priming activities. The X protein supports efficient infection and replication in vivo [11,12,16]. The core protein (HBcAg) constitutes the subunit of the viral capsid and is essential for the formation of virions. The e-antigen (HBeAg) is derived from the pre-core protein by proteolytic processing and is not part of the viral capsid. It is involved in modulating the host immune response against HBV and represents an important serological marker [11–13]. The virus encodes for three related surface (envelope) proteins (HBsAg) that share a common S-domain. They are translated from different in-frame start codons and hence are distinguished by their N-terminal extensions. The small HBsAg (HBsAgS) comprises only the S-domain with a size of 226 amino acids (aa), the middle HBsAg protein (HBsAgM) has an N-terminal extension of 55 aa (pre-S2 domain), and the large HBsAg (HBsAgL) has an additional extension of 108 or 119 aa (preS1-domain) depending on the genotype [17] (Figure 1A,B). In addition to the classification by genotypes, HBV is distinguished by four main serotypes based on the reactivity against HBsAg. All genotypes have a common serotypic reactivity against a major antigenic site called the "a"-determinant, but further express two mutually exclusive allelic antigenic determinants "d" or "y" and "w" or "r" [18–20]. The antigenic determinants of HBsAg are located in an exposed loop region of the S-domain. HBsAg and antibodies against HBsAg (anti-HBs) are important serological markers. The loss of HBsAg and seroconversion to anti-HBs antibodies are a sign of immunity and recovery from acute or chronic hepatitis B [13].

Characteristic of a HBV infection is the generation of a large quantity of HBsAg SVPs and filaments devoid of capsid and of the viral genome. SVPs exceed the presence of infectious virions in host sera by a factor between 10^2 and 10^5 [17,21–24]. SVPs are predominately composed of HBsAgS, and their presence in the sera does not seem to interfere with HBV particle entry into hepatocytes, suggesting that SVPs represent decoys by binding to virus-neutralizing antibodies [25]. HBsAgS SVPs share important immunological determinants with the mature virus, and therefore, SVPs derived from patient serum or recombinant SVPs represent effective immunogens for the induction of a protective immune response [26–28]. Vaccinated individuals develop antibodies targeting the "a"-determinant region, which provides protection against the infection of all HBV serotypes [20,29]. The discovery and characterization of "empty" genome-free virions containing HBsAg and capsid is reviewed by Hu and Liu, 2017 [30].

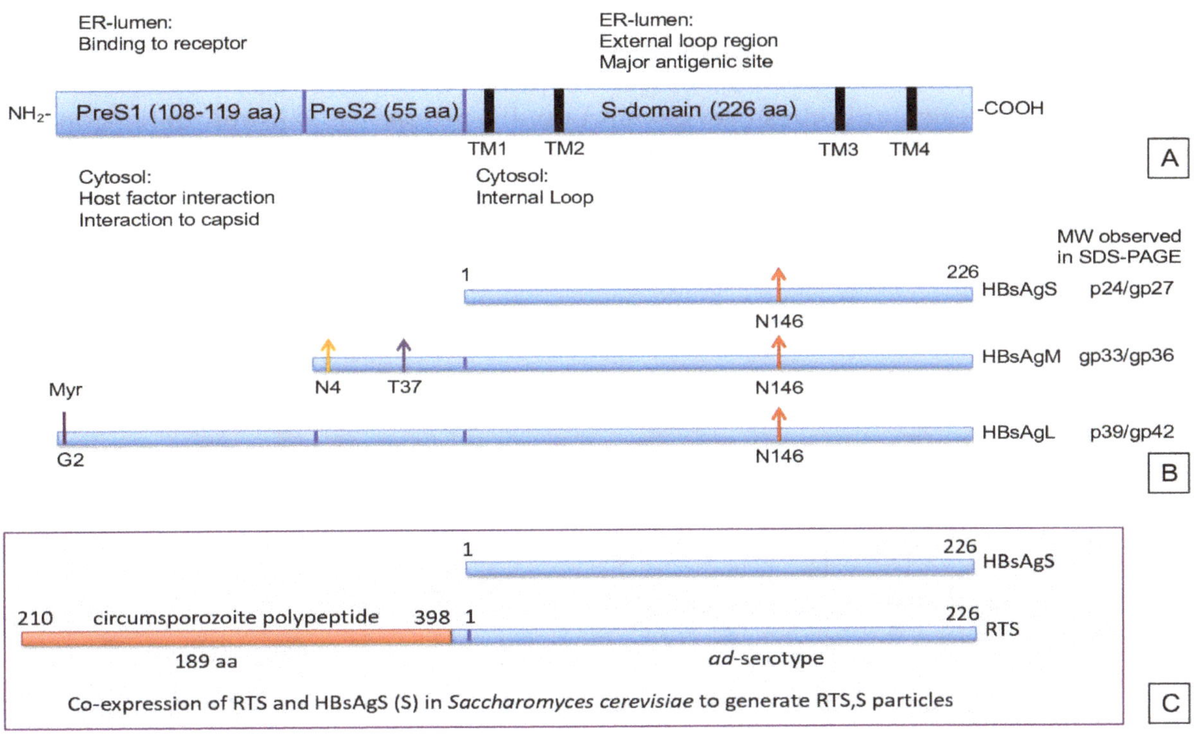

Figure 1. The surface (envelope) proteins (HBsAg) of hepatitis B virus (HBV): (**A**) The open reading frame encoding the complete hepatitis B surface antigen is depicted. The domain organization of preS1, preS2, and S, with the number of amino acids (aa) of the individual domains are specified. The four transmembrane regions (TM1–4) are indicated by the thick black lines. The function of the different domains in relation to their orientation towards the lumen of the endoplasmic reticulum (ER) or cytosol is indicated. (**B**) The individual HBsAg open reading frames for the small (HBsAgS), middle (HBsAgM), and large (HBsAgL) proteins, and their post-translational modifications are shown. The size of the HBsAgS protein is indicated by the number of amino acids. Arrows represent the utilized glycosylation sites. Red arrows mark asparagine 146 (N146) in the S-domain. Orange and purple arrows represent the N-4 and threonine 37 (T37) respectively, in the preS2 domain. The glycine residue at position 2 (G2) of the preS1 domain, indicated by a purple line, is myristolated. The observed molecular weights (MW) of the glycosylated (gp) and non-glycosylated proteins (p) separated under reducing conditions on a SDS-PAGE are indicated on the right. (**C**) Design of the RTS,S vaccine that is produced by co-expressing HBsAgS (aa 1–226) and the chimeric protein that is a fusion of the circumsporozoite polypeptide (210–398 aa) to the N-terminus of HBsAgS, including 4 aa from the preS2 domain.

3. Role of HBsAg in HBV, Filament, and SVP Formation

An essential step in the formation of virions, filaments, or SVPs is the cotranslational insertion of the HBsAgS protein into the membrane of the endoplasmic reticulum (ER) with a short luminal exposed N-terminal sequence, two transmembrane regions separated by a cytosolic loop, and a luminal domain, followed by a hydrophobic C-terminal region. The luminal domain corresponds to the external loop region of the S-domain, which contains multiple epitopes, including the immunodominant "a"-determinant region that is common to all HBV genotypes, and the allelic antigenic determinants "d/y" and "w/r" [17,31]. A conformational heparan sulfate binding site also overlaps with the "a"-determinant region and is essential to infectivity [32].

HBV virion formation depends on the presence of the viral capsid containing rcDNA and the HBsAg proteins for envelopment. The preS1 region of HBsAgL is essential for the assembly of infectious HBV particles by interacting with the capsid [17,33], possibly contributes to the binding to a proteoglycan attachment site [34,35], and is required for binding to the hepatocyte entry receptor, sodium taurochlorate cotransporting polypeptide (NTCP) [36,37]. Chaperones of the heat shock protein (hsp) 70 family facilitate the interaction of the HBsAgL preS1 domain with the capsid by retaining the preS1/preS2 sequence in the cytosolic (internal) orientation at the ER [38–40]. Virion secretion depends on host factors of the endosomal sorting complex required for transport (ESCRT) and sorting into late endosomal multivesicular bodies (MVBs), and finally, release of its intraluminal content at the hepatocyte surface [41–43]. The mature HBV virions are spherical, enveloped particles with a diameter of 42 nm with an inner capsid of 22 nm in diameter [11–13]. Due to the elevated presence of HBsAgL in virions and filaments compared to the SVPs, filaments seem to follow the secretion pathway taken by the virions (Figure 2) [44]. The filaments have a width of approximately 20 nm and are variable in length [12,23,45].

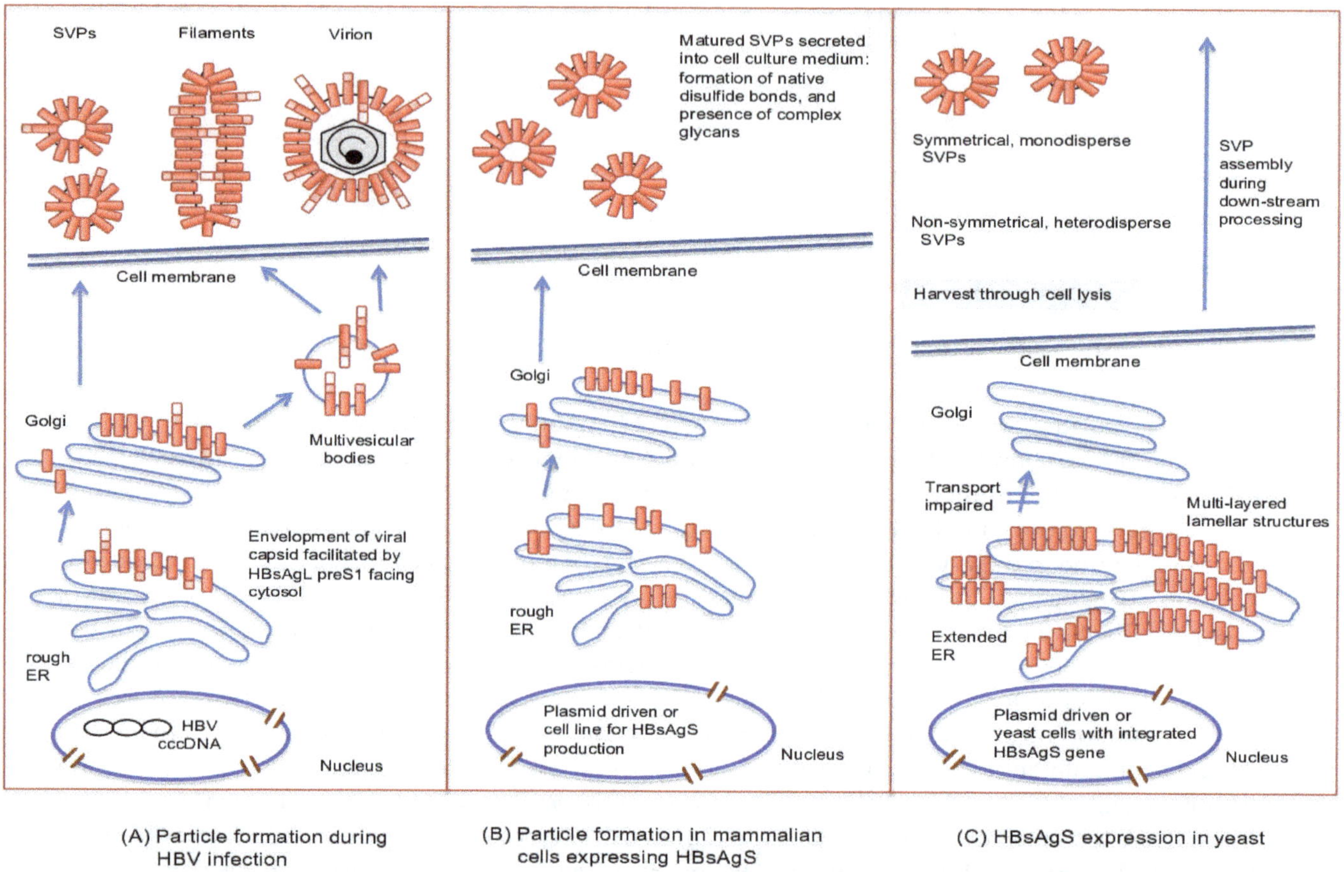

Figure 2. Illustration of HBsAg protein synthesis and assembly pathways during a natural infection (**A**), HBsAgS expression and assembly in mammalian cells in the absence of other viral gene products (**B**), or expressed in yeast (**C**). During a natural infection, virions and filaments are formed by budding from multivesicular bodies. The spherical subviral particles (SVPs) are produced and secreted through the endoplasmic reticulum (ER)-Golgi complex. The HBsAg subunits of the virions, filaments, and SVPs form intra- and intermolecular disulfide bonds, and are partially glycosylated (not shown) (**A**). Expression of the HBsAgS gene in mammalian cell lines leads to the formation of SVPs exclusively composed of HBsAgS permitting the formation of disulfide bonds and partial glycosylation (not shown) (**B**). HBsAgS protein expressed in yeast accumulates in the ER, causes an extended ER and forms multilayered lamellar structures. HBsAgS protein complexes are harvested from the cell lysate, and SVPs are assembled during down-stream processing (**C**). cccDNA: covalently closed circular DNA.

In contrast to the formation of infectious particles, the formation of SVP does not depend on the preS1 domain. HBsAgS proteins have the ability to assemble into secretion-competent SVPs and are composed solely of envelope proteins, lipids, and glycans. Contrary to virion secretion, SVP assembly follows the constitutive secretory pathway of the host cell for release [43,44]. The non-infectious SVPs are 17 to 25 nm in diameter. SVPs isolated from HBV carriers show spike-like features protruding from the surface similar to the surface projections observed on filaments and infectious virions (Dane particles) [24,45–48]. An alternative structure for recombinant SVPs expressed in transgenic mice has been proposed to possess an octahedral symmetry [49]. Mammalian cell lines expressing HBsAgS in the absence of any other viral component secrete SVPs, which are morphologically indistinguishable from serum-derived SVPs (Figure 2) [50–54]. Thus, particle morphogenesis substantially differs between SVPs and virions, but they have identical antigenic structures due to the S-domain, which is encoded by all HBV envelope proteins (Figure 1A,B).

3.1. *Topology of HBsAgS*

The correct folding of HBsAgS depends on two topogenic signal sequences, which determine the orientation of the S-domains in relation to the lipid layer. The insertion of the HBsAgS N-terminus into the ER membrane requires the presence of the topogenic N-terminal signal sequence 1 (transmembrane region 1, TM1, aa 8–22), which is not proteolytically cleaved by the host's peptidases, and allows the translocation of the N-terminus across the ER membrane. The second internal topogenic transmembrane sequence (TM2), which is located between aa 80 and 98, supports the translocation of flanking C-terminal sequences and serves as an anchor to hold the sequence in the membrane [17,55,56]. Both topogenic signal sequences are required for the correct folding of HBsAgS, resulting in the formation of a cytosolic loop (aa 23 to 79), and a loop reaching into the ER lumen (aa 99 to approximately 155), followed by a proposed amphipathic helix (aa 156 to 169) and the hydrophobic C-terminal region (aa 170 to 226) embedded in the ER membrane (Figures 1A and 3) [57]. The luminal loop region of the S-domain is located at the external surface of the mature SVPs and also infectious virions, and harbors the major HBsAg protein epitopes ("a"-determinant, and "d/y", "w/r" determinants) [13]. The hydrophobic C-terminal region (aa 170 to 226) possibly contains two additional transmembrane regions, as indicated by topological models [58,59]. The presence of transmembrane passages is supported by experimental data suggesting that the C-terminal sequences are exposed at internal and external surfaces. The sequence between residues 196 and 201 is important for packaging of hepatitis delta virus (HDV), a satellite of HBV, and therefore expected to be accessible to facilitate the interaction with the HDV ribonucleoprotein complex [60]. A second site between residue 178 and 186 is targeted by an anti-HBs monoclonal antibody, indicating surface exposure [61].

HBsAg proteins contain 14 cysteine (cys) residues located in the S-domain, which are highly conserved among different HBV genotypes; the preS1 and preS2 domains do not contain additional cysteine residues [12,17]. Eight cysteine residues are located in the external loop region, forming disulfide bonds which are important for the integrity of the major antigenic determinants [62,63], such as cys-107 in the external loop for retaining the "a"-determinant specific antigenicity [64]. The identification of HBsAgS oligomers and polymers by electrophoresis under non-reducing conditions suggests that the disulfide bonding is heterogeneous, consistent with the finding that only a fraction of HBsAgS subunits are exclusively linked by disulfide bonds formed between cys-121 and cys-147 (Figure 3) [62,63,65]. Reduction or absence of intermolecular disulfide bridges interferes with the native HBsAgS antigenicity but allows SVP formation [62,65,66].

The S-domain shared by the HBsAg proteins harbors an *N*-glycosylation site at position asparagine-146 (N146), which is partially utilized by the oligosaccharyltransferase [17,67], and hence, HBsAgS proteins are synthesized as unglycosylated p24 and *N*-glycosylated gp27 versions (Figure 1B). HBsAgS p24 and gp27 have identical transmembrane topologies and dimerize without preference for a specific pairing and form heterologous dimers with HBsAgM and HBsAgL [66]. Synthesis and secretion of HBsAgS SVPs do not depend on *N*-glycosylation at position N146 in the external loop region, in contrast to the formation and release of infectious HBV particles [67–70].

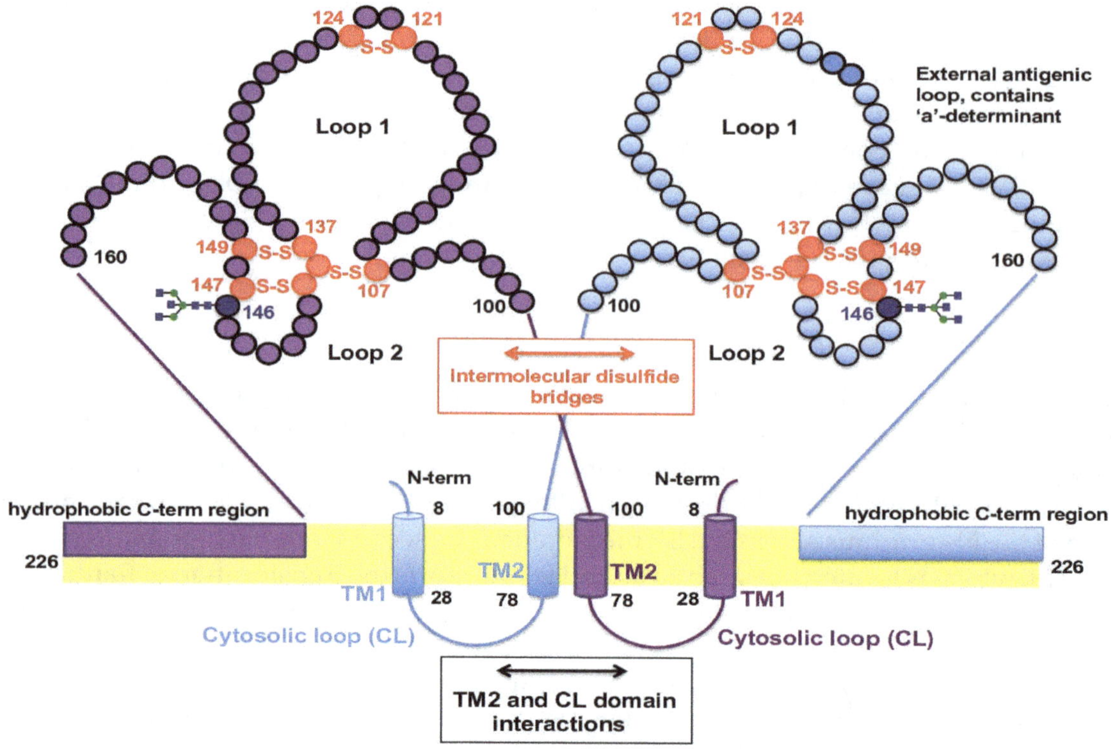

Figure 3. Proposed model for the formation of the HBsAgS homodimer based on Suffner et al. [57]. Dimerization of two HBsAgS monomers represented in purple and blue is facilitated by interactions of the transmembrane domains (TM2), cytosolic loops (CL) and intermolecular disulfide bridges (S-S) between cysteine residues (red circles) in the external loop region. The facultative *N*-glycosylation site at position N146 is indicated (dark blue). The orientation of the hydrophobic C-terminal region is illustrated in a simplified form.

3.2. Topology of HBsAgM

The middle HBsAg protein has the same transmembrane topology as HBsAgS, and hence is partly glycosylated at N146 in the S-domain. Translocation of the preS2 domain of HBsAgM is mediated by the topologic signal TM1 located in the S-domain [71]. The translocation event across the ER membrane into the lumen allows the *N*-glycosylation of the asparagine-4 (N4) residue in the preS2 domain, which is always glycosylated [72], resulting in glycoproteins with a molecular weight of 33 kDa and 36 kDa (Figure 1B). In addition to the *N*-glycosylation site in the preS2 domain, the preS2 domain can be partially *O*-glycosylated, depending on the genotype and the presence of the threonine (T37) (Figure 1B) [73]. Similar to HBsAgS, HBsAgM proteins assemble into SVPs and can be secreted independently from other viral proteins [74–77]. HBsAgM, however, is not essential for virion morphogenesis and infectivity [78].

3.3. Topology of HBsAgL

The large HBsAg protein adopts two distinguished transmembrane topologies facilitating an internal or external location of the preS1/S2 domain (Figure 1A) [17,79–81]. The internal orientation allows preS1/S2 to interact with the viral capsid, a critical step in viral morphogenesis. The preS2 region of the HBsAgL protein serves as a possible spacer to facilitate conformational changes of the preS1/S2 domain [17,81,82]. During the maturation process, the preS1/S2 domain is translocated to adopt an external orientation, which is essential for virus attachment to the host cell through a specific interaction with heparan sulfate proteoglycan [34,35] and binding to the entry receptor [36,37]. In addition, the preS1 domain is myristoylated at the N-terminus, which is required for efficient HBV entry into hepatocytes (Figure 1B) [83,84]. The potential *N*- and *O*-glycosylation sites in the HBsAgL preS1/S2 domain are not utilized due to the cytosolic orientation of the preS1/preS2 domain after translation. HBsAgL molecules have molecular weights of 39 kD (p39) or 42kD (gp42) depending on the glycosylation status at position N146 in the S-domain (Figure 1B). Expression of HBsAgL in mammalian cells in the absence of HBsAgS and HBsAgM does lead to particle formation, but not secretion, and it is retained in post-ER and pre-Golgi compartments [85]. HBsAgL causes a dose-dependent inhibition of particle release if co-expressed with HBsAgS [86,87].

Taken together, the S-domain is shared by the HBV envelope proteins and defines the backbone of the particle due to the presence of the topogenic transmembrane regions, glycans at position N146, cysteine residues to form inter- and intra-molecular disulfide bonds, and the external loop region. The correct folding of the external loop defines the HBsAg-specific antigenic determinants.

4. Biochemical Properties of SVPs

The proportion of the HBsAgL, -M, and -S proteins differ between Dane particles, filaments, and SVPs generated during a natural infection. It is estimated that the envelope of Dane particles contains HBsAgL, HBsAgM, and HBsAgS at a ratio of approximately 3:2:5, and filaments at a ratio of 1:1:4. SVPs contain less HBsAgM compared to filaments with trace amounts of HBsAgL [46,83,88]. HBsAgS SVPs have a molecular weight of 2–4 × 10^6, and are composed of protein (75% by weight), carbohydrates (in form of glycoproteins) and lipids (25% by weight) [89]. Approximately 100 HBsAgS proteins assemble with lipids into lipoprotein particles, fifty HBsAgS dimers were identified in SVPs purified from sera of transgenic mice [49,89,90]. Three different regions of the S-domain contribute to the oligomerization of the HBsAg proteins, the cytosolic loop, TM2, and the luminal loop (Figure 3) [57]. The SVPs are compact particles with a reported density of 1.21 g/mL in caesium chloride (CsCl) compared to a density of infectious virions between 1.24 and 1.26 g/mL [23,91,92]. The compact structure of the SVPs is due to the large number of intra- and inter-molecular disulfide bonds within and between the S-domains of the individual HBsAg subunits [62,65,90,93–95]. Kinetic studies demonstrated that disulfide-linked HBsAgS dimers are formed in the ER, then the immature particle precursors are transported to a post-ER, pre-Golgi compartment, which excludes the enzyme "protein disulfide isomerase" and allows the formation of HBsAgS oligomers [96]. Intracellular HBsAgS particles contain high-mannose oligosaccharide chains, and after secretion, SVPs contain complex oligosaccharide chains with terminal sialic acid *N*-acetylglucosamine residues representing glycosylation patterns conforming with the HBsAg movement from the ER through the Golgi cisternae [12,67,97].

Cryo-EM studies and biophysical analyses of the SVPs produced in cell culture or purified from sera of transgenic mice demonstrates a tight HBsAgS protein–lipid interaction. The lipid composition of HBsAgS SVPs purified from the plasma of several HBV carriers showed that phospholipids, in particular, phosphatidylcholine is a major lipid class; with palmitic, stearic, oleic, and linoleic acids being the major fatty acid components [89]. Consistently, SVPs produced in human hepatoma cell lines predominantly contain phospholipids, with phosphatidylcholine being the dominant component [98]. The tight protein–lipid interaction restricts lipid movement suggesting that the lipids are not aligned in a typical bilayer structure. HBsAg particles seem to contain the lipids in an unusual arrangement, with the lipids being closely intercalated with the proteins, located on the particle surface, and are hence likely arranged in a lipid monolayer [99,100]. HBsAg proteins contain a high content of alpha helices (45%–52%), which are lipid-associated, and provide an arrangement which allows the disposal of the loop regions in the particle interior or on its surface [100,101]. Assessing yeast (*Hansenula polymorpha*)-derived SVPs, the particles have an ordered and rigid lipid interface, possibly organized as a phospholipid monolayer, with a hydrophobic and fluid inner core. HBsAgS proteins penetrate into the lipid core, with parts of the protein protruding from the particle surface [89,102,103]. The lipids contribute to the antigenic activity of HBsAg particles [100], likely by stabilizing the proper helical structure of the HBsAg proteins and the conformation of their hydrophilic region, which contains the antigenic site. Removal of lipids decreases the helical content and reduces the antigenic activity of the particles [100]. S-domain antigenic structures seem to be strongly impacted by the lipid–protein interface, which defines the formation of alpha-helical structures and accommodates the arrangement of proper disulfide bonding patterns and the correct folding of HBsAg.

5. The First Vaccine Generation Against HBV: Vaccine Derived from Patient Plasma

The first vaccine against HBV was based on the unique approach to purify the HBsAg immunogen directly from the blood of asymptomatic HBV carriers [104]. The identification of the HBsAg as an important immune target was based on observations that anti-HBs human immunoglobulins conferred passive protection against hepatitis B [105,106]. Consistently, active immunization studies with HBsAg protected chimpanzees from hepatitis B [29,107,108], and clinical studies with recipients of blood transfusion indicated that patients who developed anti-HBs were less likely to develop hepatitis [109]. Patients on a renal dialysis unit and staff were less likely to acquire hepatitis if they had anti-HBs antibodies [110]. The first reported vaccination against hepatitis B was performed with a diluted, heat-inactivated HBsAg-positive serum in children, then the children challenged with infectious HBV, resulting in an incomplete but considerable protection [111]. For the generation of a proper vaccine, methodologies were developed to purify HBsAg using isopycnic banding and rate-zonal separation [26,27,112,113], affinity columns [114], adsorption onto colloidal silicate and desorption, differential polyethylene glycol (PEG) precipitations and gel filtration [27]. To minimize the risk of infections due to the presence of hepatitis B virions, the vaccine preparations were inactivated with formalin [112,114]. Plasma was from "ad" and "ay" donors, the SVPs mixed, then adsorbed onto aluminium hydroxide, or used in the absence of an adjuvant [26,27]. The pilot vaccines demonstrated that the plasma-derived SVPs induced anti-HBs antibody responses in different animal models [26]. Safety testing in chimpanzees, which are susceptible to HBV infection, did not provide any evidence of hepatitis in chimpanzees, which had received the inactivated plasma-derived SVP vaccine. Vaccinated chimpanzees were protected from a challenge with infectious HBV and did not show any indication of a hepatitis B infection [26,108].

The use of the first plasma-derived vaccines, Heptavax-B (Merck Sharp and Dohme, MSD) and Hevac-B (Institute Pasteur) provided good protection rates, and they were safe [114–117]. Depending on the purification and inactivation procedure, the composition of the plasma-derived HBsAg SVPs can vary, and they may or may not contain small quantities of HBsAgM, providing the preS2 domain in addition to HBsAgS. The Hevac-B vaccine contained 1%–2% HBsAgM. In contrast, the Heptavax-B vaccine did not contain preS2 proteins due to a treatment step with proteases, which however did not interfere with HBsAg-specific antigenicity [118–120]. Similar serum-derived vaccines were then produced from various manufacturers, such as Hepavax-B (Green Cross, Korea), Hepaccine-B (Cheil, Korea), and GCC VAC (Green Cross Corporation, Osaka) (Table 1). Limitations given by the supply of human plasma from chronically infected patients, and the risk associated with human-derived products due to contaminating proteins and the potential presence of other pathogens transmitted by blood, in particular a non-A non-B hepatitis virus, confronted the use of human plasma-derived HBsAg SVP vaccines [121–123]. Safety concerns about products from human sources, together with the advances in recombinant DNA technology and biotechnology, led to the development of recombinant hepatitis B vaccines.

Table 1. Key vaccines against HBV utilizing hepatitis B surface antigens.

Source	Cell type	Name	Antigen	Subtype	Manufacturer
Plasma-derived vaccines	-	Heptavax-B®	HBsAgS	ad	Merck [116]
	-	Hevac B®	HBsAgS, -M	ad *and* ay	Pasteur [120,124,125]
	-	GCC VAC	HBsAgS		Green Cross Operation, Osaka [125]
	-	Hepavax-B	HBsAgS		Korean Green Cross [126,127]
	-	Hepaccine B	HBsAgS		Cheil Foods & Chemicals Company [128]

Table 1. *Cont.*

Source	Cell type	Name	Antigen	Subtype	Manufacturer
Recombinant (yeast-derived)	*Saccharomyces cerevisiae*	Recombivax® HB HB-Vax II®	HBsAgS	adw	Merck [129]
	Saccharomyces cerevisiae	Engerix-B®	HBsAgS	adw	GlaxoSmithKline [129,130]
	Saccharomyces cerevisiae	TGP 943™	HBsAgS, -M	adr	Takeda Chemical Industries [131]
	Saccharomyces cerevisiae	Euvax B®	HBsAgS		LG Chemical Ltd, [130,132]
	Pichia pastoris	Shanvac B	HBsAgS	adw2	Shantha Biotechnics [133]
	Pichia pastoris	Heberbiovac-HB®	HBsAgS	adw2	Heber Biotech S.A., [130]
	Hansenula polymorpha	Heplisav-B®	HBsAgS	adw	Dynavax Technologies [134]
	Hansenula polymorpha	Hepavax-Gene™	HBsAgS	adr	Janssen Pharma [130,135]
Recombinant (mammalian cell-derived)	*Chinese hamster ovary cells*	Gen Hevac B®	HBsAgS, -M	ayw	Pasteur [120]
	Chinese hamster ovary cells	Sci-B-Vac/Bio-Hep-B™/Hepimmune™	HBsAgS, -M, -L	adw	VBI Vaccines [136]
	Mouse c127 clonal cell line	AG-3™ (Hepacare/Hepagene™)	HBsAgS, -M, -L	adw & ayw	Medeva [137]

6. The Second Vaccine Generation Against HBV: Yeast-Derived Recombinant HBsAgS SVPs

The identification of HBsAgS as the major HBV envelope protein of plasma-derived HBsAg SVPs and encoding the major antigenic determinants prompted the expression of HBsAgS in mammalian cell lines and yeast [13]. Yeast cell strains (*Saccharomyces cerevisiae, Pichia pastoris, Hansenula polymorpha*) were developed which express HBsAgS in high quantities. HBsAgS SVPs are isolated from yeast cell extracts with a sedimentation rate and buoyant density similar to particles from human samples or expressed in cell culture [138–140]. Yeast-derived SVPs have reduced antigenic reactivity compared to SVPs derived from human plasma but immunization studies established that yeast-derived SVPs induce anti-HBs antibody responses, which provide protection of immunized chimpanzees following a challenge with HBV. Importantly, the yeast-derived HBsAgS SVP vaccine of the "adw" subtype conferred protection against HBV subtypes "adr" and "ayw" [28]. Clinical trials using different age groups, healthy individuals, and special target populations confirmed that the yeast-derived vaccine is highly immunogenic, and generated qualitative and quantitative anti-HBs antibody responses with a protective efficacy similar to the plasma-derived vaccines [141]. The vaccines achieved 99% seroprotection rates in healthy children and adolescents but approximately 5%–7% of the adult population are non-responders and the rate can increase to 70% in elderly persons and in special risk groups [13,129,136,142]. Also, genetically determined resistance may contribute to non-responsiveness to HBsAgS SVP vaccines [143–145]. At the molecular level, yeast-derived HBsAg SVPs are not *N*-glycosylated at the N146 position within the S-domain, in contrast to SVPs produced in mammalian cell lines and harvested from the cell culture medium, or isolated from the blood of chronic hepatitis B patients. HBsAgS expressed in yeast generate SVPs [146], but experimental evidence indicates that the SVP are not formed within the yeast cell and generated during the down-stream purification procedures. HBsAgS expression in *Pichia pastoris* showed that HBsAgS assembles at the ER into multi-layered lamellar structures [147]. Monitoring SVP assembly during the purification procedure demonstrated that particulate structures are formed after eluting HBsAg bound to colloidal silica. Irregular SVP-like structures were visualized, and morphological changes observed after pH adjustment (colloidal silica eluate pH 10.8 to 8.0), ion-exchange, and size-exclusion chromatography. The monodispersity improved after potassium thiocyanate (KSCN) treatment, also the SVPs have a more-fine structured surface [148–150]. The correct disulfide bonding is the molecular basis for the formation of native epitopes as probed with an anti-HBs antibody [151]. Lipid-containing SVPs undergo KSCN-induced maturation by the formation of intra- and inter-molecular disulfide bonds to generate fully disulfide-bonded SVPs, resulting in a decreased conformational flexibility of HBsAgS in the matured particles [149,152]. Restricted conformational flexibility is possibly required for the formation of native HBsAg-specific antigenic structures, which allows epitope recognition by anti-HBs antibodies, and importantly in eliciting neutralizing antibodies [149]. The particle size (diameter) of yeast-derived SVPs is consistent with the data obtained from mammalian-cell-derived SVPs, but the size distribution can vary depending on the SVP maturation level [148,153]. Yeast-derived SVPs have a high content of alpha-helical structures, and the movement of the HBsAgS proteins is restricted due to the tight association with the lipid membrane [102,154]. Similarly, the lipid composition is characterized by high levels of phospholipids, in particular, phosphatidylcholine consistent with mammalian cell-derived SVPs [154–156]. No significant differences in the anti-HBs response induced by the plasma-derived or yeast-derived hepatitis B vaccines was observed [123,157].

The widely distributed, yeast cell-derived hepatitis B vaccines, Engerix®-B (GlaxoSmithKline) and Recombivax HB™ (Merck Sharp and Dohme) use aluminium hydroxide or aluminium hydroxyphosphate sulfate as adjuvanting substances, respectively. Aluminium-based adjuvants are widely used and activate the inflammasome pathway [158–160]. The adsorption of HBsAgS SVPs on aluminium hydroxide is mediated by binding of the phosphate groups of the HBsAgS SVPs phospholipids with hydroxyl groups of aluminium hydroxide through a ligand-exchange mechanism [161,162]. After vaccine administration, the SVPs are eluted from the aluminium adjuvant upon contact with the interstitial fluid [163,164]. Adsorption of HBsAgS SVPs derived from *Hansenula polymorpha* on an aluminium gel followed by a mild desorption step using competing phosphate anions demonstrated that the conformation of the HBsAgS protein is retained, and consistently, no significant changes of the lipid core and lipid membrane surface of the SVPs were identified [165]. To improve immunization outcomes in adults at risk of a hepatitis B infection, HBsAgS SVPs synthesized in *Hansenula polymorpha* are formulated with a Toll-like receptor 9 (TLR 9) agonist, cytidine-phosphate-guanosine oligodeoxynucleotide (CpG-ODN) 1018 as an adjuvant (Heplisav-B™, Dynavax Technologies). TLR9 is a pattern recognition receptor of the innate immune system, which induces the production of cytokines such as interleukin-12 and interferon-alpha to stimulate the adaptive immune response [134,166]. Heplisav-B™ induced earlier seroprotection rates allowing a two-dose regimen compared to three doses required for the Engerix-B vaccine, but it caused more injection-site reactions [134].

The ability of HBsAgS subunits expressed in yeast cells to form SVPs during down-stream procedures, and to reproduce native antigenic structures, allowed the development of a highly successful preventative vaccine. The advancement of the vaccine adjuvant technology allowed new HBsAgS SVP formulations and demonstrated strategies to enhance the magnitude of the anti-HBs immune response with immediate practical applications

7. Third Generation Vaccine Concepts against HBV

The development of third-generation HBsAg vaccines providing the S-domain in combination with preS1 and/or preS2 sequences was directed by the objective to enhance the protective efficacy of the human plasma-derived vaccines (which consisted predominantly of HBsAgS subunits), and the second-generation recombinant yeast-derived vaccines (which consisted exclusively of HBsAgS subunits). The third-generation vaccines attracted interest to improve the immunization outcomes in persons who do not respond to the conventional HBsAgS vaccines [13]. The importance of the preS1 domain for viral entry and assembly makes it a potential target for vaccine development, anti-preS1 antibodies protected chimpanzees from HBV infection [167]. PreS1/S2 sequences provide additional B-cell epitopes to generate protective antibody responses [167–169] and may also serve as a T cell immunogen to overcome the non-responsiveness to the S-domain [170–172]. Small quantities of HBsAgL present in the HBsAgS vaccine induced significant T-cell activation measured as in vitro proliferation specific for the preS domain [172]. In addition, preS2 peptide vaccines protect chimpanzees against a challenge with HBV [169], and the use of SVPs with preS1 and/or preS2 sequences generated anti-HBs immune responses in mouse strains, which are non-responsive to the standard yeast-derived HBsAgS SVP vaccine [173].

For the generation of third-generation vaccines, different yeast expression systems and mammalian cell lines were utilized to synthesize SVPs composed of HBsAgM and HBsAgL proteins in the presence or absence of HBsAgS. Utilizing *Saccharomyces cerevisiae*, the expression of a modified HBsAgM in the absence of HBsAgS allowed the formation of SVPs. The modified HBsAgM protein (P31c) contains a deletion of six amino acids to make it resistant to trypsin-like proteases in *S. cerevisiae*. The HBsAgM-P31c proteins assembled into SVPs with a diameter of approximately 20 nm and retained HBsAg antigenicity [174,175]. Immunization studies in BALB/c mice and guinea pigs demonstrated that anti-HBs antibody titres can be induced comparable to the plasma-derived Heptavax-B vaccine (MSD). Also, anti-preS2 antibodies were detected in animals immunized with the HBsAgM-P31c SVP vaccine. In contrast to the yeast-derived HBsAgS vaccine, the HBsAgM-P31c SVPs are glycosylated with N- and O-linked glycans located in the preS2 domain [174,175], which may facilitate interactions with lectin receptors expressed by antigen-presenting cells. In an independent study, HBsAgM SVPs induced anti-S and anti-preS2 antibodies in healthy young adults but the anti-S response was lower than in the patient group who received HBsAgS SVPs, and hence, the HBsAgM vaccine failed to achieve the objective of inducing an early and strong anti-S and anti-preS2 immune response [176]. The HBsAgM-P31c SVPs, however, were used to formulate a new vaccine (TGP-943, Takeda) and demonstrated a protective effect in the chimpanzee model and also generated protective levels of anti-preS2 antibodies in humans [177,178]. Clinical studies demonstrated that the vaccine TGP-943 induced both anti-S and anti-preS2 antibodies, approximately 50% of non-responders became positive for either or both anti-S and anti-preS2 [131].

For the development of a HBsAgL-based vaccine, HBsAgL expression during the exponential *S. cerevisiae* growth phase generated high levels of HBsAgL but did not assemble into the typical 20–25 nm SVPs, but generated a polydisperse population of small (2–3 nm) and large aggregates (15–50 nm) [179]. HBsAgL was glycosylated by *N*- and *O*-linked glycans in the preS1/S2 domain indicating that HBsAgL accessed the lumen of the ER of the yeast cell and caused morphological changes in the ER compartment [179,180]. The presence of *N*-linked and *O*-linked glycans in the preS1/S2 domain of yeast-derived HBsAgL proteins is in contrast to preS1/preS2 of HBsAgL isolated from human plasma due to the cytoplasmic exposure of the preS1/S2 domain during the orderly and regulated process of virion morphogenesis [83,88,179,180]. Particle formation using *S. cerevisiae* could be rescued providing an N-terminal signal sequence, which possibly allows a correct entry into the secretory pathway, and after purification from the yeast lysate, spheres and filaments with a diameter of 23 nm were obtained, the length of the filaments was in the range of 40 to 120 nm, visualized by negative staining electron microscopy. HBsAgL proteins expressed in the absence of the signal sequence did not form such an ordered structure [181]. The visualization of the particles by atomic force microscopy (AFM) demonstrated a heterogeneous population of rugged spherical forms between 50 and 500 nm in diameter [182]. Immunization of mice with the yeast-derived HBsAgL SVPs elicited anti-S, anti-preS2, and anti-preS1 antibodies, and the effective dose (ED_{50}) for anti-S and anti-preS2 antibodies were similar to those achieved with HBsAgM particles [182]. Using an alternative strategy, hybrid SVPs were generated in *S. cerevisiae* composed of HBsAgS and a modified HBsAgL (HBsAgL*). HBsAgL* contains a truncated preS1/S2 region with sequences relevant for the hepatocyte-binding site and immunologically important B- and T-helper epitopes but does not contain sites for proteolysis and the binding site for polymerized human serum albumin. The hybrid SVPs contained HBsAgS and HBsAgL* at a ratio of 75:25 [176]. The immunization of BALB/c mice with HBsAgL*/HBsAgS SVPs generated anti-S and anti-preS1 antibodies. The anti-S titers were similar to those found after immunization with Engerix B. Immunizations of African Green Monkeys (*Ceropithecus aethiops*) using HBsAgL*/HBsAgS SVPs induced anti-S, anti-preS2, and anti-preS1 antibodies [176]. Safety and immunogenicity studies in young, healthy adult persons, and in poor responders to hepatitis B vaccines demonstrated that the presence of the preS1/preS2 domain did not enhance the anti-S response compared to the control Engerix

B vaccine (GSK) [183,184], in spite of the preS1 sequence present as a strong T-cell immunogen [170]. The HBsAgL*/HBsAgS vaccine induced anti-preS1 antibodies in a young, healthy adult person cohort, and possibly provides additional neutralizing activity [183].

With the availability of mammalian cell culture technologies, recombinant hepatitis B vaccines composed of SVPs have been developed containing the HBsAgS and HBsAgM (GenHevacB, Sanofi Pasteur Vaccins) and the additional HBsAgL subunits (Sci-B-Vac, VBI Vaccines; Hepacare, Medeva Pharma) (Table 1). Chinese hamster ovary (CHO) cells (GenHevacB, Sci-B-Vac) [120,136] or murine cells (C1271) (Hepacare, Medeva Pharma) [137] were used to generate the vaccines. The GenHevac B vaccine is composed of HBsAgS/HBsAgM SVPs at a ratio 80:20, and compared in a clinical setting to the human plasma-derived Hevac B vaccine, both vaccines induced antibodies to the HBsAg in >90% of the participants (497 persons in the age range of 18–40 years). Compared to the plasma-derived vaccine, the recombinant vaccine produced early and high levels of anti-preS2 antibodies, which may provide an additional advantage in prevention of a HBV infection [120,185].

For Sci-B-Vac, the complete HBsAg gene encoding HBsAgS, -M, and -L, including native promoter, enhancer, and poly(A) signal, were used to establish a producer CHO cell line, which contains more than 100 HBsAg coding copies/cell [173]. Protein analysis of the secreted SVPs revealed the presence of all three HBsAg proteins and its glycosylated isoforms (HBsAgS p24 and gp27; HBsAgM gp33 and gp36, HBsAgL p39 and gp42). Sci-B-Vac induced anti-S and anti-preS1 antibody responses in BALB/c mice, and also in mouse strains which are resistant to immunizations with HBsAgS SVPs and/or HBsAgM [136,173]. Sci-B-Vac demonstrated an excellent safety record in clinical studies, which included healthy individuals, children, and neonates. In comparison with yeast-derived hepatitis B vaccines, more than 50% of vaccinees receiving Sci-B-Vac developed earlier seroprotection against HBV [136]. Sci-B-Vac performed superior to yeast-derived HBsAgS vaccines in specific patient risk groups and provided vaccine boosts in persons with no or low response to preceding immunizations with the conventional yeast-derived HBV vaccine. Specific risk groups including patients with renal failure, with overweight and immune-suppressed patients responded with higher seroprotection rates compared to conventional yeast derived vaccines. The Sci-B-Vac vaccine is widely used in Israel and licensed in various countries [136].

8. HBsAgS SVPs as Platforms for Medically Relevant Antigenic Sequences

SVPs display an array of antigenic sequences to the innate immune system facilitating the subsequent activation of the adaptive system [8,10,186,187]. The ability to accept foreign inserts into the SVP structure provides the basis for advanced delivery platforms for medically relevant sequences, such as malaria antigens. Chimeric SVPs can be constructed from viral capsid proteins, such as capsids from HBV, human papilloma virus, and Qβ phage that have been re-engineered to express foreign antigenic sequences at a high antigenic density [8,187]. Similarly, SVPs derived from the HBV envelope assemble into highly compact lipid-containing particles, and have been exploited as carrier platforms for foreign antigenic sequences by introducing N- or C-terminal extensions [188–191], N-terminal extensions in addition to substitutions of the HBsAgS N-terminal sequence [192], by replacing the HBsAgM preS2-domain [193,194], by insertions into the external loop region including replacing antigenic determinants [195–201], or by replacing HBsAgS-specific cytotoxic T lymphocyte (CTL) epitopes [202] (Table 2). The insertion of a poliovirus-specific epitope with a length of 11 amino acids into the external loop region of HBsAgS allowed the expression of the chimeric, assembly and secretion competent HBsPolioAg proteins in a mouse cell line [201,203]. The chimeric SVPs contained glycosylated and non-glycosylated HBsPolioAg subunits and formed particles with 22 nm in diameter, similar to wild-type HBsAgS proteins. HBsPolioAg SVPs were used in mouse immunization studies and induced anti-poliovirus peptide-specific antibodies with neutralizing activity and a low level of anti-HBs antibodies, possibly due to a partial loss of HBsAg-specific antigenicity. The co-expression of both wild-type HBsAgS proteins and HBsPolioAg generated hybrid SVPs composed of both proteins, which facilitated the induction of anti-HBs and anti-poliovirus epitope antibodies [203].

Similar studies inserting heterologous B-cell epitopes in an exposed site in the external loop region reduced HBsAg-specific antigenicity depending on the length of the insert, but the recombinant proteins retained the ability to induce anti-HBs antibodies [195,196,198,204]. Chimeric SVPs composed of subunits distinguished by the number of inserted epitope repeats from the *Plasmodium falciparum* circumsporozoite (CS) protein demonstrated that the CS epitope number influenced the activity of the anti-CS epitope antibodies. The effect of the epitope-specific density on the antibody quality may instruct chimeric SVP designs to optimize immunological outcomes and vaccine efficacy [195]. The RTS,S/AS01 vaccine (Mosquirix™) is the most advanced vaccine with a heterologous antigenic sequence arrayed on SVPs. The RTS,S vaccine is based on the fusion of a *Plasmodium falciparum* CS polypeptide of 189 aa with selected tandem repeats of B-cell and T-cell epitopes to the HBsAgS N-terminus (RTS) (Figure 1C). The CS-protein is expressed on the *Plasmodium* sporozoite surface, and essential for hepatocyte invasion and for establishing a productive infection, and therefore an important target for the development of a pre-erythrocyte vaccine [205]. The genes for HBsAgS and RTS are integrated into the genome of *S. cerevisiae* and co-expressed at a ratio RTS:HBsAgS of 1:4 to generate non-glycosylated mixed (hybrid) lipoprotein particles [190,191]. The RTS,S vaccine is well-tolerated, safe, and immunogenic, and is considered to be the first advanced vaccine against the pre-erythrocyte stage of the malaria parasite, and induces both anti-HBs and anti-CS protein antibodies. The anti-malaria RTS,S/AS01 vaccine in children of five months or older reduced clinical malaria episodes by 39% and life-threatening severe malaria episodes by 29%. The vaccine is licensed in three African countries [5,6,206]. Mosquirix™ (RTS,S/AS01) is adjuvanted with AS01, which is a liposome formulation and contains monophosphoryl lipid A (MPL) and the saponin QS-21. RTS,S in combination with AS01 resulted in higher anti-CS protein immune responses than AS02, which is an oil-in-water emulsion-based adjuvant [7,205–207]. To enhance the vaccine efficacy against malaria, a RTS,S-related vaccine (R21) with an increased proportion of CS-polypeptides was developed. CS-polypeptide-HBsAg fusion proteins were expressed in *Pichia pastoris*, and SVPs were obtained after caesium chloride density ultracentrifugation and gel filtration [208]. The R21 vaccine induces a sterile protection in mice against a challenge with transgenic sporozoites. The induction of anti-HBs antibodies is compromised, possibly because the high content of the CS-polypeptide blocks access to the HBsAg external loop region, which contains the antigenic "a"-determinant [208].

Table 2. Selection of chimeric HBsAg SVP platforms and vaccines.

Antigen	Target	Delivery Site	Expression System	Name	Study/Manufacturer
CS-HBsAg/HBsAgS	Malaria	N-terminal	*Saccharomyces cerevisiae*	RTS,S/AS01 Mosquirix™	GlaxoSmithKline [5,6,190]
CS-HBsAgS	Malaria	N-terminal	*Pichia pastoris*	R21	[208]
DENV-EDIII-HBsAgS/HBsAgS	Dengue virus	N-terminal	*Pichia pastoris*	DSV4	[188]
HBsAgS-gp120 (HIV-1)	HIV-1	C-terminal	CV-1 cell line	MR15, MR23	[189]
Env1-, Env2-HBsAgS	Hepatitis C virus	Substitution/N-terminal extension	CHO cells		[192,209]
HBsAgS-NANP repeats	Malaria	Insertion	HEK293F cell line	M-HBsAg-N4, -N9	[195]
HBsAgS-HCV env epitopes	Hepatitis C virus	Insertion	HEK293T cell line		[196,198]
HBsAgS-catalase epitope	*Helicobacter pylori*	Insertion	HuH-7	VLP-KatA	[197]
HBsAgS-VP1 capsid epitope	Poliovirus	Insertion	Mouse L cells	HBsPolioAg	[201,203]
HBsAgS-matrix CTL epitope	Influenza A virus	Insertion/Substitution	HEK293T cell line		[202]
Polyepitope-HBsAgS;	HIV	Substitution preS2 sequence	SW480 cells		[193]

CS—circumsporozoite polypeptide; DENV-EDIII—Dengue virus envelope domain III; env—envelope protein; HCV—hepatitis C virus; HIV—Human immunodeficiency virus; CTL—cytotoxic T lymphocyte. VLP—virus-like particle.

Preexisting immunity against vaccine vectors can impose a negative effect on the outcome of the vaccination [210–213]. HBsAgS SVPs are widely used in immunization programs to combat HBV, and therefore, the use of chimeric SVPs could pose a problem for recipients previously immunized against hepatitis B. Immunization studies in mice using chimeric SVPs with a foreign epitope inserted into the external loop of HBsAgS or fused to the N-terminus of HBsAgS demonstrated that pre-existing anti-HBs antibodies do not compromise the immunogenicity of the foreign antigenic sequence presented by the chimeric HBsAgS SVPs [214,215]. Consistently, clinical studies with human volunteers to assess the RTS,S malaria vaccine did not provide any evidence that a pre-existing anti-HBs status prevented an anti-CS-protein immune response [190]. In relation to a HBV chronic carrier status and the use of the RTS,S vaccine, there was no evidence that chronic HBV carriers (HBsAg positive) and HBsAg-negative individuals respond differently regarding an antibody response to the CS-protein [216].

9. Enhancement of Platform Immunogenicity through Biochemical Modifications

Based on the importance of SVPs as medical tools and platforms for the presentation of native viral antigenic sequences, it is critical to understand their immunogenicity in relation to antigen structure in order to enhance or to modulate their immunogenicity. Depending on the SVP type, targeted biochemical modifications of the SVP subunits may allow the generation of SVP variants with enhanced immunogenicity. HBsAgS SVPs are glycosylated lipoprotein particles and are stabilized by extensive intra- and inter-molecular disulfide bonds, which allows targeted modifications of the glycan content and level of disulphide bonding.

Changing disulfide bonding impacts on antigen processing and epitope selection by modifying the conformational flexibility [217]. The three-dimensional structure guides processing and presentation of T helper (Th) and CTL epitopes, and subtle changes in antigen structure can modulate T cell responses due to qualitative and quantitative differences in protein processing [217–220]. Distinct Th cell epitope profiles emerged from human immunodeficiency virus type 1 (HIV-1) gp120 molecules after destabilizing the three-dimensional structure as a consequence of deleted cysteine residues [221]. In an attempt to enhance immunogenicity, HBsAgS SVPs with a reduced level of disulfide bonds were generated. The biochemically modified SVPs showed a higher protease sensitivity, potentially due to introducing structural changes associated with enhanced cellular immunogenicity [65]. Altering SVP structure may represent an attractive strategy to modulate proteolytic sensitivity to influence antigen processing and promoting an enhanced immune response and/or a changed hierarchy of epitope presentation [218,222].

Manipulation of protein glycosylation represents an alternative strategy to promote antigen internalization and antigen presentation via MHC class I and class II molecules to enhance the adaptive immune responses [223,224]. The glycosylation status and glycan density of the immunogen impacts on its interaction with antigen-presenting cells and recognition by lectins [224]. Glycan-mediated interactions with immunocompetent cells impact on protein uptake and can enhance or modulate cell-mediated and humoral immune responses [225–229]. Contrarily, glycans can shield protein epitopes to evade recognition by antibodies and can block antigen processing [230]. Mannosylation provided an efficient strategy to improve uptake and processing of a SVP derived from the rabbit hemorrhagic disease virus [225]. Consistently, mannosylated solid lipid nanoparticles loaded with HBsAg induced stronger cellular responses than nanoparticles devoid of mannose [229]. Mutant HBsAgS subunits with additional *N*-glycosylation sites assembled into hyperglycosylated SVP. Antigenic fingerprints indicated that additional glycans do not extensively shield HBsAg-specific antigenic sites. Immunization studies demonstrated that the hyperglycosylated SVPs induced earlier and longer-lasting antibody responses than hypoglycosylated SVPs or wild type SVPs [231]. The ability of biochemically modified SVPs to promote immune responses possibly due to differences in their glycosylation-related interaction with cells of the innate immune system illustrates approaches for the design of immunogens with superior immunological characteristics.

10. Concluding Remarks

The development of preventative vaccines against hepatitis B resulted in remarkable advances in reducing HBV associated liver diseases. However, chronic hepatitis B is still difficult to control due to continuous viral replication driven by the episomal cccDNA present in the nuclei of infected hepatocytes. Novel strategies to generate vaccines based on structurally modified subunits to enhance immunogenicity and/or to modify antigen processing to change the hierarchy of epitope presentation may represent a pathway to overcome chronic viral infections or may complement a vaccine based on native proteins [65,218,224–226,231]. HBsAgS SVPs have been used as carrier platforms for various antigenic sequences to induce anti-foreign humoral and cellular immune responses [8,186]. One of the most advanced chimeric vaccines with a foreign antigenic sequence arrayed on a particulate carrier is based on the HBsAgS backbone fused to a *P. falciparum* CS-polypeptide [5,6]. For the design of next generation vaccines with therapeutic capabilities, formulations based on antigen combinations, such as mixtures of HBsAgS SVPs and SVPs composed of the HBV nucleocapsid antigen (HBcAg), may allow the induction of broad CD4 and CD8 T-cell responses suitable for therapeutic outcomes [232]. Alternatively, the assessment of synergistic effects between biochemically modified immunogens and adjuvant compounds possibly represent an avenue for the generation of optimized vaccines and delivery platforms, which may be suitable for therapeutic applications to overcome established chronic infections.

Author Contributions: H.-J.N. wrote the original draft version; J.K.-T.H. and B.J.-R. edited and reviewed the manuscript. All authors have read and agreed to the published version of the manuscript.

References

1. Huzair, F.; Sturdy, S. Biotechnology and the transformation of vaccine innovation: The case of the hepatitis B vaccines 1968–2000. *Stud. Hist. Philos. Biol. Biomed. Sci.* **2017**, *64*, 11–21. [CrossRef]
2. Millman, I. The development of the hepatitis B vaccine. In *Hepatitis B. The Virus, the Disease, and the Vaccine*; Millman, I., Eisenstein, T.K., Blumberg, B.S., Eds.; Plenum Publishing Corp.: New York, NY, USA, 1984; pp. 137–147.
3. World Health Organization. *Hepatitis B. Key Facts*; World Health Organization: Geneva, Switzerland, 2019.
4. World Health Organization. *Prevention and Control of Viral Hepatitis Infection. Framework for Global Action*; World Health Organization: Geneva, Switzerland, 2012.
5. Adepoju, P. RTS, S malaria vaccine pilots in three African countries. *Lancet* **2019**, *393*, 1685. [CrossRef]
6. Schuerman, L. RTS, S malaria vaccine could provide major public health benefits. *Lancet* **2019**, *394*, 735–736. [CrossRef]
7. Cohen, J.; Nussenzweig, V.; Nussenzweig, R.; Vekemans, J.; Leach, A. From the circumsporozoite protein to the RTS, S/AS candidate vaccine. *Hum. Vaccines* **2010**, *6*, 90–96. [CrossRef] [PubMed]
8. Mohsen, M.O.; Zha, L.; Cabral-Miranda, G.; Bachmann, M.F. Major findings and recent advances in virus-like particle (VLP)-based vaccines. *Semin. Immunol.* **2017**, *34*, 123–132. [CrossRef]
9. López-Sagaseta, J.; Malito, E.; Rappuoli, R.; Bottomley, M.J. Self-assembling protein nanoparticles in the design of vaccines. *Comput. Struct. Biotechnol. J.* **2016**, *14*, 58–68. [CrossRef] [PubMed]
10. Tan, M.; Jiang, X. Recent advancements in combination subunit vaccine development. *Hum. Vaccines Immunother.* **2017**, *13*, 180–185. [CrossRef] [PubMed]
11. Yuen, M.-F.; Chen, D.-S.; Dusheiko, G.M.; Janssen, H.L.A.; Lau, D.T.Y.; Locarnini, S.A.; Peters, M.G.; Lai, C.-L. Hepatitis B virus infection. *Nat. Rev. Dis. Primers* **2018**, *4*, 18035. [CrossRef] [PubMed]
12. Seeger, C.; Mason, W.S. Molecular biology of hepatitis B virus infection. *Virology* **2015**, *479–480*, 672–686. [CrossRef]
13. Gerlich, W.H. Medical virology of hepatitis B: How it began and where we are now. *Virol. J.* **2013**, *10*, 239. [CrossRef]
14. Kramvis, A. Genotypes and genetic variability of hepatitis B virus. *Intervirology* **2014**, *57*, 141–150. [CrossRef] [PubMed]

15. Norder, H.; Couroucé, A.M.; Coursaget, P.; Echevarria, J.M.; Lee, S.D.; Mushahwar, I.K.; Robertson, B.H.; Locarnini, S.; Magnius, L.O. Genetic diversity of hepatitis B virus strains derived worldwide: Genotypes, subgenotypes and HBsAg subtypes. *Intervirology* **2004**, *47*, 289–309. [CrossRef] [PubMed]
16. Slagle, B.L.; Bouchard, M.J. Role of HBx in hepatitis B virus persistence and its therapeutic implications. *Curr. Opin. Virol.* **2018**, *30*, 32–38. [CrossRef]
17. Bruss, V. Hepatitis B virus morphogenesis. *World J. Gastroenterol.* **2007**, *13*, 65–73. [CrossRef] [PubMed]
18. Le Bouvier, G.L. The heterogeneity of Australia antigen. *J. Infect. Dis.* **1971**, *123*, 671–675. [CrossRef] [PubMed]
19. Bancroft, W.H.; Mundon, F.K.; Russell, P.K. Detection of additional antigenic determinants of hepatitis B antigen. *J. Immunol.* **1972**, *109*, 842–848.
20. Jazayeri, S.M.; Alavian, S.M.; Dindoost, P.; Thomas, H.C.; Karayiannis, P. Molecular variants of hepatitis B surface antigen (HBsAg). In *Viral Hepatitis*, 4th ed.; Thomas, H.C., Lok, A.S.F., Locarnini, S.A., Zuckerman, A.J., Eds.; John Wiley & Sons Ltd.: Hoboken, NJ, USA, 2014; pp. 107–126.
21. Désiré, N.; Ngo, Y.; Franetich, J.-F.; Dembele, L.; Mazier, D.; Vaillant, J.-C.; Poynard, T.; Thibault, V. Definition of an HBsAg to DNA international unit conversion factor by enrichment of circulating hepatitis B forms. *J. Viral Hepat.* **2015**, *22*, 718–726.
22. Brunetto, M.R. A new role for an old marker, HBsAg. *J. Hepatol.* **2010**, *52*, 475–477. [CrossRef]
23. Dreesman, G.R.; Hollinger, F.B.; Suriano, J.R.; Fujioka, R.S.; Brunschwig, J.P.; Melnick, J.L. Biophysical and biochemical heterogeneity of purified hepatitis B antigen. *J. Virol.* **1972**, *10*, 469–476. [CrossRef]
24. Dane, D.S.; Cameron, C.H.; Briggs, M. Virus-like particles in serum of patients with Australia-antigen associated hepatitis. *Lancet* **1970**, *1*, 695–698. [CrossRef]
25. Rydell, G.E.; Prakash, K.; Norder, H.; Lindh, M. Hepatitis B surface antigen on subviral particles reduces the neutralizing effect of anti-HBs antibodies on hepatitis B viral particles in vitro. *Virology* **2017**, *509*, 67–70. [CrossRef] [PubMed]
26. Hilleman, M.R.; Bertland, A.U.; Buynak, E.B.; Lampson, G.P.; McAleer, W.J.; McLean, A.A.; Roehm, R.R.; Tytell, A.A. Clinical and laboratory studies of HBsAg vaccine. In *Viral Hepatitis*; Vyas, G.N., Cohen, S.N., Schmid, R., Eds.; The Franklin Institute Press: Philadelphia, PA, USA, 1978; pp. 525–537.
27. Maupas, P.; Goudeau, A.; Coursaget, P.; Drucker, J.; Barin, F.; André, M. Immunization against hepatitis B in man: A pilot study of two years' duration. In *Viral Hepatitis*; Vyas, G.N., Cohen, S.N., Schmid, R., Eds.; The Franklin Institute Press: Philadelphia, PA, USA, 1978; pp. 539–556.
28. McAleer, W.J.; Buynak, E.B.; Maigetter, R.Z.; Wampler, D.E.; Miller, W.J.; Hilleman, M.R. Human hepatitis B vaccine from recombinant yeast. *Nature* **1984**, *307*, 178–180. [CrossRef] [PubMed]
29. Murphy, B.L.; Maynard, J.E.; Le Bouvier, G.L. Viral subtypes and cross-presentation in hepatitis B virus infections of chimpanzees. *Intervirology* **1974**, *3*, 378–381. [CrossRef] [PubMed]
30. Hu, J.; Liu, K. Complete and incomplete hepatitis B virus particles: Formation, function, and application. *Viruses* **2017**, *9*, 56. [CrossRef]
31. Selzer, L.; Zlotnick, A. Assembly and release of hepatitis B virus. *Cold Spring Harb. Perspect. Med.* **2015**, *5*, a021394. [CrossRef]
32. Sureau, C.; Salisse, J. A conformational heparan sulfate binding site essential to infectivity overlaps with the conserved hepatitis B virus a-determinant. *Hepatology* **2013**, *57*, 985–994. [CrossRef]
33. Bruss, V.; Vieluf, K. Functions of the internal pre-S domain of the large surface protein in hepatitis B virus particle morphogenesis. *J. Virol.* **1995**, *69*, 6652–6657. [CrossRef]
34. Schulze, A.; Gripon, P.; Urban, S. Hepatitis B virus infection initiates with a large surface protein-dependent binding to heparan sulfate proteoglycans. *Hepatology* **2007**, *46*, 1759–1768. [CrossRef]
35. Leistner, C.M.; Gruen-Bernhard, S.; Glebe, D. Role of glycosaminoglycans for binding and infection of hepatitis B virus. *Cell. Microbiol.* **2008**, *10*, 122–133. [CrossRef]
36. Neurath, A.R.; Kent, S.B.H.; Strick, N.; Parker, K. Identification and chemical synthesis of a host cell receptor binding site on hepatitis B virus. *Cell* **1986**, *46*, 429–436. [CrossRef]
37. Yan, H.; Zhong, G.; Xu, G.; He, W.; Jing, Z.; Gao, Z.; Huang, Y.; Qi, Y.; Peng, B.; Wang, H.; et al. Sodium taurocholate cotransporting polypeptide is a functional receptor for human hepatitis B and D virus. *eLife* **2012**, *1*, e00049. [CrossRef]

38. Lambert, C.; Prange, R. Chaperone action in the posttranslational topological reorientation of the hepatitis B virus large envelope protein: Implications for translocational regulation. *Proc. Natl. Acad. Sci. USA* **2003**, *100*, 5199–5204. [CrossRef] [PubMed]
39. Cho, D.Y.; Yang, G.H.; Ryu, C.J.; Hong, H.J. Molecular chaperone GRP78/BiP interacts with the large surface protein of hepatitis B virus in vitro and in vivo. *J. Virol.* **2003**, *77*, 2784–2788. [CrossRef] [PubMed]
40. Löffler-Mary, H.; Werr, M.; Prange, R. Sequence-specific repression of cotranslational translocation of the hepatitis B virus envelope proteins coincides with binding of heat shock protein Hsc70. *Virology* **1997**, *235*, 144–152. [CrossRef] [PubMed]
41. Stieler, J.T.; Prange, R. Involvement of ESCRT-II in hepatitis B virus morphogenesis. *PLoS ONE* **2014**, *9*, e91279. [CrossRef]
42. Lambert, C.; Döring, T.; Prange, R. Hepatitis B virus maturation is sensitive to functional inhibition of ESCRT-III, Vps4, and γ2-Adaptin. *J. Virol.* **2007**, *81*, 9050–9060. [CrossRef]
43. Watanabe, T.; Sorensen, E.M.; Naito, A.; Schott, M.; Kim, S.; Ahlquist, P. Involvement of host cellular multivesicular body functions in hepatitis B virus budding. *Proc. Natl. Acad. Sci. USA* **2007**, *104*, 10205–10210. [CrossRef]
44. Jiang, B.; Himmelsbach, K.; Ren, H.; Boller, K.; Hildt, E. Subviral hepatitis B virus filaments, like infectious viral particles, are released via multivesicular bodies. *J. Virol.* **2016**, *90*, 3330–3341. [CrossRef]
45. Chairez, R.; Hollinger, F.B.; Melnick, J.L.; Dreesman, G.R. Biophysical properties of purified morphologic forms of hepatitis B antigen. *Intervirology* **1974**, *3*, 129–140. [CrossRef]
46. Short, J.M.; Chen, S.; Roseman, A.M.; Butler, P.J.G.; Crowther, R.A. Structure of hepatitis B surface antigen from subviral tubes determined by electron cryomicroscopy. *J. Mol. Biol.* **2009**, *390*, 135–141. [CrossRef]
47. Dryden, K.A.; Wieland, S.F.; Whitten-Bauer, C.; Gerin, J.L.; Chisari, F.V.; Yeager, M. Native hepatitis B virions and capsids visualized by electron cryomicroscopy. *Mol. Cell* **2006**, *22*, 843–850. [CrossRef]
48. Cao, J.; Zhang, J.; Lu, Y.; Luo, S.; Zhang, J.; Zhu, P. Cryo-EM structure of native spherical subviral particles isolated from HBV carriers. *Virus Res.* **2019**, *259*, 90–96. [CrossRef]
49. Gilbert, R.J.C.; Beales, L.; Blond, D.; Simon, M.N.; Lin, B.Y.; Chisari, F.V.; Stuart, D.I.; Rowlands, D.J. Hepatitis B small surface antigen particles are octahedral. *Proc. Natl. Acad. Sci. USA* **2005**, *102*, 14783–14788. [CrossRef] [PubMed]
50. Crowley, C.W.; Liu, C.-C.; Levinson, A.D. Plasmid-directed synthesis of hepatitis B surface antigen in monkey cells. *Moll. Cell. Biol.* **1983**, *3*, 44–55. [CrossRef] [PubMed]
51. Liu, C.-C.; Yansura, D.; Levinson, A.D. Direct expression of hepatitis B surface antigen in monkey cells from an SV40 vector. *DNA* **1982**, *1*, 213–221. [CrossRef] [PubMed]
52. Moriarty, A.M.; Hoyer, B.H.; Shih, J.W.K.; Gerin, J.L.; Hamer, D.H. Expression of the hepatitis B virus surface antigen gene in cell culture by using a simian virus 40 vector. *Proc. Natl. Acad. Sci. USA* **1981**, *78*, 2606–2610. [CrossRef] [PubMed]
53. Dubois, M.F.; Pourcel, C.; Rousset, S.; Chany, C.; Tiollais, P. Excretion of hepatitis B surface antigen particles from mouse cells transformed with cloned viral DNA. *Proc. Natl. Acad. Sci. USA* **1980**, *77*, 4549–4553. [CrossRef] [PubMed]
54. Lee, Y.S.; Kim, B.K.; Choi, E.-C. Physiochemical properties of recombinant hepatitis B surface antigen expressed in mammalian cell (C127). *Arch. Pharm. Res.* **1998**, *21*, 521–526. [CrossRef]
55. Eble, B.E.; Lingappa, V.R.; Ganem, D. Hepatitis B surface antigen: An unusual secreted protein initially synthesized as a transmembrane polypeptide. *Mol. Cell. Biol.* **1986**, *6*, 1454–1463. [CrossRef]
56. Eble, B.E.; MacRae, D.R.; Lingappa, V.R.; Ganem, D. Multiple topogenic sequences determine the transmembrane orientation of hepatitis B surface antigen. *Mol. Cell. Biol.* **1987**, *7*, 3591–3601. [CrossRef]
57. Suffner, S.; Gerstenberg, N.; Patra, M.; Ruibal, P.; Orabi, A.; Schindler, M.; Bruss, V. Domains of the hepatitis B virus small surface protein S mediating oligomerization. *J. Virol.* **2018**, *92*, e02232-17. [CrossRef] [PubMed]
58. Stirk, H.J.; Thornton, J.M.; Howard, C.R. A topological model for hepatitis B surface antigen. *Intervirology* **1992**, *33*, 148–158. [CrossRef] [PubMed]
59. Berting, A.; Hahnen, J.; Kröger, M.; Gerlich, W.H. Computer-aided studies on the spatial structure of the small hepatitis B surface protein. *Intervirology* **1995**, *38*, 8–15. [CrossRef] [PubMed]

60. Komla-Soukha, I.; Sureau, C. A tryptophan-rich motif in the carboxyl terminus of the small envelope protein of hepatitis B virus is central to the assembly of hepatitis delta virus particles. *J. Virol.* **2006**, *80*, 4648–4655. [CrossRef] [PubMed]
61. Paulij, W.P.; de Wit, P.L.M.; Sünnen, C.M.G.; van Roosmalen, M.H.; Petersen-van Ettekoven, A.; Cooreman, M.P.; Heijtink, R.A. Localization of a unique hepatitis B virus epitope sheds new light on the structure of hepatitis B virus surface antigen. *J. Gen. Virol.* **1999**, *80*, 2121–2126. [CrossRef] [PubMed]
62. Mangold, C.M.T.; Unckell, F.; Werr, M.; Streeck, R.E. Analysis of intermolecular disulfide bonds and free sulfhydryl groups in hepatitis B surface antigen particles. *Arch. Virol.* **1997**, *142*, 2257–2267. [CrossRef] [PubMed]
63. Mangold, C.M.T.; Streeck, R.E. Mutational analysis of the cysteine residues in the hepatitis B virus small envelope protein. *J. Virol.* **1993**, *67*, 4588–4597. [CrossRef]
64. Mangold, C.M.T.; Unckell, F.; Werr, M.; Streeck, R.E. Secretion and antigenicity of hepatitis B virus small envelope proteins lacking cysteines in the major antigenic region. *Virology* **1995**, *211*, 535–543. [CrossRef]
65. Cheong, W.S.; Hyakumura, M.; Yuen, L.; Warner, N.; Locarnini, S.; Netter, H.J. Modulation of the immunogenicity of virus-like particles composed of mutant hepatitis B virus envelope subunits. *Antivir. Res.* **2012**, *93*, 209–218. [CrossRef]
66. Wunderlich, G.; Bruss, V. Characterization of early hepatitis B virus surface protein oligomers. *Arch. Virol.* **1996**, *141*, 1191–1205. [CrossRef]
67. Patzer, E.J.; Nakamura, G.R.; Yaffe, A. Intracellular transport and secretion of hepatitis B surface antigen in mammalian cells. *J. Virol.* **1984**, *51*, 346–353. [CrossRef]
68. Lu, X.; Mehta, A.; Dwek, R.; Butters, T.; Block, T. Evidence that N-linked glycosylation is necessary for hepatitis B virus secretion. *Virology* **1995**, *213*, 660–665. [CrossRef] [PubMed]
69. Ito, K.; Qin, Y.; Guarnieri, M.; Garcia, T.; Kwei, K.; Mizokami, M.; Zhang, J.; Li, J.; Wands, J.R.; Tong, S. Impairment of hepatitis B virus virion secretion by single-amino-acid substitutions in the small envelope protein and rescue by a novel glycosylation site. *J. Virol.* **2010**, *84*, 12850–12861. [CrossRef] [PubMed]
70. Julithe, R.; Abou-Jaoudé, G.; Sureau, C. Modification of the hepatitis B virus envelope protein glycosylation pattern interferes with secretion of viral particles, infectivity, and susceptibility to neutralizing antibodies. *J. Virol.* **2014**, *88*, 9049–9059. [CrossRef] [PubMed]
71. Eble, B.E.; Lingappa, V.R.; Ganem, D. The N-terminal (pre-S2) domain of a hepatitis B virus surface glycoprotein is translocated across membranes by downstream signal sequences. *J. Virol.* **1990**, *64*, 1414–1419. [CrossRef] [PubMed]
72. Stibbe, W.; Gerlich, W.H. Characterization of pre-s gene products in hepatitis B surface antigen. *Dev. Biol. Stand.* **1983**, *54*, 33–43.
73. Schmitt, S.; Glebe, D.; Tolle, T.K.; Lochnit, G.; Linder, D.; Geyer, R.; Gerlich, W.H. Structure of pre-S2 *N*- and *O*-linked glycans in surface proteins from different genotypes of hepatitis B virus. *J. Gen. Virol.* **2004**, *85*, 2045–2053. [CrossRef]
74. Cheng, K.-C.; Moss, B. Selective synthesis and secretion of particles composed of the hepatitis B virus middle surface protein directed by a recombinant vaccinia virus: Induction of antibodies to pre-S and S epitopes. *J. Virol.* **1987**, *61*, 1286–1290. [CrossRef]
75. McLachlan, A.; Milich, D.R.; Raney, A.K.; Riggs, M.G.; Hughes, J.L.; Sorge, J.; Chisari, F.V. Expression of hepatitis B virus surface and core antigens: Influences of pre-S and precore sequences. *J. Virol.* **1987**, *61*, 683–692. [CrossRef]
76. Molnar-Kimber, K.L.; Jarocki-Witek, V.; Dheer, S.K.; Vernon, S.K.; Conley, A.J.; Davis, A.R.; Hung, P.P. Distinctive properties of the hepatitis B virus envelope proteins. *J. Virol.* **1988**, *62*, 407–416. [CrossRef]
77. Sheu, S.Y.; Lo, S.J. Biogenesis of the hepatitis B viral middle (M) surface protein in a human hepatoma cell line: Demonstration of an alternative secretion pathway. *J. Gen. Virol.* **1994**, *75*, 3031–3039. [CrossRef] [PubMed]
78. Fernholz, D.; Galle, P.R.; Stemler, M.; Brunetto, M.; Bonino, F.; Will, H. Infectious hepatitis B virus variant defective in pre-S2 protein expression in a chronic carrier. *Virology* **1993**, *194*, 137–148. [CrossRef] [PubMed]
79. Ostapchuk, P.; Hearing, P.; Ganem, D. A dramatic shift in the transmembrane topology of a viral envelope glycoprotein accompanies hepatitis B viral morphogenesis. *EMBO J.* **1994**, *13*, 1048–1057. [CrossRef] [PubMed]
80. Prange, R.; Streeck, R.E. Novel transmembrane topology of the hepatitis B virus envelope proteins. *EMBO J.* **1995**, *14*, 247–256. [CrossRef]

81. Seitz, S.; Iancu, C.; Volz, T.; Mier, W.; Dandri, M.; Urban, S.; Bartenschlager, R. A slow maturation process renders hepatitis B virus infectious. *Cell Host Microbe* **2016**, *20*, 25–35. [CrossRef]
82. Ni, Y.; Sonnabend, J.; Seitz, S.; Urban, S. The pre-S2 domain of the hepatitis B virus is dispensable for infectivity but serves a spacer function for L-protein-connected virus assembly. *J. Virol.* **2010**, *84*, 3879–3888. [CrossRef]
83. Bruss, V.; Gerhardt, E.; Vieluf, K.; Wunderlich, G. Functions of the large hepatitis B virus surface protein in viral particle morphogenesis. *Intervirology* **1996**, *39*, 23–31. [CrossRef]
84. Gripon, P.; Le Seyec, J.; Rumin, S.; Guguen-Guillouzo, C. Myristylation of the hepatitis B virus large surface protein is essential for viral infectivity. *Virology* **1995**, *213*, 292–299. [CrossRef]
85. Xu, Z.; Bruss, V.; Yen, T.S.B. Formation of intracellular particles by hepatitis B virus large surface protein. *J. Virol.* **1997**, *71*, 5487–5494. [CrossRef]
86. Persing, D.H.; Varmus, H.E.; Ganem, D. Inhibition of secretion of hepatitis B surface antigen by a related presurface polypeptide. *Science* **1986**, *234*, 1388–1391. [CrossRef]
87. Ou, J.H.; Rutter, W.J. Regulation of secretion of the hepatitis B virus major surface antigen by the preS-1 protein. *J. Virol.* **1987**, *61*, 782–786. [CrossRef] [PubMed]
88. Heermann, K.H.; Goldmann, U.; Schwartz, W.; Seyffarth, T.; Baumgarten, H.; Gerlich, W.H. Large surface proteins of hepatitis B virus containing the pre-s sequence. *J. Virol.* **1984**, *52*, 396–402. [CrossRef] [PubMed]
89. Gavilanes, F.; Gonzalez-Ros, J.M.; Peterson, D.L. Structure of hepatitis B surface antigen. *J. Biol. Chem.* **1982**, *257*, 7770–7777. [PubMed]
90. Peterson, D.L. The structure of hepatitis B surface antigen and its antigenic sites. *BioEssays* **1987**, *6*, 258–262. [CrossRef]
91. Shih, C.; Li, L.S.; Roychoudhury, S.; Ho, M.H. In vitro propagation of human hepatitis B virus in a rat hepatoma cell line. *Proc. Natl. Acad. Sci. USA* **1989**, *86*, 6323–6327. [CrossRef]
92. Hruska, J.F.; Robinson, W.S. The proteins of hepatitis B Dane particle cores. *J. Med. Virol.* **1977**, *1*, 119–131. [CrossRef]
93. Sukeno, N.; Shirachi, R.; Yamaguchi, J.; Ishida, N. Reduction and reoxidation of Australia antigen: Loss and reconstitution of particle structure and antigenicity. *J. Virol.* **1972**, *9*, 182–183. [CrossRef]
94. Vyas, G.N.; Rao, K.R.; Ibrahim, A.B. Australia antigen (hepatitis B antigen): A conformational antigen dependent of disulfide bonds. *Science* **1972**, *178*, 1300–1301. [CrossRef]
95. Imai, M.; Gotoh, A.; Nishioka, K.; Kurashina, S.; Miyakawa, Y.; Mayumi, M. Antigenicity of reduced and alkylated Australia antigen. *J. Immunol.* **1974**, *112*, 416–419.
96. Huovila, A.-P.J.; Eder, A.M.; Fuller, S.D. Hepatitis B surface antigen assembles in a post-ER, pre-Golgi compartment. *J. Cell Biol.* **1992**, *118*, 1305–1320. [CrossRef]
97. Patzer, E.J.; Nakamura, G.R.; Simonsen, C.C.; Levinson, A.D.; Brands, R. Intracellular assembly and packaging of hepatitis B surface antigen particles occur in the endoplasmic reticulum. *J. Virol.* **1986**, *58*, 884–892. [CrossRef] [PubMed]
98. Satoh, O.; Umeda, M.; Imai, H.; Tunoo, H.; Inoue, K. Lipid composition of hepatitis B surface antigen particles and the particle-producing human hepatoma cell lines. *J. Lipid Res.* **1990**, *31*, 1293–1300. [PubMed]
99. Satoh, O.; Imai, H.; Yoneyama, T.; Miyamura, T.; Utsumi, H.; Inoue, K.; Umeda, M. Membrane structure of the hepatitis B virus surface antigen particle. *J. Biochem.* **2000**, *127*, 543–550. [CrossRef] [PubMed]
100. Gavilanes, F.; Gomez-Gutierrez, J.; Aracil, M.; Gonzales-Ros, J.M.; Ferragut, J.A.; Guerrero, E.; Peterson, D.L. Hepatitis B surface antigen. Role of lipids in maintaining the structural and antigenic properties of protein components. *Biochem. J.* **1990**, *265*, 857–864. [CrossRef]
101. Guerrero, E.; Gavilanes, F.; Peterson, D.L. Model for the protein arrangement in HBsAg particles based on physical and chemical studies. In *Viral Hepatitis and Liver Disease*; Zuckerman, A.J., Ed.; Alan, R. Liss Inc.: New York, NY, USA, 1988; pp. 606–613.
102. Greiner, V.J.; Egelé, C.; Oncul, S.; Ronzon, F.; Manin, C.; Klymchenko, A.; Mély, Y. Characterization of the lipid and protein organization in HBsAg viral particles by steady-state and time-resolved fluorescence spectroscopy. *Biochimie* **2010**, *92*, 994–1002. [CrossRef]
103. Milhiet, P.-E.; Dosset, P.; Godefroy, C.; Le Grimellec, C.; Guigner, J.M.; Larquet, E.; Ronzon, F.; Manin, C. Nanoscale topography of hepatitis B antigen particles by atomic force microscopy. *Biochimie* **2011**, *93*, 254–259. [CrossRef]
104. Blumberg, B.S. Australia antigen and the biology of hepatitis B. *Science* **1977**, *197*, 17–25. [CrossRef]

105. Courroucé-Pauty, A.M.; Delons, S.; Soulier, J.P. Attempt to prevent hepatitis by using specific anti-HBs immunoglobulin. *Am. J. Med. Sci.* **1975**, *270*, 375–383.
106. Iwarson, S.; Kjellman, H.; Ahlmén, J.; Ljunggren, C.; Eriksson, E.; Selander, D.; Hermodsson, S. Hepatitis B immune serum globulin and standard gamma globulin in prevention of hepatitis B infection among hospital staff: A preliminary report. *Am. J. Med. Sci.* **1975**, *270*, 385–389. [CrossRef]
107. Hilleman, M.R.; Buynak, E.B.; Roehm, R.R.; Tytell, A.A.; Bertland, A.U.; Lampson, G.P. Purified and inactivated human hepatitis B vaccine: Progress report. *Am. J. Med. Sci.* **1975**, *270*, 401–404. [CrossRef]
108. Purcell, R.H.; Gerin, J.L. Hepatitis B subunit vaccine: A preliminary report of safety and efficacy tests in chimpanzees. *Am. J. Med. Sci.* **1975**, *270*, 395–399. [CrossRef] [PubMed]
109. Okochi, K.; Murakami, S.; Ninomiya, K.; Kaneko, M. Australia antigen, transfusion and hepatitis. *Vox Sang.* **1970**, *18*, 289–300. [CrossRef]
110. London, W.T.; Drew, J.S.; Lustbader, E.D.; Werner, B.G.; Blumberg, B.S. Host responses to hepatitis B infection in patients in a chronic hemodialysis unit. *Kidney Int.* **1977**, *12*, 51–58. [CrossRef] [PubMed]
111. Krugman, S.; Giles, J.P.; Hammond, J. Viral Hepatitis, type B (MS-2 strain). Studies on active immunization. *JAMA* **1971**, *217*, 41–45. [CrossRef]
112. Buynak, E.B.; Roehm, R.R.; Tytell, A.A.; Bertland, A.U., II; Lampson, G.P.; Hilleman, M.R. Vaccine against human hepatitis B. *J. Am. Med. Assoc.* **1976**, *235*, 2832–2834. [CrossRef]
113. Gerin, J.L.; Holland, P.V.; Purcell, R.H. Australia antigen: Large-scale purification from human serum and biochemical studies of its proteins. *J. Virol.* **1971**, *7*, 569–576. [CrossRef]
114. Maupas, P.; Goudeau, A.; Coursaget, P.; Drucker, J.; Bagros, P. Immunisation against hepatitis B in man. *Lancet* **1976**, *307*, 1367–1370. [CrossRef]
115. McMahon, B.J.; Helminiak, C.; Wainwright, R.B.; Bulkow, L.; Trimble, B.A.; Wainwright, K. Frequency of adverse reactions to hepatitis B vaccine in 43,618 persons. *Am. J. Med.* **1992**, *92*, 254–256. [CrossRef]
116. Szmuness, W.; Stevens, C.E.; Zang, E.A.; Harley, E.J.; Kellner, A. A controlled clinical trial of the efficacy of the hepatitis B vaccine (Heptavax B): A final report. *Hepatol* **1981**, *1*, 377–385. [CrossRef]
117. Shaw, F.E.; Graham, D.J.; Guess, H.A.; Milstien, J.B.; Johnson, J.M.; Schatz, G.C.; Hadler, S.C.; Kuritsky, J.N.; Hiner, E.E.; Bregman, D.J.; et al. Postmarketing surveillance for neurologic adverse events reported after hepatitis B vaccination. Experience of the first three years. *Am. J. Epidemiol.* **1988**, *127*, 337–352. [CrossRef]
118. Neurath, A.R.; Strick, N.; Kent, S.B.H.; Offensperger, W.; Wahl, S.; Christman, J.K.; Acs, G. Enzyme-linked immunoassay of pre-S gene-coded sequences in hepatitis B vaccines. *J. Virol. Method* **1985**, *12*, 185–192. [CrossRef]
119. Neurath, A.R.; Kent, S.B.H.; Strick, N.; Taylor, P.; Stevens, C.E. Hepatitis B virus contains pre-S gene-encoded domains. *Nature* **1985**, *315*, 154–156. [CrossRef] [PubMed]
120. Coursaget, P.; Bringer, L.; Sarr, G.; Bourdil, C.; Fritzell, B.; Blondeau, C.; Yvonnet, B.; Chiron, J.P.; Jeannée, E.; Guindo, S.; et al. Comparative immunogenicity in children of mammalian cell-derived recombinant hepatitis B vaccine and plasma-derived hepatitis B vaccine. *Vaccine* **1992**, *10*, 379–382. [CrossRef]
121. Zuckerman, A.J. Hepatitis-B vaccine. Safety criteria and non-B infection. *Lancet* **1976**, *307*, 1396–1397. [CrossRef]
122. Hilleman, M.R.; Ellis, R. Vaccines made from recombinant yeast cells. *Vaccine* **1986**, *4*, 75–76. [CrossRef]
123. Stephenne, J. Recombinant versus plasma-derived hepatitis B vaccines: Issues of safety, immunogenicity and cost-effectiveness. *Vaccine* **1988**, *6*, 299–303. [CrossRef]
124. Coursaget, P.; Adamowicz, P.; Bourdil, C.; Yvonnet, B.; Buisson, Y.; Barrès, J.L.; Saliou, P.; Chiron, J.P.; Diop Mar, I. Anti-preS2 antibodies in natural hepatitis B virus infection and after immunization. *Vaccine* **1988**, *6*, 357–361. [CrossRef]
125. Lau, J.Y.N.; Lai, C.L.; Wu, P.C.; Lin, H.J. Comparison of two plasma-derived hepatitis B vaccines: Long-term report of a prospective, randomized trial. *J. Gastroenterol. Hepatol.* **1989**, *4*, 331–337. [CrossRef]
126. Lee, H.S.; Kim, C.Y. Seroepidemiology of HBV and HCV in Korea: The decreasing prevalence rate of HBV infection after launching HB vaccination program. *Int. Hepatol. Commun.* **1996**, *5*, 53–61. [CrossRef]
127. Kalayanarooj, S.; Vaughn, D.W.; Ariyasriwatana, C.; Snitbhan, R. Protective antibody after a 'one dollar' hepatitis B vaccine. *Southeast Asian J. Trop. Med. Public Health* **1996**, *27*, 659–663.
128. Schoub, B.D.; Matai, U.; Singh, B.; Blackburn, N.K.; Levin, J.B. Universal immunization of infants with low doses of a low-cost, plasma-derived hepatitis B vaccine in South Africa. *Bull. World Health Organ.* **2002**, *80*, 277–281. [PubMed]

129. Coates, T.; Wilson, R.; Patrick, G.; André, F.; Watson, V. Hepatitis B vaccines: Assessment of the seroprotective efficacy of two recombinant DNA vaccines. *Clin. Ther.* **2001**, *23*, 392–403. [CrossRef]
130. Hernández-Bernal, F.; Aguilar-Betancourt, A.; Aljovin, V.; Arias, G.; Valenzuela, C.; de Alejo, K.P.; Hernández, K.; Oquendo, O.; Figueredo, N.; Figueroa, N.; et al. Comparison of four recombinant hepatitis B vaccines applied on an accelerated schedule in healthy adults. *Hum. Vaccine* **2011**, *7*, 1026–1036. [CrossRef] [PubMed]
131. Suzuki, H.; Iino, S.; Shiraki, K.; Akahane, Y.; Okamoto, H.; Domoto, K.; Mishiro, S. Safety and efficacy of a recombinant yeast-derived pre-S2 + S-containing hepatitis B vaccine (TGP-943): Phase 1, 2 and 3 clinical testing. *Vaccine* **1994**, *12*, 1090–1096. [CrossRef]
132. Teles, S.A.; Martins, R.M.B.; Lopes, C.L.R.; dos Santos Carneiro, M.A.; Souza, K.P.; Yoshida, C.F.T. Immunogenicity of a recombinant hepatitis B vaccine (Euvax-B) in haemodialysis patients and staff. *Eur.J. Epidemiol.* **2001**, *17*, 145–149. [CrossRef]
133. Abraham, P.; Mistry, F.P.; Bapat, M.R.; Sharma, G.; Reddy, G.R.; Prasad, K.S.N.; Ramanna, V. Evaluation of a new recombinant DNA hepatitis B vaccine (*Shanvac-B*). *Vaccine* **1999**, *17*, 1125–1129. [CrossRef]
134. Anonymous. A two-dose hepatitis B vaccine for adults (Heplisav-B). *Med. Lett. Drugs Ther.* **2018**, *60*, 17–18.
135. Zhu, F.; Deckx, H.; Roten, R.; Michiels, B.; Sarnecki, M. Comparative efficacy, safety and immunogenicity of Hepavax-Gene TF and Engerix-B recombinant hepatitis B vaccines in neonates in China. *Pediatr. Infect. Dis. J.* **2017**, *36*, 94–101. [CrossRef]
136. Shouval, D.; Roggendorf, H.; Roggendorf, M. Enhanced immune response to hepatitis B vaccination through immunization with a Pre-S1/Pre-S2/S vaccine. *Med. Microbiol. Immunol.* **2015**, *204*, 57–68. [CrossRef]
137. Young, M.D.; Schneider, D.L.; Zuckerman, A.J.; Du, W.; Dickson, B.; Maddrey, W.C. Adult hepatitis B vaccination using a novel triple antigen recombinant vaccine. *Hepatology* **2001**, *34*, 372–376. [CrossRef]
138. Valenzuela, P.; Medina, A.; Rutter, W.J.; Ammerer, G.; Hall, B.D. Synthesis and assembly of hepatitis B virus surface antigen particles in yeast. *Nature* **1982**, *298*, 347–350. [CrossRef] [PubMed]
139. Harford, N.; Cabezon, T.; Crabeel, M.; Simoen, E.; Rutgers, A.; De Wilde, M. Expression of hepatitis B surface antigen in yeast. *Dev. Biol. Stand.* **1983**, *54*, 125–130. [PubMed]
140. Miyanohara, A.; Toh-e, A.; Nozaki, C.; Hamada, F.; Ohtomo, N.; Matsubara, K. Expression of hepatitis B surface antigen gene in yeast. *Proc. Natl. Acad. Sci. USA* **1983**, *80*, 1–5. [CrossRef] [PubMed]
141. André, F.E. Overview of a 5-year clinical experience with a yeast-derived hepatitis B vaccine. *Vaccine* **1990**, *8* (Suppl. 1), S74–S78.
142. Wolters, B.; Junge, U.; Dziuba, S.; Roggendorf, M. Immunogenicity of combined hepatitis A and B vaccine in elderly persons. *Vaccine* **2003**, *21*, 3623–3628. [CrossRef]
143. Zhang, Z.; Wang, C.; Liu, Z.; Zou, G.; Li, J.; Lu, M. Host genetic determinants of hepatitis B virus infection. *Front. Genet.* **2019**, *10*, 696. [CrossRef]
144. Li, Z.K.; Nie, J.J.; Li, J.; Zhuang, H. The effec t of HLA on immunological response to hepatitis B vaccine in healthy people: A meta-analysis. *Vaccine* **2013**, *31*, 4355–4361. [CrossRef]
145. Milich, D.R.; Leroux-Roels, G.G. Immunogenetics of the response to HBsAg vaccination. *Autoimmun. Rev.* **2003**, *2*, 248–257. [CrossRef]
146. Cregg, J.M.; Tschopp, J.F.; Stillman, C.; Siegel, R.; Akong, M.; Craig, W.S.; Buckholz, R.G.; Madden, K.R.; Kellaris, P.A.; Davis, G.R.; et al. High-level expression and efficient assembly of hepatitis B surface antigen in the methylotrophic yeast, Pichia pastoris. *Biotechnology* **1987**, *5*, 479–485. [CrossRef]
147. Lünsdorf, H.; Gurramkonda, C.; Adnan, A.; Khanna, N.; Rinas, U. Virus-like particle production with yeast: Ultrastructural and immunocytochemical insights into *Pichia pastoris* producing high levels of the hepatitis B surface antigen. *Microb. Cell Factories* **2011**, *10*, 48. [CrossRef]
148. Zahid, M.; Lünsdorf, H.; Rinas, U. Assessing stability and assembly of the hepatitis B surface antigen into virus-like particles during down-stream processing. *Vaccine* **2015**, *33*, 3739–3745. [CrossRef] [PubMed]
149. Zhao, Q.; Wang, Y.; Freed, D.; Fu, T.-M.; Gimenez, J.A.; Sitrin, R.D.; Washabaugh, M.W. Maturation of recombinant hepatitis B virus surface antigen particles. *Hum. Vaccines* **2006**, *2*, 174–180. [CrossRef] [PubMed]
150. Gurramkonda, C.; Zahid, M.; Nemani, S.K.; Adnan, A.; Gudi, S.K.; Khanna, N.; Ebensen, T.; Lünsdorf, H.; Guzmán, C.A.; Rinas, U. Purification of hepatitis B surface antigen virus-like particles from recombinant *Pichia pastoris* and *in vivo* analysis of their immunogenic properties. *J. Chromatogr. B* **2013**, *940*, 104–111. [CrossRef] [PubMed]

151. Zhao, Q.; Towne, V.; Brown, M.; Wang, Y.; Abraham, D.; Oswald, C.B.; Gimenez, J.A.; Washabaugh, M.W.; Kennedy, R.; Sitrin, R.D. In-depth process understanding of RECOMBIVAX HB® maturation and potential epitope improvements with redox treatment: Multifaceted biochemical and immunochemical characterization. *Vaccine* **2011**, *29*, 7936–7941. [CrossRef] [PubMed]
152. Wampler, D.E.; Lehman, E.D.; Boger, J.; McAleer, W.J.; Scolnick, E.M. Multiple chemical forms of hepatitis B surface antigen produced in yeast. *Proc. Natl. Acad. Sci. USA* **1985**, *82*, 6830–6834. [CrossRef]
153. Yamaguchi, M.; Sugahara, K.; Shiosaki, K.; Mizokami, H.; Takeo, K. Fine structure of hepatitis B virus surface antigen produced by recombinant yeast: Comparison with HBsAg of human origin. *FEMS Microbiol. Lett.* **1998**, *165*, 363–367. [CrossRef]
154. Sonveaux, N.; Conrath, K.; Capiau, C.; Brasseur, R.; Goormaghtigh, E.; Ruysschaert, J.M. The topology of the S protein in the yeast-derived hepatitis B surface antigen particles. *J. Biol. Chem.* **1994**, *269*, 25637–25645.
155. Van der Meeren, P.; Van Criekinge, W.; Vanderdeelen, J.; Baert, L. Phospholipid composition of r-DNA hepatitis B surface antigens. *Int. J. Pharm.* **1994**, *106*, 89–92. [CrossRef]
156. Diminsky, D.; Schirmbeck, R.; Reimann, J.; Barenholz, Y. Comparison between hepatitis B surface antigen (HBsAg) particles derived from mammalian cells (CHO) and yeast cells (*Hansenula polymorpha*): Composition, structure and immunogenicity. *Vaccine* **1997**, *15*, 637–647. [CrossRef]
157. Brown, S.E.; Stanley, C.; Howard, C.R.; Zuckerman, A.J.; Steward, M.W. Antibody responses to recombinant and plasma derived hepatitis B vaccines. *Br. Med. J.* **1986**, *292*, 159–161. [CrossRef]
158. Franchi, L.; Núñez, G. The Nlrp3 inflammasome is critical for aluminium hydroxide-mediated IL-1β secretion but dispensible for adjuvant activity. *Eur. J. Immunol.* **2008**, *38*, 2085–2089. [CrossRef] [PubMed]
159. Li, H.; Willingham, S.B.; Ting, J.P.-Y.; Re, F. Cutting Edge: Inflammasome activation by alum and alum's adjuvant effect are mediated by NLRP3. *J. Immunol.* **2008**, *181*, 17–21. [CrossRef] [PubMed]
160. Kool, M.; Pétrilli, V.; De Smedt, T.; Rolaz, A.; Hammad, H.; van Nimwegen, M.; Bergen, I.M.; Castillo, R.; Lambrecht, B.N.; Tschopp, J. Cutting edge: Alum adjuvant stimulates inflammatory dendritic cells through activation of the NALP3 inflammasome. *J. Immunol.* **2008**, *181*, 3755–3759. [CrossRef] [PubMed]
161. HogenEsch, H. Mechanism of immunopotentiation and safety of aluminum adjuvants. *Front. Immunol.* **2013**, *3*, 406. [CrossRef] [PubMed]
162. Iyer, S.; Robinett, R.S.R.; HogenEsch, H.; Hem, S.L. Mechanism of adsorption of hepatitis B surface antigen by aluminum hydroxide adjuvant. *Vaccine* **2004**, *22*, 1475–1479. [CrossRef] [PubMed]
163. Hansen, B.; Belfast, M.; Soung, G.; Song, L.; Egan, P.M.; Capen, R.; HogenEsch, H.; Mancinelli, R.; Hem, S.L. Effect of the strength of adsorption of hepatitis B surface antigen to aluminum hydroxide adjuvant on the immune response. *Vaccine* **2009**, *27*, 888–892. [CrossRef] [PubMed]
164. Shi, Y.; HogenEsch, H.; Hem, S.L. Change in the degree of adsorption of proteins by aluminum-containing adjuvants following exposure to interstitial fluid: Freshly prepared and aged model vaccines. *Vaccine* **2002**, *20*, 80–85. [CrossRef]
165. Greiner, V.J.; Ronzon, F.; Larquet, E.; Desbat, B.; Estèves, C.; Bonvin, J.; Gréco, F.; Manin, C.; Klymchenko, A.S.; Mély, Y. The structure of HBsAg particles is not modified upon their adsorption on aluminium hydroxide gel. *Vaccine* **2012**, *30*, 5240–5245. [CrossRef]
166. Jackson, S.; Lentino, J.; Kopp, J.; Murray, L.; Ellison, W.; Rhee, M.; Shockey, G.; Akella, L.; Erby, K.; Heyward, W.L.; et al. Immunogenicity of a two-dose investigational hepatitits B vaccine, HBsAg-1018, using a toll-like receptor 9 agonist adjuvant compared with a licensed hepatitis B vaccine in adults. *Vaccine* **2018**, *36*, 668–674. [CrossRef]
167. Neurath, A.R.; Seto, B.; Strick, N. Antibodies to synthetic peptides from the preS1 region of the hepatitis B virus (HBV) envelope (env) protein are virus-neutralizing and protective. *Vaccine* **1989**, *7*, 234–236. [CrossRef]
168. Neurath, A.R.; Kent, S.B.H.; Parker, K.; Prince, A.M.; Strick, N.; Brotman, B.; Sproul, P. Anrtibodies to a synthetic peptide from the preS 120-145 region of the hepatitis B virus envelope are virus-neutralizing. *Vaccine* **1986**, *4*, 35–37. [CrossRef]
169. Itoh, Y.; Takai, E.; Ohnuma, H.; Kitajima, K.; Tsuda, F.; Machida, A.; Mishiro, S.; Nakamura, T.; Miyakawa, Y.; Mayumi, M. A synthetic peptide vaccine involving the product of the pre-S(2) region of hepatitis B virus DNA: Protective efficacy in chimpanzees. *Proc. Natl. Acad. Sci. USA* **1986**, *83*, 9174–9178. [CrossRef] [PubMed]

170. Ferrari, C.; Penna, A.; Bertoletti, A.; Cavalli, A.; Valli, A.; Schianchi, C.; Fiaccadori, F. The preS1 antigen of hepatitis B virus is highly immunogenic at the T cell level in man. *J. Clin. Investig.* **1989**, *84*, 1314–1319. [CrossRef] [PubMed]
171. Milich, D.R. T- and B-cell recognition of hepatitis B viral antigens. *Immunol. Today* **1988**, *9*, 380–386. [CrossRef]
172. Milich, D.R.; McLachlan, A.; Chisari, F.V.; Kent, S.B.H.; Thornton, G.B. Immune response to the pre-S(1) region of the hepatitis B surface antigen (HBsAg): A pre-S(1)-specific T cell response can bypass nonresponsiveness to the pre-S(2) and S regions of HBsAg. *J. Immunol.* **1986**, *137*, 315–322.
173. Shouval, D.; Ilan, Y.; Adler, R.; Deepen, R.; Panet, A.; Even-Chen, Z.; Gorecki, M.; Gerlich, W.H. Improved immunogenicity in mice of a mammalian cell-derived recombinant hepatitis B vaccine containing pre-S_1 and pre-S_2 antigens as compared with conventional yeast-derived vaccines. *Vaccine* **1994**, *12*, 1453–1459. [CrossRef]
174. Kobayashi, M.; Asano, T.; Utsunomiya, M.; Itoh, Y.; Fijisawa, Y.; Nishimura, O.; Kato, K.; Kakinuma, A. Recombinant hepatitis B virus surface antigen carrying the pre-S2 region derived from yeast: Purification and characterization. *J. Biotechnol.* **1988**, *8*, 1–22. [CrossRef]
175. Itoh, Y.; Fujisawa, Y. Synthesis in yeast of hepatitis B virus surface antigen modified P31 particles by gene modification. *Biochem. Biophys. Res. Commun.* **1986**, *141*, 942–948. [CrossRef]
176. De Wilde, M.; Rutgers, T.; Cabezon, T.; Hauser, P.; van Opstal, O.; Harford, N.; van Wijnendaele, F.; Desmons, P.; Comberbach, M.; Roelants, P.; et al. PreS-containing HBsAg particles from *Saccharomyces cerevisiae*: Production, antigenicity, and immunogenicity. In *Viral Hepatitis and Liver Disease*; Hollinger, F.B., Lemon, S.M., Margolis, H., Eds.; Williams & Wilkins: Baltimore, MD, USA, 1991; pp. 732–736.
177. Kuroda, S.; Fujisawa, Y.; Iino, S.; Akahane, Y.; Suzuki, H. Induction of protection level of anti-pre-S2 antibodies in humans immunized with a novel hepatitis B vaccine consisting of M (pre-S2+S) protein particles (a third generation vaccine). *Vaccine* **1991**, *9*, 163–169. [CrossRef]
178. Fujisawa, Y.; Kuroda, S.; Van Eerd, P.M.C.A.; Schellekens, H.; Kakinuma, A. Protective efficacy of a novel hepatitis B vaccine consisting of M (pre-S2+S) protein particles (a third generation vaccine). *Vaccine* **1990**, *8*, 192–198. [CrossRef]
179. Kniskern, P.J.; Hagopian, A.; Burke, P.; Dunn, N.; Emini, E.A.; Miller, W.J.; Yamazaki, S.; Ellis, R.W. A candidate vaccine for hepatitis B containing the complete viral surface protein. *Hepatology* **1988**, *8*, 82–87. [CrossRef] [PubMed]
180. Biemans, R.; Thines, D.; Rutgers, T.; de Wilde, M.; Cabezon, T. The large surface protein of hepatitis B virus is retained in the yeast endoplasmic reticulum and provokes its unique enlargement. *DNA Cell Biol.* **1991**, *10*, 191–200. [CrossRef] [PubMed]
181. Kuroda, S.; Otaka, S.; Miyazaki, T.; Nakao, M.; Fujisawa, Y. Hepatitis B virus envelope L protein particles. *J. Biol. Chem.* **1992**, *267*, 1953–1961. [PubMed]
182. Yamada, T.; Iwabuki, H.; Kanno, T.; Tanaka, H.; Kawai, T.; Fukuda, H.; Kondo, A.; Seno, M.; Tanizawa, K.; Kuroda, S. Physicochemical and immunological characterization of hepatitis B virus envelope particels exclusively consisting of the entire L (pre-S1+pre-S2+S) protein. *Vaccine* **2001**, *19*, 3154–3163. [CrossRef]
183. Leroux-Roels, G.; Desombere, I.; De Tollenaere, G.; Petit, M.A.; Desmons, P.; Hauser, P.; Delem, A.; De Grave, D.; Safary, A. Hepatitis B vaccine containing surface antigen and selected preS1 and preS2 sequences. 1. Safety and immunogenicity in young, healthy adults. *Vaccine* **1997**, *15*, 1724–1731. [CrossRef]
184. Leroux-Roels, G.; Desombere, I.; Cobbaut, L.; Petit, M.A.; Desmons, P.; Hauser, P.; Delem, A.; De Grave, D.; Safary, A. Hepatitis B vaccine containing surface antigen and selected preS1 and preS2 sequences. 2. Immunogenicity in poor responders to hepatitis B vaccines. *Vaccine* **1997**, *15*, 1732–1736. [CrossRef]
185. Tron, F.; Degos, F.; Bréchot, C.; Couroucé, A.M.; Goudeau, A.; Marie, F.N.; Adamowicz, P.; Saliou, P.; Laplanche, A.; Benhamou, J.P.; et al. Randomized dose range study of a recombinant hepatitis B vaccine produced in mammalian cells and containing the S and preS2 sequences. *J. Infect. Dis.* **1989**, *160*, 199–204. [CrossRef]
186. Yan, D.; Wei, Y.Q.; Guo, H.C.; Sun, S.Q. The application of virus-like particles as vaccines and biological vehicles. *Appl. Microbiol. Biotechnol.* **2015**, *99*, 10415–10432. [CrossRef]
187. Pushko, P.; Pumpens, P.; Grens, E. Development of virus-like particle technology from small highly symmetric to large complex virus-like particle structures. *Intervirology* **2013**, *56*, 141–165. [CrossRef]

188. Ramasamy, V.; Arora, U.; Shukla, R.; Poddar, A.; Shanmugam, R.K.; White, L.J.; Mattocks, M.M.; Raut, R.; Perween, A.; Tyagi, P.; et al. A tetravalent virus-like particle vaccine designed to display domain III of dengue envelope proteins induces multi-serotype neutralizing antibodies in mice and macaques which confer protection against antibody dependent enhancement in AG129 mice. *PLoS Negl. Trop. Dis.* **2018**, *12*, 0006191. [CrossRef]
189. Berkower, I.; Raymond, M.; Muller, J.; Spadaccini, A.; Aberdeen, A. Assembly, structure, and antigenic properties of virus-like particles rich in HIV-1 envelope gp120. *Virology* **2004**, *321*, 75–86. [CrossRef] [PubMed]
190. Gordon, D.M.; McGovern, T.W.; Krzych, U.; Cohen, J.C.; Schneider, I.; LaChance, R.; Heppner, D.G.; Yuan, G.; Hollingdale, M.; Slaoui, M.; et al. Safety, immunogenicity, and efficacy of a recombinantly produced *Plasmodium falciparum* circumsporozoite protein-hepatitis B surface antigen subunit vaccine. *J. Infect. Dis.* **1995**, *171*, 1576–1585. [CrossRef] [PubMed]
191. Rutgers, T.; Gordon, D.; Gathoye, A.M.; Hollingdale, M.; Hockmeyer, W.; Rosenberg, M.; De Wilde, M. Hepatitis B surface antigen as carrier matrix for the repetitive epitope of the circumsporozoite protein of *Plasmodium falciparum*. *Bio/Technology* **1988**, *6*, 1065–1070. [CrossRef]
192. Beaumont, E.; Patient, R.; Hourioux, C.; Dimier-Poisson, I.; Roingeard, P. Chimeric hepatitis B virus/hepatitis C virus envelope proteins elicit broadly neutralizing antibodies and constitute a potential bivalent prophylactic vaccine. *Hepatology* **2013**, *57*, 1303–1313. [CrossRef] [PubMed]
193. Cervantes Gonzalez, M.; Kostrzak, A.; Guetard, D.; Pniewski, T.; Sala, M. HIV-1 derived peptides fused to HBsAg affects its immunogenicity. *Virus Res.* **2009**, *146*, 107–114. [CrossRef] [PubMed]
194. Schlienger, K.; Mancini, M.; Rivière, Y.; Dormont, D.; Tiollais, P.; Michel, M.L. Human immunodeficiency virus type 1 major nautralizing determinant exposed on hepatitis B surface antigen particles is highly immunogenic in primates. *J. Virol.* **1992**, *66*, 2570–2576. [CrossRef]
195. Kingston, N.J.; Kurtovic, L.; Walsh, R.; Joe, C.; Lovrecz, G.; Locarnini, S.; Beeson, J.G.; Netter, H.J. Hepatitis B virus-like particles expressing *Plasmodium falciparum* epitopes induce complement-fixing antibodies against the circumsporozoite protein. *Vaccine* **2019**, *37*, 1674–1684. [CrossRef]
196. Wei, S.; Lei, Y.; Yang, J.; Wang, X.; Shu, F.; Wei, X.; Lin, F.; Li, B.; Cui, Y.; Zhang, H.; et al. Neutralization effects of antibody elicited by chimeric HBV S antigen viral-like particles presenting HCV neutralization epitopes. *Vaccine* **2018**, *36*, 2273–2281. [CrossRef]
197. Kotiw, M.; Johnson, M.; Pandey, M.; Fry, S.; Hazell, S.L.; Netter, H.J.; Good, M.F.; Olive, C. Immunological response to parenteral vaccination with recombinant hepatitis B virus surface antigen virus-like particles expressing *Helicobacter pylori* KatA epitopes in a murine *H. pylori* challenge model. *Clin. Vaccine Immunol.* **2012**, *19*, 268–276. [CrossRef]
198. Vietheer, P.T.K.; Boo, I.; Drummer, H.E.; Netter, H.J. Immunizations with chimeric hepatitis B virus-like particles to induce potential anti-hepatitis C virus neutralizing antibodies. *Antivir. Ther.* **2007**, *12*, 477–487.
199. Pumpens, P.; Razanskas, R.; Pushko, P.; Renhof, R.; Gusars, I.; Skrastina, D.; Ose, V.; Borisova, G.; Sominskaya, I.; Petrovskis, I.; et al. Evaluation of HBs, HBc, and frCP virus-like particles for expression of human papillomavirus 16 E7 oncoprotein epitopes. *Intervirology* **2002**, *45*, 24–32. [CrossRef]
200. von Brunn, A.; Früh, K.; Müller, H.M.; Zentgraf, H.W.; Bujard, H. Epitopes of the human malaria parasite *P. falciparum* carried on the surface of HBsAg particles elicit an immune response against the parasite. *Vaccine* **1991**, *9*, 477–484. [CrossRef]
201. Delpeyroux, F.; Chenciner, N.; Lim, A.; Malpièce, Y.; Blondel, B.; Crainic, R.; van der Werf, S.; Streeck, R.E. A poliovirus neutralization epitope expressed on hybrid hepatitis B surface antigen particles. *Science* **1986**, *233*, 472–475. [CrossRef] [PubMed]
202. Cheong, W.S.; Reiseger, J.; Turner, S.J.; Boyd, R.; Netter, H.J. Chimeric virus-like particles for the delivery of an inserted influenza A-specific CTL epitope. *Antivir. Res.* **2009**, *81*, 113–122. [CrossRef] [PubMed]
203. Delpeyroux, F.; Peillon, N.; Blondel, B.; Crainic, R.; Streeck, R.E. Presentation and immunogenicity of the hepatitis B surface antigen and a poliovirus neutralization antigen on mixed empty envelope particles. *J. Virol.* **1988**, *62*, 1836–1839. [CrossRef]
204. Netter, H.J.; Macnaughton, T.B.; Woo, W.P.; Tindle, R.; Gowans, E.J. Antigenicity and immunogenicity of novel chimeric hepatitis B surface antigen particles with exposed hepatitis C virus epitopes. *J. Virol.* **2001**, *75*, 2130–2141. [CrossRef]
205. Casares, S.; Brumeanu, T.D.; Richie, T.L. The RTS, S malaria vaccine. *Vaccine* **2010**, *28*, 4880–4894. [CrossRef]

206. RTS,S Clinical Trials Partnership. Efficacy and safety of RTS,S/AS01 malaria vaccine with or without a booster dose in infants and children in Africa: Final results of a phase 3, individually randomised, controlled trial. *Lancet* **2015**, *386*, 31–45. [CrossRef]
207. Kester, K.E.; Cummings, J.F.; Ofori-Anyinam, O.; Ockenhouse, C.F.; Krzych, U.; Moris, P.; Schwenk, R.; Nielsen, R.A.; Debebe, Z.; Pinelis, E.; et al. Randomized, double-blind, phase 2a trial of falciparum malaria vaccines RTS,S/AS01B and RTS,S/AS02A in malaria-naive adults: Safety, efficacy, and immunologic associates of protection. *J. Infect. Dis.* **2009**, *200*, 337–346. [CrossRef]
208. Collins, K.A.; Snaith, R.; Cottingham, M.G.; Gilbert, S.C.; Hill, A.V.S. Enhancing protective immunity to malaria with a highly immunogenic virus-like particle vaccine. *Sci. Rep.* **2017**, *7*, 46621. [CrossRef]
209. Patient, R.; Hourioux, C.; Vaudin, P.; Pagès, J.C.; Roingeard, P. Chimeric hepatitis B and C viruses envelope proteins can form subviral particles: Implications for the design of new vaccine strategies. *New Biotechnol.* **2009**, *25*, 226–234. [CrossRef] [PubMed]
210. McCluskie, M.J.; Evans, D.M.; Zhang, N.; Benoit, M.; McElhiney, S.P.; Unnithan, M.; DeMarco, S.C.; Clay, B.; Huber, C.; Deora, A.; et al. The effect of pre-existing anti-carrier immunity on subsequent responses to CRM197 or Qb-VLP conjugate vaccines. *Immunopharmacol. Immunotoxicol.* **2016**, *38*, 184–196. [CrossRef] [PubMed]
211. Saxena, M.; Van, T.T.H.; Baird, F.J.; Coloe, P.J.; Smooker, P.M. Pre-existing immunity against vaccine vectors—Friend or foe? *Microbiology* **2013**, *159*, 1–11. [CrossRef] [PubMed]
212. Jegerlehner, A.; Wiesel, M.; Dietmeier, K.; Zabel, F.; Gatto, D.; Saudan, P.; Bachmann, M.F. Carrier induced epitopic suppression of antibody responses induced by virus-like particles is a dynamic phenomenon caused by carrier-specific antibodies. *Vaccine* **2010**, *28*, 5503–5512. [CrossRef]
213. Schutze, M.P.; Leclerc, C.; Jolivet, M.; Audibert, F.; Chedid, L. Carrier-induced epitopic suppression, a major issue for future synthetic vaccines. *J. Immunol.* **1985**, *135*, 2319–2322.
214. Beaumont, E.; Roingeard, P. Chimeric hepatitis B virus (HBV)/hepatitis C virus (HCV) subviral envelope particles induce efficient anti-HCV antibody production in animals pre-immunized with HBV vaccine. *Vaccine* **2015**, *33*, 973–976. [CrossRef]
215. Netter, H.J.; Woo, W.P.; Tindle, R.; Macfarlan, R.I.; Gowans, E.J. Immunogenicity of recombinant HBsAg/HCV particles in mice pre-immunised with hepatitis B virus-specific vaccine. *Vaccine* **2003**, *21*, 2692–2697. [CrossRef]
216. Bojang, K.A.; Milligan, P.J.M.; Pinder, M.; Vigneron, L.; Alloueche, A.; Kester, K.E.; Ballou, W.R.; Conway, D.J.; Reece, W.H.H.; Gothard, P.; et al. Efficacy of RTS,S/AS02 malaria vaccine against *Plasmodium falciparum* infection in semi-immune adult men in The Gambia: A randomised trial. *Lancet* **2001**, *358*, 1927–1934. [CrossRef]
217. Li, P.; Haque, M.A.; Blum, J.S. Role of disulfide bonds in regulating antigen processing and epitope selection. *J. Immunol.* **2002**, *169*, 2444–2450. [CrossRef]
218. Carmicle, S.; Steede, N.K.; Landry, S.J. Antigen three-dimensional structure guides the processing and presentation of helper T-cell epitopes. *Mol. Immunol.* **2007**, *44*, 1159–1168. [CrossRef] [PubMed]
219. Prato, S.; Fleming, J.; Schmidt, C.W.; Corradin, G.; Lopez, J.A. Cross-presentation of a human malaria CTL epitope is conformation dependent. *Mol. Immunol.* **2006**, *43*, 2031–2036. [CrossRef] [PubMed]
220. Dai, G.; Carmicle, S.; Steede, N.K.; Landry, S.J. Structural basis for helper T-cell and antibody epitope immunodominance in bacteriophage T4 Hsp10. *J. Biol. Chem.* **2002**, *277*, 161–168. [CrossRef] [PubMed]
221. Mirano-Bascos, D.; Steede, N.K.; Robinson, J.E.; Landry, S.J. Influence of disulfide-stabilized structure on the specificity of helper T-cell and antibody responses to HIV envelope glycoprotein gp120. *J. Virol.* **2010**, *84*, 3303–3311. [CrossRef] [PubMed]
222. Landry, S.J. Three-dimensional structure determines the pattern of CD4+ T-cell epitope dominance in influenza virus hemagglutinin. *J. Virol.* **2008**, *82*, 1238–1248. [CrossRef]
223. Wolfert, M.A.; Boons, G.J. Adaptive immune activation: Glycosylation does matter. *Nat. Chem. Biol.* **2013**, *9*, 776–784. [CrossRef]
224. Dam, T.K.; Brewer, C.F. Lectins as pattern recognition molecules: The effects of epitope density in innate immunity. *Glycobiology* **2010**, *20*, 270–279. [CrossRef]
225. Al-Barwani, F.; Young, S.L.; Baird, M.A.; Larsen, D.S.; Ward, V.K. Mannosylation of virus-like particles enhances internalization by antigen-presenting cells. *PLoS ONE* **2014**, *9*, e104523. [CrossRef]

226. Freire, T.; Zhang, X.; Dériaud, E.; Ganneau, C.; Vichier-Guerre, S.; Azria, E.; Launay, O.; Lo-Man, R.; Bay, S.; Leclerc, C. Glycosidic Tn-based vaccines targeting dermal dendritic cells favor germinal center B-cell development and potent antibody response in the absence of adjuvant. *Blood* **2010**, *116*, 3526–3536. [CrossRef]
227. Sheng, K.C.; Kalkanidis, M.; Pouniotis, D.S.; Esparon, S.; Tang, C.K.; Apostolopoulos, V.; Pietersz, G.A. Delivery of antigen using a novel mannosylated dendrimer potentiates immunogenicity in vitro and in vivo. *Eur. J. Immunol.* **2008**, *38*, 424–436. [CrossRef]
228. Doe, B.; Steimer, K.S.; Walker, C.M. Induction of HIV-1 envelope (gp120)-specific cytotoxic T lymphocyte responses in mice by recombinant CHO cell-derived gp120 is enhanced by enzymatic removal of N-linked glycans. *Eur. J. Immunol.* **1994**, *24*, 2369–2376. [CrossRef]
229. Mishra, H.; Mishra, D.; Mishra, P.K.; Nahar, M.; Dubey, V.; Jain, N.K. Evaluation of solid lipid nanoparticles as carriers for delivery of hepatitis B surface antigen for vaccination using subcutaneous route. *J. Pharm. Pharm. Sci.* **2010**, *13*, 495–509. [CrossRef] [PubMed]
230. Vigerust, D.J.; Shepherd, V.L. Virus glycosylation: Role in virulence and immune interactions. *Trends Microbiol.* **2007**, *15*, 211–218. [CrossRef] [PubMed]
231. Hyakumura, M.; Walsh, R.; Thaysen-Andersen, M.; Kingston, N.J.; La, M.; Lu, L.; Lovrecz, G.; Packer, N.H.; Locarnini, S.; Netter, H.J. Modification of asparagine-linked glycan density for the design of hepatitis B virus virus-like particles with enhanced immunogenicity. *J. Virol.* **2015**, *89*, 11312–11322. [CrossRef] [PubMed]
232. Lopez, M.; Rodriguez, E.N.; Lobaina, Y.; Musacchio, A.; Falcon, V.; Guillen, G.; Aguilar, J.C. Characterization of the size distribution and aggregation of virus-like nanoparticles used as active ingredients of the HeberNasvac therapeutic vaccine against chronic hepatitis B. *Adv. Nat. Sci. Nanosci. Nanotechnol.* **2017**, *8*, 025009. [CrossRef]

8

Immunization of Cats against Fel d 1 Results in Reduced Allergic Symptoms of Owners

Franziska Thoms [1,2], Stefanie Haas [1,2], Aline Erhart [3], Claudia S. Nett [4], Silvia Rüfenacht [5], Nicole Graf [6], Arnis Strods [7], Gauravraj Patil [7], Thonur Leenadevi [7], Michael C. Fontaine [7], Lindsey A. Toon [7], Gary T. Jennings [1,2], Gabriela Senti [8], Thomas M. Kündig [9] and Martin F. Bachmann [10,11,*]

1 Department of Dermatology, Zurich University Hospital, Wagistrasse 12, 8952 Schlieren/Zurich, Switzerland; franziskazabel@hotmail.com (F.T.); haasstefanie206@hotmail.com (S.H.); Gary.jennings@usz.ch (G.T.J.)
2 HypoPet AG, Moussonstrasse 2, 8091 Zurich, Switzerland
3 Clinical Trials Center Zurich, University Hospital Zurich, Moussonstrasse 2, 8044 Zurich, Switzerland; alineerhart@hotmail.com
4 vetderm.ch, Ennetseeklink für Kleintiere, Rothusstrasse 2, 6331 Hünenberg, Switzerland; cnett@vetderm.ch
5 dermaVet, Tierklinik Aarau West AG, Muhenstrasse 56, 5036 Oberentfelden, Switzerland; s.ruefenacht@dermavet.ch
6 Graf Biostatistics, Amelenweg 5, 8400 Winterthur, Switzerland; graf@biostatistics.ch
7 Benchmark Animal Health, Benchmark Holdings Plc, 8 Smithy Wood Dr, Sheffield S35 1QN, UK; arnis.strods@bmkvaccines.com (A.S.); gauravraj.patil@bmkvaccines.com (G.P.); thonur.leenadevi@bmkvaccines.com (T.L.); michael.fontaine@bmkanimalhealth.com (M.C.F.); lindsey.toon@bmkanimalhealth.com (L.A.T.)
8 Director Research and Education, University Hospital Zurich, Rämistrasse 100, 8091 Zurich, Switzerland; Gabriela.senti@usz.ch
9 Department of Dermatology, University Hospital Zurich, Gloriastrasse 31, 8091 Zurich, Switzerland; Thomas.kuendig@usz.ch
10 Department of Immunology, Inselspital, University of Bern, Salihaus 2, 3007 Bern, Switzerland
11 Jenner Institute, University of Oxford, Old Road Campus, Roosevelt Drive, Oxford OX3 7BN, UK
* Correspondence: martin.bachmann@me.com

Abstract: An innovative approach was tested to treat cat allergy in humans by vaccinating cats with Fel-CuMV (HypoCat™), a vaccine against the major cat allergen Fel d 1 based on virus-like particles derived from cucumber mosaic virus (CuMV-VLPs). Upon vaccination, cats develop neutralizing antibodies against the allergen Fel d 1, which reduces the level of reactive allergen, thus lowering the symptoms or even preventing allergic reactions in humans. The combined methodological field study included ten cat-allergic participants who lived together with their cats ($n = 13$), that were immunized with Fel-CuMV. The aim was to determine methods for measuring a change in allergic symptoms. A home-based provocation test (petting time and organ specific symptom score (OSSS)) and a general weekly (or monthly) symptom score (G(W)SS) were used to assess changes in allergic symptoms. The petting time until a pre-defined level of allergic symptoms was reached increased already early after vaccination of the cats and was apparent over the course of the study. In addition, the OSSS after provocation and G(W)SS recorded a persistent reduction in symptoms over the study period and could serve for long-term assessment. Hence, the immunization of cats with HypoCat™ (Fel-CuMV) may have a positive impact on the cat allergy of the owner, and changes could be assessed by the provocation test as well as G(W)SS.

Keywords: cat allergy; vaccination; Fel d 1; HypoCat™; virus-like particle

---

1. Introduction

Cats are among the most popular and common pets worldwide and are a significant source of indoor allergens [1]. Hence, allergies to cats are widespread, with a prevalence of 10%–30% in the Western population [2]. A total number of 10 *Feline domesticus* (Fel d) allergens, that are recognized by human IgEs, have been identified [3–9]. Fel d 1, an uteroglobin-like protein, is considered to be the major cat allergen. In fact, 94% of patients allergic to cats have Fel d 1-specific IgE [10]. Fel d 1 belongs to the family of secretoglobins with homologies to uteroglobin. Its function is unknown but it has been postulated to play a potential role in skin protection and pelt conditioning or have an involvement in the transport of steroids, hormones and pheromones [11,12]. Fel d 1 is produced in sebaceous, salivary, lacrimal, and anal glands and is present in the saliva, tears, skin and fur [13–16]. It is shed from the cat to the environment through airborne dander and if inhaled by humans may result in sensitization and induction of cat allergy [17].

The immune response against innocuous cat allergens is characterized as type I and IV hypersensitivity, involving Th2 cells shaping the environment for production of IgE antibodies by B and plasma cells and recruitment of additional inflammatory cells [18–20]. Affected patients suffer from mild symptoms, e.g., sneezing, itchiness of skin and eyes, to severe symptoms ranging from conjunctivitis, rhinitis to asthma, which, upon direct exposure to cats, can lead to life-threatening conditions. There are several recommendations for dealing with cat allergy [21]. Allergic people are advised to avoid allergen exposure by removal of all potential allergen-containing or contaminated objects in the households, e.g., pillows, blankets, carpets, rugs. Environmental cleaning and the use of air humidifiers and HEPA filters can also contribute to the relief of symptoms. Another approach is to remove the cat. However, the bond between owners and their cats is often so strong that they are more likely to accept the risk to their health, which they may not even be fully aware of, than give up their pet [22].

Cat allergic subjects usually treat their allergic symptoms with antihistamines and corticosteroids. Another possibility is allergen specific immunotherapy (AIT), which is the only disease-modifying option, but carries the risk of inducing serious side effects and may take years. In fact, AIT can require 30–80 injections over a duration of three to five years with a low chance of success. New approaches explore different routes of administration (e.g., epicutaneous, sublingual, intralymphatic), different formulations of allergens with adjuvants (e.g., MPL, MCT), the introduction of mutations into the protein sequence which delete T cell or IgE epitopes, and finally the use of short peptides instead of full-length allergens [23–31]. The challenge for the development of new therapies is exemplified by the recent failure of a phase III clinical study testing a peptide-based vaccine to treat cat allergy [32]. Orengo et al. are developing a monoclonal IgG antibody therapy targeting Fel d 1 in humans that aims to increase the allergen-specific IgG/IgE ratio and relieve symptoms and showed good clinical impact [33].

An alternative approach to the problem of cat allergy, and one that does not involve separation of the cat from its owner, is to lower Fel d 1 on the animal itself. One recently described method is the addition of anti-Fel d 1 IgY harvested from chicken eggs to cat food. A reduction in active Fel d 1 in saliva and fur has been reported but whether this will result in clinically significant reductions in allergy still needs to be addressed [34,35].

Another approach to lowering allergenic Fel d 1 levels on the cat is active immunization with the aim of inducing anti-Fel d 1 antibodies in the animal itself. Towards this end, a feline vaccine targeting Fel d 1 in cats to treat cat allergy in humans is being developed [36]. The vaccine is based on a recombinantly expressed Fel d 1 protein covalently linked to a virus-like particle (VLP) derived from the Cucumber mosaic virus (CuMV) [37]. The VLP consists of the CuMV coat protein, without any viral genetic information, which serves as a carrier and induces, due to its particulate and repetitive structure, strong and sustained antibody responses, even against self molecules like the Fel d 1 protein in cats [38,39]. To date, vaccination with Fel-CuMV (HypoCat^{TM}) has been tested in 70 cats and was well tolerated without short- or long-term (two years) side effects. Furthermore, vaccination induced strong neutralizing anti-Fel d 1 IgG responses lowering levels of reactive allergen in tear extracts of study cats tested with human basophils from cat allergic subjects [36].

In the current manuscript, we report the results of a first field trial with ten cat allergic participants living together with their cats, and the cats were vaccinated with Fel-CuMV. The aim of this exploratory methodology study was 1) to determine a suitable method for measuring a change in the allergic symptoms of the owner and 2) quantify changes in the interactions between the cat and the owner. These methods may then be used in a larger trials in the future. Three parameters were monitored over a duration of almost two years. A home-based provocation test determined the petting time, defined as the time during which the owner was able to interact with the cat until a certain level of symptoms using a visual analogue scale (VAS score of 5) was reached and their organ-specific symptoms score (OSSS) after petting their cats. In addition, a general weekly or monthly symptom score (GWSS and GSS, respectively) assessed overall changes in allergic symptoms in human subjects without interaction with the cat. The provocation test was assessed as a parameter of the acute allergic reaction, comparable to a hospital-based provocation test (e.g., nasal or conjunctival test), whereas the G(W)SS served as readout of chronic symptoms. As observed in previous studies [36], vaccination with Fel-CuMV was well-tolerated by cats and induced strong serum antibody responses. Changes in symptoms of cat owners and interaction times with their cats were observed after vaccination of the pets. Thus, both tests, the provocation test and the G(W)SS, are suitable to detect changes in the symptoms of cat allergic patients. In particular, the petting time may serve as an early efficacy read-out following vaccination of the cats, whereas the OSSS and G(W)SS seem to be more appropriate for long-term monitoring.

2. Materials and Methods

2.1. Study Population

The study participants were recruited from March till July 2017 and the study commenced in April 2017. Upon completion in February 2018, an extension study with seven of the study participants was conducted from May 2018 until April 2019. Males or females aged 18-65 with a history of cat allergy that were cohabitating with cat(s) were eligible for study inclusion. An understanding of the nature, meaning and scope of the study and signing of an informed consent were also required. Participants were also required to test positive for skin prick tests performed with histamine dihdrochloride and cat allergen extract. In order to confirm the cat allergy to their own cat, participants were also tested positive by a screening scratch test to fur of their own cat.

Participants were not enrolled if they suffered from immunosuppression or anemias, leukemia or other hematological diseases. Additional exclusion criteria were: pregnancy, breast feeding or intent to become pregnant during the course of the study; a positive skin prick test with the negative control; a known history of anaphylactic reactions to pet allergens; the use of Beta-blockers, neuroleptic drugs and tricyclic anti-depressants.

Medications like ACE-inhibitors and Beta2-agonists as well as anti-histamines and corticosteroids could influence the study results and were therefore prohibited within 3 days prior to the application of allergen extracts or the provocation test.

Main study: Ten cat allergic participants ranging from 21 to 51 years old, including eight women and two men, were screened and enrolled in the study at the University Hospital Zurich, Switzerland (Table 1). A total of 13 cats (two participants had two or three cats, respectively) were enrolled in the animal part of the study.

Extension study: Seven participants, including six women and one man, aged between 22 and 52 years old continued in the extension study. A total of nine cats (one participant had three cats) were enrolled in the animal part of the study.

2.2. Study Design

The study was a single-center, open-label, non-placebo controlled, combined, methodological field trial to determine (a) method(s) for measuring cat allergy symptoms in participants that have immunized their cats with Fel-CuMV.

Human part: *Main study*—Screening visits took place at the Clinical Trials Center, University Hospital Zurich (USZ), CH in collaboration with the Department of Dermatology (USZ). After the informed consent was given, the participants underwent two tests to confirm their cat allergy. A skin-prick test was performed using a standard cat allergen and a scratch-test was performed with fur from the own cat. Home-based provocation tests were performed in study weeks 1–3 before vaccination of the cat(s), and in weeks 4, 8, 12, 16, 20 and 24 after vaccination of the cat(s). The provocation test assessed two parameters, the petting time and organ-specific symptoms score (OSSS). The test was only valid if participants had not taken medication containing anti-histamines less than 3 days before the test, otherwise they had to reschedule the test accordingly. If the rescheduling did not happen, the test for that timepoint was invalid and not considered in the statistical analysis. Once a week, the participants filled in a questionnaire retrospectively recording their organ-specific symptoms of the previous week (i.e., general weekly symptom score GWSS). A close-out phone call at the end of the study in week 29 was done to follow up on the well-being and health of the study participant.

Extension study - Seven of ten participants of the main study signed the informed consent form and were enrolled in the extension study. They performed a provocation test before the booster injection of their cat(s) in study week 1 (or week 54 in the combined schedule of main and extension study including the intervening time) followed by four additional tests in study weeks 5, 9, 25 and 45 (weeks 58, 62, 78 and 98, respectively). Again, a provocation test was only valid if participants had not taken medication containing anti-histamines less than 3 days before the test. In the event of a breach, the procedure was followed as described in the main study. In addition, participants recorded their general organ-specific symptoms without provocation monthly (i.e., general specific symptoms GSS). The study finished with a close-out phone call by the clinical study team in study week 45 (week 98, respectively).

Animal part: All interventions for the cats were performed by study veterinarians at the "Kleintierpraxis Schwäntenmos" in Zumikon, Zurich, "Ennetseeklinik für Kleintiere AG" in Hünenberg, Zug and "Tierklinik Aarau West AG" in Aarau, Aargau.

Main study—Thirteen cats were enrolled and received three subcutaneous injections of 100 μg Fel-CuMV formulated in 1 mL in study weeks 4, 7, and 10. Sera were collected in study weeks 4, 10, and 27 and analyzed for specific antibody responses.

Extension study—Nine cats received a subcutaneous booster injection of 100 μg Fel-CuMV formulated in 1 mL in week 3 (or week 56 in the combined study schedule). Sera were collected before the boost (week 56), 6 weeks after the boost (week 62) and at the end of the extension cat study (week 78).

2.3. Ethics Approvals

The protocol, participant information and consent form, as well as other study-specific documents, were submitted to the Zurich-based properly constituted cantonal ethic committee (KEK) in agreement with local legal requirements for formal study approval. The decision of the KEK concerning the conduct of the study had been made in writing to the Sponsor-Investigator before commencement of this study. The KEK decided the trial could be conducted without its approval, as the law for human research was judged to be not applicable. From an ethical perspective, the extension study was considered the same and was conducted without particular approval of the KEK. However, both studies were conducted in accordance with ICH/GCP Guidelines and registered with CLINICALTRIALS.gov as NCT03089788.

The Veterinary Offices of the participating cantons Zurich, Zug and Aargau approved the animal study ZH245/16 (19th March 2016). All cat owners signed informed consent for their cats. All interventions and examinations performed by the study veterinarians were in accordance to the Swiss Animal Welfare Ordinance and Animal Welfare Act on Animal Experimentation (2005, TSchG; 2008, TschV). The animal study was designed as an open-label, non-placebo controlled, multi-center, tolerability and immunogenicity study.

2.4. Study Objective

The objective of the study was to determine if the methods tested herein (provocation test and G(W)SS) were suitable to measure changes in allergy symptoms and interaction of the participants with their cats following immunization with Fel-CuMV (HypoCat^{TM}). The change in symptoms was assessed at baseline versus week 24 at the end of the main study and over the course of the entire study (main and extension study). The selected method(s) could be used in future clinical trials.

2.5. Provocation Test

In an earlier study "ZU_Hyposcore-001" (NCT02399579. https://clinicaltrials.gov/ct2/show/results/NCT02399579) the validity of the provocation test (i.e., HypoScore), a new self-assessed, home-based score specific for cat allergy, was evaluated in cat-allergic participants without vaccination of their cats. In the current study, the provocation test was used to observe changes in allergic symptoms upon vaccination of cats with Fel-CuMV. The test assessed two parameters: the petting time and organ-specific symptoms score (OSSS). The test was performed by petting the cat in order to measure the time until the participant reached a defined symptom strength level (self-assessed, 5 on a VAS ranging from 0–10). If the participant did not reach a symptom level of 5, the petting was stopped at 45 min. When symptom severity of 5 was not reached but provocation time was <45 min (e.g., did not tolerate further petting), for data analysis the time of the last provocation test was carried forward (LOCF). The petting times were measured at baseline on three occasions (week 1–3) before immunization of the cat and over the course of main and extension study. After the provocation test, the participants filled in an OSSS questionnaire on a 4-point scale (0 = no symptoms up to 3 = severe symptoms) regarding their symptoms of eyes, nose, bronchia, lung and palate. Values of the OSSS could be between 0 and 30. The baseline of the HypoScore was measured weekly on three occasions before vaccination of the cats and was compared to the end (week 24) and over the course of the study (weeks 8, 12, 16, 20 and 24 in the main study and weeks 54, 58, 62, 78 and 98 in the extension study) after vaccination of the cats in weeks 4, 7, 10 and booster injection in week 56.

2.6. General Weekly or Monthly Specific Symptoms (GWSS or GSS)

Changes in the general organ specific symptoms on a 4-point scale (0 = no symptoms up to 3 = severe symptoms) of eyes, nose, bronchia, lung, and palate were assessed weekly in the main study (GWSS) or monthly in the extension study (GSS) before and after vaccination of cats with Fel-CuMV. The test was performed without provocation (i.e., direct interaction with their cat). Values of the G(W)SS could be between 0 and 30. The baseline of the general symptoms was determined on three occasions (week 1–3) before vaccination and on 22 occasions during the main study (week 4–25) and 12 occasions during the extension study (week 54-98) after vaccination of the cats in study weeks 4, 7, 10 and booster injection in week 56.

2.7. Cat Population

The cats which participated in the study were privately owned and included 13 cats of six breeds including; British Shorthair, European Shorthair, Russian Blue, Ragdoll, Abyssinian, and Egyptian Mau of both sexes (7 ♀; 6 ♂). The age ranged from 4 to 13 years and body weights of 2.5 to 7.4 kg. Thirteen animals were enrolled in the main and nine cats in the extension study. Where several cats lived in the same household, all cats were immunized, but only one cat was designated as the study cat. The cat owner performed the provocation tests and answered all questionnaires regarding the single study cat.

2.8. Vaccination of Cats

The vaccine Fel-CuMV and the vaccine production was described previously [36]. A vaccine dose contained 100 μg Fel-CuMV (HypoCat^{TM}) formulated in 1 mL aqueous buffer solution. Subcutaneous injections were applied in study weeks 4, 7 and 10 (main study) and 56 (extension study). The vaccine used in this study was produced by Benchmark Vaccines Limited, UK using a GMP-like production process. Prior to each vaccination, the cats were thoroughly examined by one of the participating veterinarians for their general health status, including a routine physical exam with measurement of the body weight and temperature, checking the site of injection, pulse and breathing rate, abdomen palpation and general appearance. During the course of the study, the owners regularly checked the health of their animal. Twenty-four hours after every injection the owners were called by the study personnel to enquire after the well-being of the cat.

2.9. Antibody Responses in Cats

Blood for serum antibody measurements was collected from the vena jugularis or cephalica using serum tubes (Sarstedt, Germany). Sampling was done in the study weeks 4, 7, 10, 27, 56, 62, and 78. After clotting (30 min) and centrifugation (1000 $\times g$, 5 min) of blood samples, sera were transferred to labeled polypropylene tubes (Eppendorf tubes, 1.5 mL, Germany) and stored at ≤ -15 °C until thawed for antibody analyses.

A validated ELISA (developed by HypoPet AG) was performed to determine anti-Fel d 1 IgG in cat sera previously described [36]. ELISA titers are given as the reciprocals of the dilutions needed to achieve 50% of the optical density of the maximal signal measured at saturation (OD50). The geometric mean titers were calculated from the individual titers of the cats from each group.

2.10. Data and Statistical Analyses

The analysis for the human part included data from 9 out of 10 participants and was performed according to the "per protocol" (PP) analysis. Analyses were conducted in this way because one participant had urticaria, accompanied by pruritus and wheal formation, on two occasions during the study. The participant was unable to distinguish urticaria symptoms from the symptoms of cat allergy and was thus excluded from analysis. The analyses of cat data included all 13 cats, whereas the correlation of antibody responses in cats with measurements of human allergic symptoms included data from 9 out of 10 participants with their respective study cats ($n = 9$).

Statistical analyses were performed with Excel, Graph Pad Prism and R. Data were summarized by descriptive statistics: mean, standard deviation, median, first and third quartile, minimum, and maximum. This study was classified as a pilot study because there was no pre-existing information available concerning the expected change in symptoms of allergic cat owners before and after immunization of their cats (the effect size). The changes in the symptoms of the main study were evaluated using an exact Wilcoxon matched-paired signed rank test. Hypotheses were tested at a two-sided significance level of $\alpha = 0.05$. For comparison between baseline and course of study, the mean of all values was computed.

3. Results

3.1. Study Design and Population

This trial was an open-label, non-placebo controlled, single-center, exploratory study involving both cat-allergic humans and their cats (Figure 1). The aim of this methodology field trial was to assess different tests to measure allergic symptoms and to monitor possible changes in allergic symptoms in the study participants after their cats were immunized with the cat vaccine Fel-CuMV.

The study included 10 human participants (Table 1), ranging from 21 to 51 years old, and 13 cats (one participant had two cats and another three cats), ranging from 4 to 13 years old, of both sexes and six different breeds. All ten participants who were screened were enrolled in the study. There were no drop-outs and 10 of 10 participants completed the study. One participant suffered from recurrent chronic urticaria of unknown origin, but exhibited no symptoms at the beginning of the study. However, the urticaria occurred in study week 2 and again in week 16. On each occasion the urticaria lasted for 4–5 weeks until recovery. The participant was not able to distinguish symptoms of urticaria from those of cat allergy and was excluded from the analysis. Data are thus presented as "per protocol" (PP) analysis.

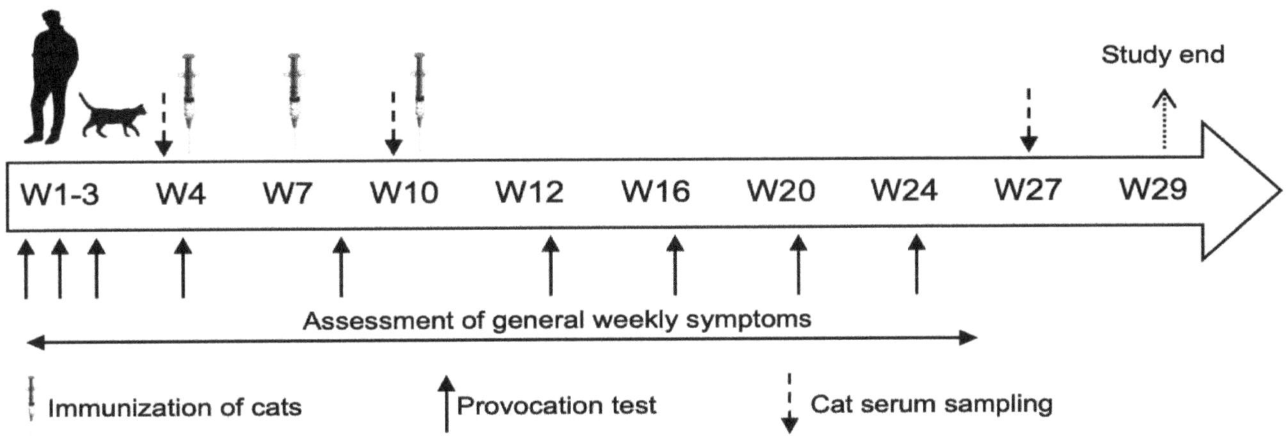

Figure 1. Study design of the combined human and animal trial. Prior to immunization of their cats, participants performed a baseline assessment of their allergic symptoms using the HypoScore (OSSS and petting time) and GWSS. In the course of the study, they performed the provocation test every four weeks and recorded their general symptoms weekly without provocation using the GWSS. Cats received three injections of 100 μg Fel-CuMV (HypoCat^{TM}) at intervals of three weeks (in study weeks 4, 7 and 10) subcutaneously. Cat sera were collected at baseline, week 10, and week 27.

3.2. Adverse Events

Since there was no treatment of the participants, the risk of inducing study-related adverse events was considered low. Nevertheless, some adverse events were recorded and included a cat bite during a veterinary visit, chronic urticaria, erythema, common cold, and pruritus (Table 2). The participant bitten by their cat during an immunization procedure at the veterinary practice was referred to their doctor and received prophylactic antibiotic treatment. They fully recovered from the wound after 1 week. Another participant #10 (excluded from analysis) suffered from an urticaria and presented with strong pruritus and wheal formation. The symptoms were treated with topical urea, macrogol-6-laurylether and fexofenadine-hydrochloride.

There were no severe adverse events observed in the cat population. Several minor clinical signs were noted upon immunization with Fel-CuMV and were judged to be normal vaccination reactions in cats. They disappeared within 72 h of administration. All reactions during and after injection of Fel-CuMV were less frequent on the second and third dosing occasions. There were no treatment related changes in body weight or temperature observed over the study period. Cat owners reported no change in the behavior or appearance (e.g., fur condition) of the cats.

Table 1. Study population.

Participant#	Age	Sex	Age When Allergy Was Observed the First Time	Affected Organs				Baseline VAS Score (0–10) Without Direct Interaction with Cat	Maximal VAS score (0 –10) After direct interaction with cat	Continued in Follow up Study
				Eyes	Nose	Lungs/Bronchia	Palate			
1	50	female	10	x			x	2.5	8.8	x
2	29	female	8	x	x	x		3.5	9.2	x
3	21	male	21	x	x	x		3.9	7.2	x
4	43	female	28	x		x		1.1	7	x
5	24	female	22	x	x		x	3.7	7.2	x
6	45	male	23	x		x		4.2	9	-
7	40	female	10	x	x			1.3	5.6	x
8	28	female	12	x	x			0.3	7.7	x
9	51	female	41	x	x	x		1.4	8.5	-
10	37	female	23		x	x		1.9	4.9	-
Mean/Aver.	**36.8 ±10.8**	**8 ♀; 2 ♂**	**19.0 ± 11.3**	**9/10**	**7/10**	**6/10**	**2/10**	**2.4 ± 1.4**	**7.5 ± 1.4**	**7/10**

Table 2. Adverse events.

Adverse Event	Severity	Participant #	Total Number	Percentage of All AEs	Related to Intervention
Erythema and pruritus	mild	9	3	17.6%	Possible
Tooth infection	moderate	9	1	5.9%	No
Common cold	mild	2, 4, 6, 8	6	35.2%	No
Nausea with vomiting	moderate	10	1	5.9%	No
Nettle rash	moderate	10	1	5.9%	No
Cat allergy reactions	mild	24	1	5.9%	No
Swollen lips	mild	10	1	5.9%	No
Gastroenteritis	moderate	8	1	5.9%	No
Cat bite (hand)	severe	2	1	5.9%	Possible
Chronic urticaria (strong pruritus and wheal formation)	moderate	10	1	5.9%	Possible

3.3. Assessment of the OSSS after Provocation

Seven of nine participants showed lower OSSS at week 24 compared to baseline (Figure 2A) demonstrating a change in the OSSS after provocation. The change from mean 11.7 at baseline to mean 7.3 at week 24 was not significant (p = 0.098). The change in the OSSS over the course of the study was also assessed (Figure 2B–D). There was a significant reduction in the mean OSSS from week 8 to 24 (mean OSSS ranging from 6.4–9.1) compared to baseline (mean OSSS 11.7) (Figure 2B). The reduction in the OSSS in seven of nine participants over the study period compared to baseline was statistically significant (p = 0.03) (Figure 2C,D), demonstrating a sustained reduction in organ-specific symptoms after vaccination of the cat observed from week 8 to week 24.

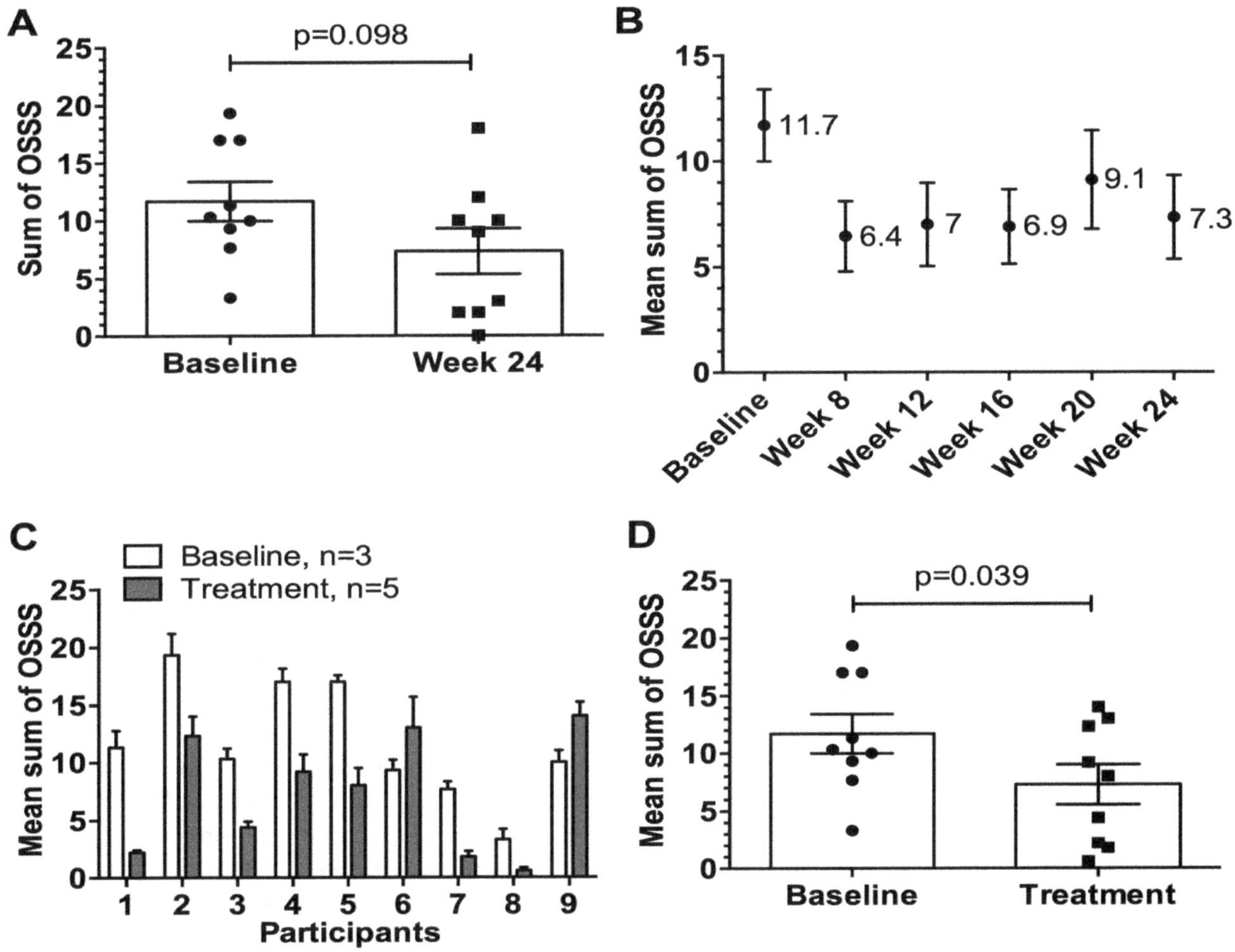

Figure 2. Organ specific symptom score (OSSS) after provocation. (**A**) Individual OSSS with SEM of participants (n = 9) at baseline versus week 24 at the end of the study. (**B**) Mean OSSS with SEM of participants (n = 9) at baseline and over the course of the study. (**C**) Individual mean OSSS with SEM comparing baseline (weeks 1–3, n = 3) vs. treatment period (weeks 8, 12, 16, 20 and 24, n = 5). (**D**) Individual mean OSSS (n = 9) with SEM comparing baseline (n = 3, weeks 1–3) vs. treatment period (n = 5, weeks 8, 12, 16, 20 and 24). Statistical significances were obtained by an exact Wilcoxon matched-paired signed rank test. Possible OSSS values from 0–30.

3.4. Petting Time

There were eight out of nine possible successes, meaning that the time of interaction with their cats to reach a defined level of allergic symptoms for eight participants was greater at week 24 than the mean baseline of weeks 1–3 (Figure 3A). The change from mean 16.9 min (1016 s) at baseline to mean

27.7 min (1659 s) was statistically significant ($p = 0.02$). Of note, three participants had reached the maximum interaction time of 45 min by the end of the study.

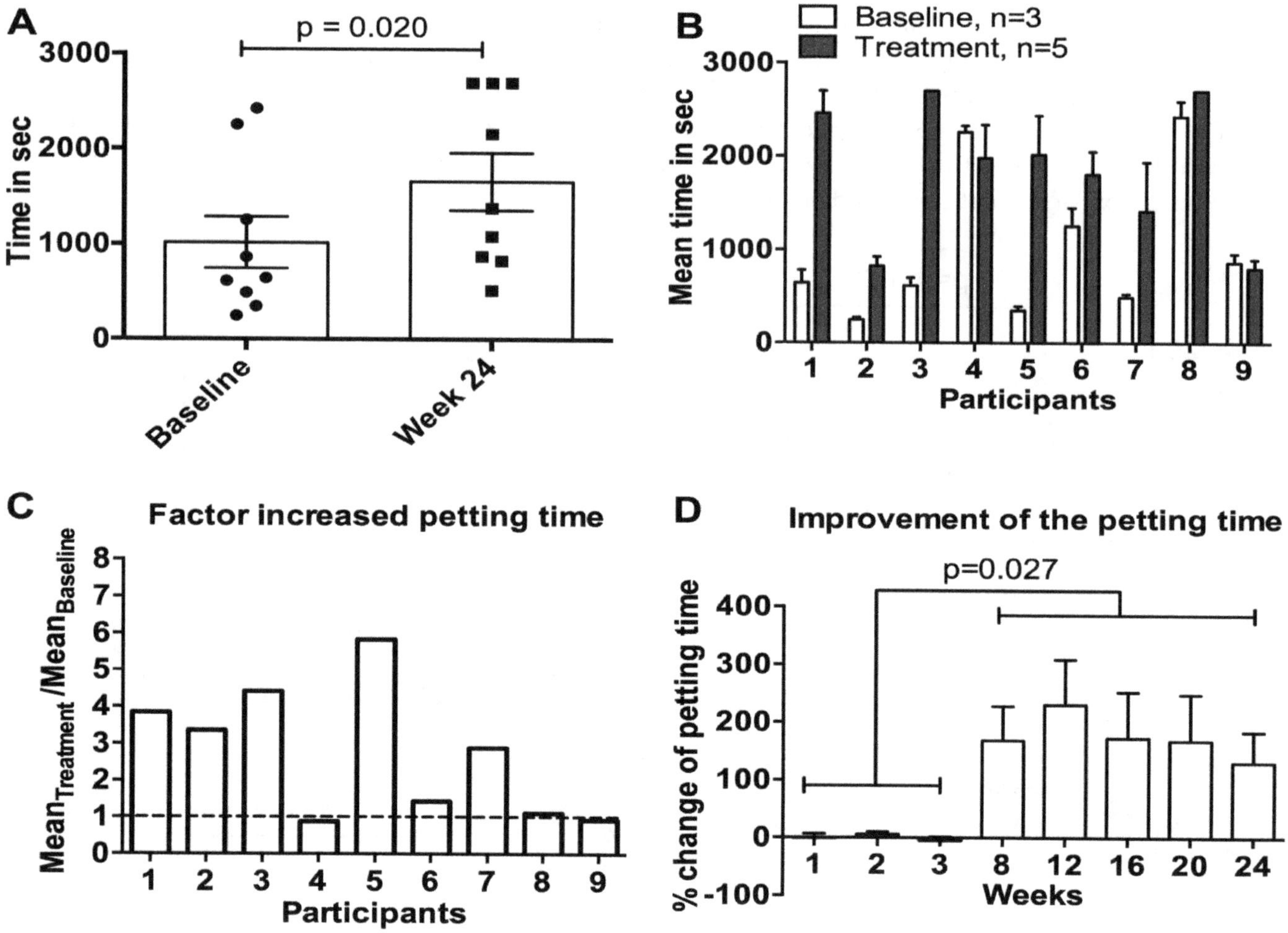

Figure 3. Time of petting as part of the provocation test. (**A**) Mean petting time with SEM in seconds of nine participants comparing baseline ($n = 3$) versus week 24 at the end of the study. (**B**) Individual mean petting time with SEM in seconds at baseline ($n = 3$, weeks 1–3) compared to treatment period ($n = 5$, weeks 8, 12, 16, 20 and 24). (**C**) Factor of changed petting time for each participant shown as ratio of the mean timepoints during treatment ($n = 5$, weeks 8, 12, 16, 20 and 24) to mean baseline time ($n = 3$, weeks 1–3). (**D**) Change in % of the mean petting time with SEM of nine participants during the treatment period in weeks 8, 12, 16, 20 and 24 compared to mean baseline in weeks 1–3. Statistical significances were obtained by an exact Wilcoxon matched-paired signed rank test.

The improved petting time was apparent over the entire course of the study after vaccination of the cats in weeks 4, 7 and 10 (Figure 3B–D). On a per participant basis, the petting time was increased in seven of nine participants up to 6-fold (Figure 3B,C), which corresponded to an average improvement of 100%–230% across weeks 8, 12, 16, 20, and 24 compared to baseline (Figure 3D).

3.5. General Weekly Symptom Score

There were eight of possible nine successes, meaning that the GWSS of eight participants were lower at week 24 compared to baseline (Figure 4A). The mean GWSS at baseline compared to week 24 was significantly reduced from 7.2 to 4.4 ($p = 0.023$).

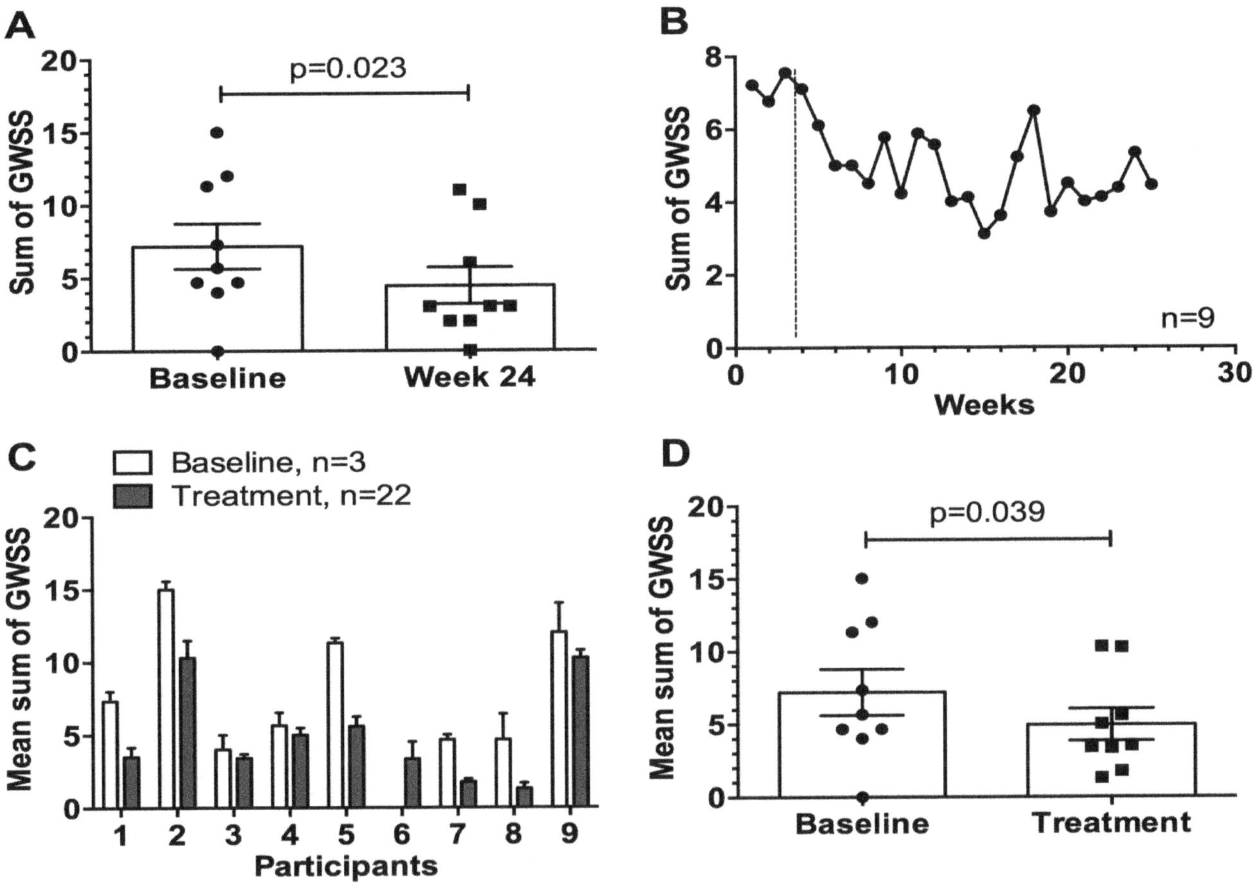

Figure 4. General weekly symptom score GWSS. (**A**) Mean GWSS with SEM of participants ($n = 9$) at baseline ($n = 3$, mean of weeks 1–3) versus week 24 at the end of the study. (**B**) Mean GWSS with SEM of participants ($n = 9$) at baseline ($n = 3$, weeks 1–3) and over the course of the study ($n = 22$, weeks 4–25). (**C**) Individual mean GWSS with SEM at baseline ($n = 3$, weeks 1–3) compared to treatment period ($n = 22$, weeks 4–25). (**D**) Mean GWSS with SEM of nine participants comparing baseline ($n = 3$, weeks 1–3) vs. treatment period ($n = 22$, weeks 4–25). Statistical significances were obtained by an exact Wilcoxon matched-paired signed rank test. Possible GWSS values from 0–30.

The average GWSS of all participants over the entire study period was also assessed (Figure 4B–D). Towards the end of the study, the mean GWSS was consistently lower than the baseline values (Figure 4B). Comparing the average baseline with the average treatment values of the GWSS, a change in the general allergic symptoms ($p = 0.039$) was observed in eight of nine participants, demonstrating a persistent improvement in symptoms upon immunization of the cats (Figure 4C,D).

3.6. Induction of Anti-Fel d 1 IgG Antibody Responses in Cats upon Vaccination with Fel-CuMV

Subcutaneous injection of Fel-CuMV vaccine was considered to be well-tolerated and safe, as only mild and transient side reactions were noted. Cat sera were assessed for Fel d 1-specific IgG antibody responses throughout the course of the study (Figure 5). Participant #8 had three cats, identified as cats 8.1, 8.2, and 8.3. There are no serological data available for cat 8.3 because it rejected the sampling procedure. There was a significant increase in anti-Fel d 1 IgG in all vaccinated cats ($p < 0.001$) detectable after two immunizations at week 10. By the end of the study at week 27, the anti-Fel d 1-specific antibody response in sera ($p = 0.001$) was still significantly increased compared to baseline.

The antibody responses of the study cats were compared with the OSSS and petting time of the provocation test and the GWSS of the participants at the corresponding timepoints (Figure 5C–E). The parameters for assessing the allergic symptoms of the participants correlated well with the antibody responses in cats. Petting time showed a direct correlation with the anti-Fel d 1 IgG titers, whereas the OSSS and the GWSS measurements were inversely correlated with the anti-Fel d 1 IgG titers.

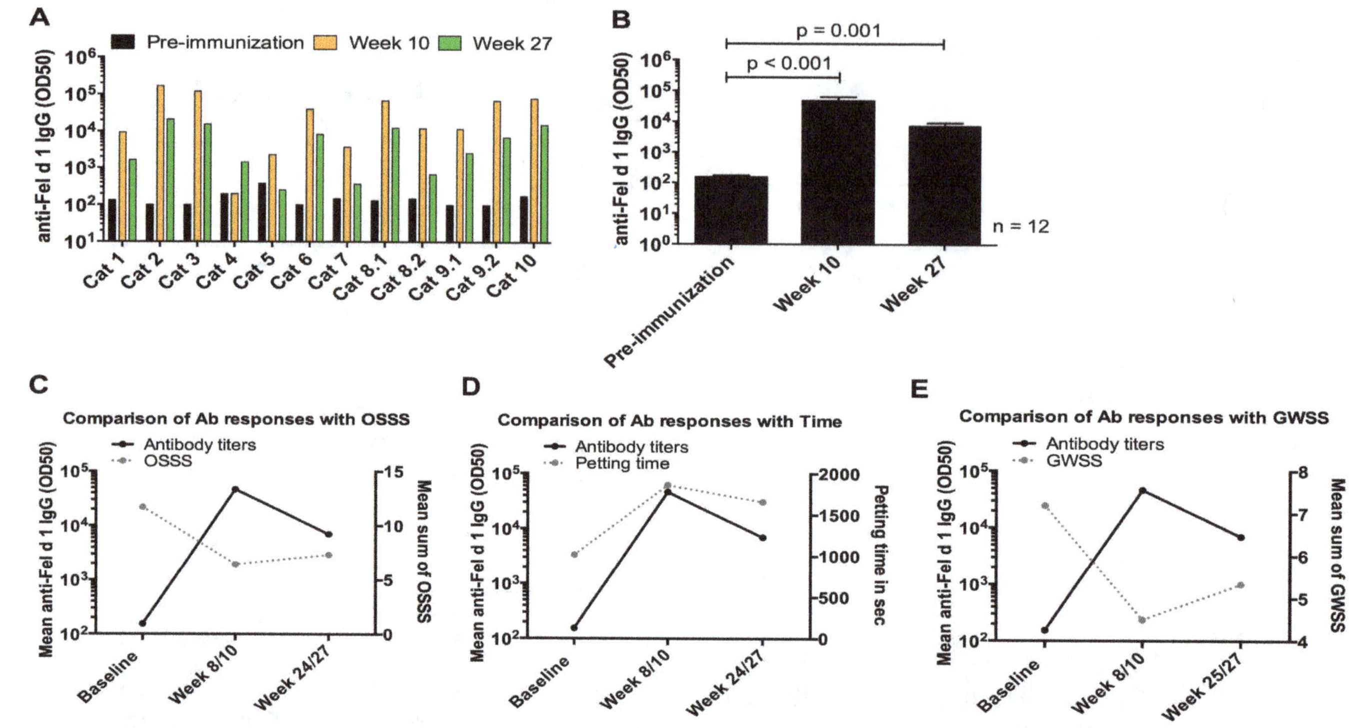

Figure 5. Antibody responses in cat sera. (**A**) Anti-Fel d 1 IgG antibody titers in cats before and after immunization, $n = 12$. (**B**) Mean anti-Fel d 1 IgG antibody titers with SEM, $n = 12$. (**C**) Anti-Fel d 1 IgG antibody titers in cats at baseline (before immunization), week 10 and 27 vs. OSSS at corresponding timepoints baseline (before immunization), week 8 and 24. (**D**) Anti-Fel d 1 IgG antibody titers in cats at baseline (before immunization), week 10 and 27 vs. petting time at corresponding timepoints baseline (before immunization), week 8 and 24. (**E**) Anti-Fel d 1 IgG antibody titers in cats at baseline (before immunization), week 10 and 27 vs. GWSS at corresponding timepoints baseline (before immunization), week 8 and 25. (C-E) Data included from participants ($n = 9$) with corresponding study cats ($n = 9$). Statistical significances were obtained by an exact Wilcoxon matched-paired signed rank test.

3.7. Data of the Extension Study

After completion of the main study, an extension study was conducted with seven of the original participants (Figure 6A). Reasons for the discontinuation of three participants were the exclusion of the urticaria patient, the cat of one participant died due to a study-unrelated icterus, and personal preferences of one participant.

The analysis presented in Figure 6 includes the data obtained from the seven participants and their respective cats (seven study cats plus two cats; one participant had three cats), who participated in both studies.

As described above, there was a reduction in the OSSS from week 8 to 24 (mean OSSS ranging from 4.3 to 5.6) compared to baseline (mean OSSS 12.3). The mean OSSS increased to 9.3 in the intervening period between both studies (i.e., from week 24 to 54). After the boost immunization in week 56, there was a small decrease in mean OSSS observed in study weeks 58 to 98 ranging from 6.0 to 7.4. Although the reduction in the OSSS over both study periods compared to baseline was not statistically significant, a trend of reduced OSSS was observed over the entire study period of almost 2 years (94 weeks) after vaccination of the cats.

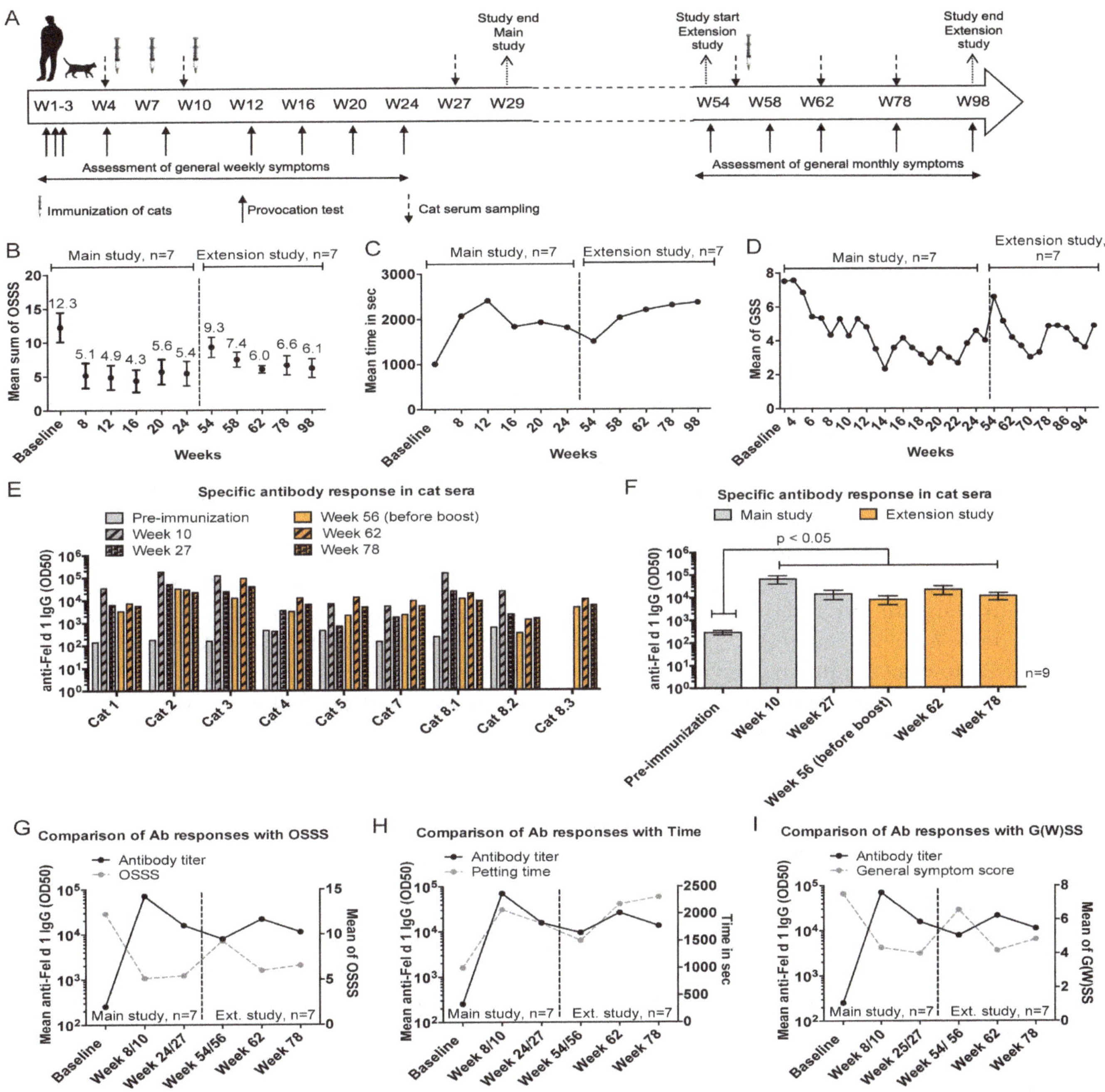

Figure 6. Extension study: Changes in allergic symptoms of participants after booster injection of cats. (**A**) Study design of the main and extension study including seven participants and nine cats. In addition to the main study, the participants performed a provocation test before the boost (week 56) followed by four additional provocation tests in study weeks 58, 62, 78, and 98. Participants also recorded their general organ specific symptoms (GSS) without provocation at monthly intervals during the extension study. The cats received a boost immunization of 100 µg Fel-CuMV subcutaneously in week 56. In addition to the collected serum samples of the main study, cat sera were also collected in study weeks 56, 62, and 78. (**B**) Mean OSSS with SEM over the course of the main and extension study of seven participants. (**C**) Mean petting time over the course of the main and extension study of seven participants. (**D**) Mean general symptoms (G(W)SS) over the course of the main (assessed weekly) and extension (assessed monthly) study of seven participants. (**E**) Measurement of anti-Fel d 1 IgG in cat sera of nine cats participating in the main and extension study. (**F**) Mean anti-Fel d 1 IgG antibody titers with SEM in cat sera. (**G**) Mean anti-Fel d 1 IgG antibody titers in cats vs. mean OSSS over the course of the main (baseline (before immunization), week 8/10 and 24/27) and extension study (week 54/56 (before boost), week 62 and 78). (**H**) Mean anti-Fel d 1 IgG antibody titers in cats vs. mean petting time

over the course of the main (baseline (before immunization), week 8/10 and 24/27) and extension study (week 54/56 (before boost), week 62 and 78). (**I**) Mean anti-Fel d 1 IgG antibody titers in cats vs. mean G(W)SS over the course of the main (baseline (before immunization), week 8/10 and 24/27) and extension study (week 54/56 (before boost), week 62 and 78). (**G-I**) Data included from participants (n = 7) with corresponding study cats (n = 7). Statistical significances were obtained by an exact Wilcoxon matched-paired signed rank test.

The GSS followed a consistent trend of lower symptoms from week 5 to 25 after the initial cat immunizations in weeks 4, 7 and 10 (Figure 6D). The mean GSS at baseline (weeks 1–3) of 7.5 improved to a mean score of 6.8, which was already detectable in week 5, and further improved to 2.3 in study week 14. By the end of the main study in week 25, the mean GSS of 4 was still lower compared to baseline (i.e., GSS 7.5). Before cats received the boost injection in week 56, the mean GSS increased to 6.5 but was still lower compared to baseline (i.e., GSS 7.5 of weeks 1–3). Upon booster injection, allergic symptoms improved again, reaching the lowest mean GSS of 3 in week 70. Clinical improvement was still evident by the end of the study in week 98 (i.e., GSS 4.8). Notably, the participants had reduced GSS at any timepoint after the first vaccination of their cats in study week 4, as the mean GSS over both study periods was always lower compared to baseline (weeks 1–3).

Cat sera were assayed for Fel d 1-specific IgG antibodies throughout both study periods (Figure 6E,F). The mean Fel d 1-specific IgG titers increased ~300-fold measured after two injections in week 10 and were still on a high level at the end of the main study at week 27 (Figure 6F). Specific antibodies declined between weeks 27 and 56 (before the boost) compared to the peak response detected in week 10. Following administration of a booster injection in week 56, the specific IgG levels increased again in eight of nine cats when measured by week 62, 6 weeks after the boost. Almost 4 months later, by the end of the study in week 78, the anti-Fel d 1 IgG responses were still significantly higher compared to baseline and were slightly above the antibody level measured before boost (week 56).

The antibody responses were inversely related to the OSSS and G(W)SS over the period of the main and extension studies (Figure 6G,I). In contrast, antibody responses directly correlated to the petting time of the provocation test (Figure 6H), indicating that specific antibodies reduced symptoms and increased petting time. Specifically, after the induction of anti-Fel d 1 antibodies detected in week 10, the OSSS decreased from a mean score of 12.5 at baseline to 5.1 and 5.4, measured in week 8 and 24, respectively. During the intervening phase of the main and extension study, the antibody titers declined and the mean OSSS increased to 9.3, detected in week 54. After the boost injection which caused an increase in specific antibodies, the mean OSSS decreased to a mean score of 6.0 and 6.6 in study weeks 62 and 78, respectively. Similar observations were made for G(W)SS.

The antibody titers also showed a correlation with petting time. Relative to baseline (week 1–3), mean petting time and anti-Fel d 1 IgG, determined in week 8 and 10, increased the mean petting time by a factor of 2, demonstrating that owners were found to be able to interact with their cats twice as long before they developed an allergic symptom strength of 5 according to VAS. The subsequent decrease in specific antibodies was associated with a decrease in petting time observed in weeks 24 and 54, although still above baseline. Upon the increase in specific antibodies after the booster injection, petting time increased again by a factor of 2.3 compared to baseline.

4. Discussion

Allergy is the most common chronic disease in Europe and U.S and often manifests with chronic conditions including rhinitis, conjunctivitis and asthma, which is associated with individual morbidity and high socio-economic costs. In fact, more than 150 million Europeans are affected by chronic allergic diseases (EAACI, 2016). The danger of developing chronic asthma is particularly high, especially in allergies, which are caused by air-borne allergens such as hay fever and cat allergy. One in five patients with allergies lives with the constant fear of getting an asthmatic or anaphylactic shock at any time or even dying as a result of a severe allergic reaction upon allergen encounter. The World Health Organization estimates that approximately 300 million individuals currently suffer from asthma worldwide and expect an increasing incidence to 400 million by 2025 [21,40]. This development is worrisome, threatening health and economies alike, and demands action of the global community for the development of new therapies, medications and diagnostic tools to address this major challenge [7,41]. Cat allergy contributes to a significant proportion of the allergic disease burden.

There are several new therapeutic developments to treat cat allergy that are currently pursued by various research groups and clinicians. Our novel approach of vaccinating the cat against Fel d 1, offers a cost-effective therapy without the risk of inducing severe side effects in cat-allergic patients, as they often occur during AITs, and without adversely affecting the cat. The vaccine targets Fel d 1, the major cat allergen for humans. By immunizing cats, the reactive allergen level can be lowered, thereby alleviating the symptoms of cat allergic patients. Here, we present clinical data of a first combined human and animal field trial conducted as an open-label, exploratory methodological study. The aim of the study was to assess different methods of measuring the allergic symptoms and determine if those methods could detect changes in allergic symptoms after vaccination of cats with Fel-CuMV (HypoCat^{TM}).

The collection of clinical research data must be reproducible, valid and traceable using standardized procedures [42,43]. However, the selection and combination of various tests and scoring systems for monitoring allergic symptoms and their changes usually have a significant impact on the outcome of clinical trials and the development of innovative medications. Therefore, it is advisable to select as few questionnaires, tests and scoring systems as possible to capture the changes that best reflect the effect of the treatment [44,45]. To this end, we developed a new method to record allergic symptoms by a self-assessed, home-based symptom score, the provocation test. The validity of the test was evaluated in a previously conducted human clinical trial involving non-immunized cats (NCT02399579). The test consists of two elements: an assessment of organ-specific symptom score (OSSS) after petting—a standardized score—and measurement of the time of petting the cat until a defined level of allergy symptom was reached (level of 5 on a VAS). Both parameters, the OSSS and the time, are analyzed separately. In addition to the provocation test, another self-assessed, home-based standard method was investigated in this study: a general symptom score (G(W)SS) assessing the allergic symptoms without provocation.

The mean OSSS as part of the provocation test at week 24 was reduced in seven of nine participants compared to baseline. Moreover, the change in the OSSS was apparent throughout the course of the main study (weeks 8, 12, 16, 20 and 24 vs. baseline) and showed a variable yet sustained reduction in seven of nine participants. It should be noted that a reduction in the OSSS was not necessarily expected to be large, since the cat owners were required to record their symptoms after petting the cat until they had reached a symptom strength of 5 on the VAS. Hence, upon cessation of the provocation test (i.e., petting), the OSSS would have been similar on each occasion. A reason why a substantial decrease in OSSS in the main study was achieved may have been due to the fact that three participants, at week 24, were able to pet their cat for the maximum time of 45 min. In this circumstance, the VAS score of 5 was not reached, and thus the OSSS was lower. Regarding the extension study, several participants at several occasions could pet their cat to the maximum petting time of 45 min and did not reach the symptom strength of 5 on a VAS. Thus, the allergic symptoms were not as pronounced, resulting in lower OSSS.

The second parameter of the provocation test was the petting time. Relative to baseline, an increased time of petting was observed in eight of the nine participants at week 24 and over the entire period of the main study in seven of the nine. The increase in petting time was even more pronounced in the extension study. Several participants could pet their cat to the maximum time of 45 min on several occasions. The average petting time increased by a factor of two upon immunization of the cats and showed a sustained improvement over the period of the main and extension studies, demonstrating that the participants could interact longer with their cats.

A change in general allergic symptoms without provocation assessed by the G(W)SS was noted upon vaccination of the cats. Relative to baseline, a reduction in the GWSS at week 24 and over the period of the main study was observed in eight of nine participants. Moreover, the GSS measured throughout the course of the extension study showed a variable yet sustained reduction in seven of seven participants. Of note, the improvement in general allergic symptoms of the participants recorded without direct interaction with their cats at all timepoints after immunization of the cats over the period of the main and extension studies indicates that the participants generally felt better and suffered less from allergic symptoms.

Subcutaneous injection of three doses of Fel-CuMV vaccine followed by a single boost injection a year later was considered to be well tolerated in several breeds of privately owned adult cats. No serious adverse event occurred during the study. The clinical signs and reactions upon vaccination with Fel-CuMV were mild and reversible. No related effects on body weight, food consumption, behavior and appearance were observed. Moreover, the intended immunological response in cats immunized with Fel-CuMV, i.e., induction of anti-Fel d 1 IgG antibodies, was achieved. Anti-Fel d 1 antibodies were measured in sera at week 10, three weeks after the second immunization. Previous studies in cats ($n > 60$) with Fel-CuMV have shown that about 50% of immunized animals achieved peak titers 2–3 weeks after the second immunization [36]. This would correspond to week 10 of the current study. These findings support the observation of the improved symptoms assessed by the provocation test and G(W)SS of the participants from week 8 and 6, respectively onwards, as Fel d 1-specific antibodies were present and had the potential to neutralize Fel d 1 as previously shown [36]. The improvement of symptoms had lessened by the end of the main study, which may be related to the kinetics of the antibody response, which showed a decline from week 10 to week 27. Upon administration of a booster injection, the symptoms and petting time improved again.

However, the results and conclusions of this open label, exploratory methodology study with a small sample size ($n = 9$ in main and $n = 7$ in extension study) must be taken with caution. There was no pre-existing information available regarding the expected change in symptoms of the participants before and after immunization of their cats. As a consequence, no sample size calculation could be done beforehand. Nevertheless, it is interesting to note that several parameters measured in the study were suggestive that targeting the major cat allergen Fel d 1 by immunization of cats with Fel-CuMV had a positive impact on the allergic sensation of the participant. In particular, the time that participants were able to interact with their cats before a particular level of allergic symptoms was reached increased significantly.

Improvements of the organ specific symptoms with (OSSS) and without provocation (G(W)SS) over the course of the study were also noted. Notably, it was observed that the improvement in these measures had lessened at the end of the main study but increased again after the booster injection. This observation of the kinetics is valuable for planning and conducting further studies. Therefore, all measured parameters (i.e., provocation test and GSS) are suitable to assess changes in allergic symptoms of the cat owners.

Finally, from a veterinary perspective, targeting Fel d 1, the major cat allergen in humans, by active vaccination has, to date, been well-tolerated. The general health status of the cats was not compromised by the induction of auto-antibodies against Fel d 1. However, allergic symptoms of the cat allergic owners were alleviated. As a result of the owner being less burdened by their allergy, the quality of life of their cat may be improved. The ability of allergic cat owners to better tolerate and increase the duration of their interactions with their pet can benefit the animal through better training and socialization and awareness of the animals' overall health. Moreover, the likelihood of abandonment and subsequent euthanasia in animal shelters could be decreased.

Author Contributions: Conceptualization, F.T., G.T.J., S.H., G.S., T.M.K. and M.F.B.; methodology, F.T., S.H., G.T.J., G.S., T.M.K. and M.F.B.; software, F.T., S.H., N.G.; validation, F.T., S.H., G.T.J., T.M.K. and M.B.F.; formal analysis, F.T., S.H., A.E., N.G., G.T.J. and M.F.B.; investigation, G.S., T.M.K. and M.F.B.; resources, F.T., G.T.J., S.H., G.S., T.M.K., A.S., G.P., T.L., M.C.F., L.A.T., C.S.N., S.R., and M.F.B.; data curation, F.T., S.H., N.G., G.T.J. and M.F.B.; writing—original draft preparation, F.T., G.T.J., S.H., G.S., C.S.N., S.R., N.G., T.M.K. and M.F.B; writing—review and editing, A.S., G.P., T.L., M.C.F. and L.A.T.; visualization, F.T. and S.H.; supervision, N.G., G.T.J., T.M.K. and M.F.B.; project administration, F.T., G.T.J.; funding acquisition, M.C.F., L.A.T., G.S., T.M.K. and M.F.B. All authors have read and agreed to the published version of the manuscript.

Acknowledgments: We thank Antonia Gabriel-Fettelschoss, Monique Vogel and Pål Johansen for scientific discussion or careful reading of the manuscript.

Abbreviations

Ab	Antibody
AE	Adverse Event
CSR	Clinical Study Report
eCRF	Electronic Case Report Form
ELISA	Enzyme-linked immunosorbent assay
Fel d 1	Felis domesticus 1 allergen
Fel-CuMV	Fel d 1 - Cucumber mosaic virus-like particle conjugate vaccine
GCP	Good Clinical Practice
GSS	General montly Symptom Score
GWSS	General Weekly Symptom Score
ICH	International Conference on Harmonization
IEC	Independent Ethics Committee
ITT	Intention to Treat
KEK	Cantonal Ethics Committee Zürich
LOCF	Last Observation Carried Forward
LPLV	Last Patient Last Visit
OSSS	Organ Specific Symptom Score
PP	Per Protocol
SAE	Serious Adverse Event
VAS	Visual Analogue Scale

References

1. Platts-Mills, T.A.; Carter, M.C. Asthma and indoor exposure to allergens. *N. Engl. J. Med.* **1997**, *336*, 1382–1384. [CrossRef] [PubMed]
2. Rance, F. Animal dander allergy in children. *Arch. Pediatr.* **2006**, *13*, 584–586. [PubMed]
3. Anderson, M.C.; Baer, H. Allergenically active components of cat allergen extracts. *J. Immunol.* **1981**, *127*, 972–975. [PubMed]
4. Lowenstein, H.; Lind, P.; Weeke, B. Identification and clinical significance of allergenic molecules of cat origin. Part of the DAS 76 Study. *Allergy* **1985**, *40*, 430–441. [CrossRef] [PubMed]
5. Smith, W.; O'Neil, S.E.; Hales, B.J.; Chai, T.L.; Hazell, L.A.; Tanyaratsrisakul, S.; Piboonpocanum, S.; Thomas, W.R. Two newly identified cat allergens: The von Ebner gland protein Fel d 7 and the latherin-like protein Fel d 8. *Int. Arch. Allergy Immunol.* **2011**, *156*, 159–170. [CrossRef]
6. Smith, W.; Butler, A.J.; Hazell, L.A.; Chapman, M.D.; Pomes, A.; Nickels, D.G.; Thomas, W.R. Fel d 4, a cat lipocalin allergen. *Clin. Exp. Allergy* **2004**, *34*, 1732–1738. [CrossRef]
7. Konradsen, J.R.; Fujisawa, T.; van Hage, M.; Hedlin, G.; Hilger, C.; Kleine-Tebbe, J.; Matsui, E.C.; Roberts, G.; Ronmark, E.; Platts-Mills, T.A. Allergy to furry animals: New insights, diagnostic approaches, and challenges. *J. Allergy Clin. Immunol.* **2015**, *135*, 616–625. [CrossRef]
8. Ohman, J.L.; Lowell, F.C.; Bloch, K.J. Allergens of mammalian origin: Characterization of allergen extracted from cat pelts. *J. Allergy Clin. Immunol.* **1973**, *52*, 231–241. [CrossRef]
9. Bonnet, B.; Messaoudi, K.; Jacomet, F.; Michaud, E.; Fauquert, J.L.; Caillaud, D.; Evrard, B. An update on molecular cat allergens: Fel d 1 and what else? Chapter 1: Fel d 1, the major cat allergen. *Allergy Asthma Clin. Immunol.* **2018**, *14*, 14. [CrossRef]

10. Ukleja-Sokolowska, N.; Gawronska-Ukleja, E.; Zbikowska-Gotz, M.; Socha, E.; Lis, K.; Sokolowski, L.; Kuzminski, A.; Bartuzi, Z. Analysis of feline and canine allergen components in patients sensitized to pets. *Allergy Asthma Clin. Immunol.* **2016**, *12*, 61. [CrossRef]
11. Kaiser, L.; Gronlund, H.; Sandalova, T.; Ljunggren, H.G.; van Hage-Hamsten, M.; Achour, A.; Schneider, G. The crystal structure of the major cat allergen Fel d 1, a member of the secretoglobin family. *J. Biol. Chem.* **2003**, *278*, 37730–37735. [CrossRef] [PubMed]
12. Karn, R.C. The mouse salivary androgen-binding protein (ABP) alpha subunit closely resembles chain 1 of the cat allergen Fel dI. *Biochem. Genet.* **1994**, *32*, 271–277. [CrossRef] [PubMed]
13. Charpin, C.; Mata, P.; Charpin, D.; Lavaut, M.N.; Allasia, C.; Vervloet, D. Fel d I allergen distribution in cat fur and skin. *J. Allergy Clin. Immunol.* **1991**, *88*, 77–82. [CrossRef]
14. Dabrowski, A.J.; Van der Brempt, X.; Soler, M.; Seguret, N.; Lucciani, P.; Charpin, D.; Vervloet, D. Cat skin as an important source of Fel d I allergen. *J. Allergy Clin. Immunol.* **1990**, *86*, 462–465. [CrossRef]
15. De Andrade, A.D.; Birnbaum, J.; Magalon, C.; Magnol, J.P.; Lanteaume, A.; Charpin, D.; Vervloet, D. Fel d I levels in cat anal glands. *Clin. Exp. Allergy* **1996**, *26*, 178–180. [CrossRef]
16. van Milligen, F.J.; Vroom, T.M.; Aalberse, R.C. Presence of Felis domesticus allergen I in the cat's salivary and lacrimal glands. *Int. Arch. Allergy Appl. Immunol.* **1990**, *92*, 375–378. [CrossRef]
17. Custovic, A.; Simpson, B.M.; Simpson, A.; Hallam, C.L.; Marolia, H.; Walsh, D.; Campbell, J.; Woodcock, A.; National Asthma Campaign Manchester Asthma and Allergy Study Group. Current mite, cat, and dog allergen exposure, pet ownership, and sensitization to inhalant allergens in adults. *J. Allergy Clin. Immunol.* **2003**, *111*, 402–407. [CrossRef]
18. Platts-Mills, T.A. The role of immunoglobulin E in allergy and asthma. *Am. J. Respir. Crit. Care Med.* **2001**, *164*, S1–S5. [CrossRef]
19. Platts-Mills, T.; Vaughan, J.; Squillace, S.; Woodfolk, J.; Sporik, R. Sensitisation, asthma, and a modified Th2 response in children exposed to cat allergen. A population-based cross-sectional study. *Lancet* **2001**, *357*, 752–756. [CrossRef]
20. Anderson, G.P.; Coyle, A.J. TH2 and 'TH2-like' cells in allergy and asthma: Pharmacological perspectives. *Trends Pharmacol. Sci.* **1994**, *15*, 324–332. [CrossRef]
21. Pawankar, R.; Canonica, G.W.; Holgate, S.T.; Lockey, R.F.; Blaiss, M.S. *WAO The White Book on Allergy*; World Allergy Organization: Milwaukee, WI, USA, 2013.
22. Turner, D.C. A review of over three decades of research on cat-human and human-cat interactions and relationships. *Behav. Processes* **2017**, *141*, 297–304. [CrossRef] [PubMed]
23. Leuthard, D.S.; Duda, A.; Freiberger, S.N.; Weiss, S.; Dommann, I.; Fenini, G.; Contassot, E.; Kramer, M.F.; Skinner, M.A.; Kundig, T.M.; et al. Microcrystalline Tyrosine and Aluminum as Adjuvants in Allergen-Specific Immunotherapy Protect from IgE-Mediated Reactivity in Mouse Models and Act Independently of Inflammasome and TLR Signaling. *J. Immunol.* **2018**, *200*, 3151–3159. [CrossRef]
24. Zubeldia, J.M.; Ferrer, M.; Davila, I.; Justicia, J.L. Adjuvants in Allergen-Specific Immunotherapy: Modulating and Enhancing the Immune Response. *J. Investig. Allergol. Clin. Immunol.* **2019**, *29*, 103–111. [CrossRef] [PubMed]
25. Klimek, L.; Willers, J.; Hammann-Haenni, A.; Pfaar, O.; Stocker, H.; Mueller, P.; Renner, W.A.; Bachmann, M.F. Assessment of clinical efficacy of CYT003-QbG10 in patients with allergic rhinoconjunctivitis. A phase IIb study. *Clin. Exp. Allergy* **2011**, *41*, 1305–1312. [CrossRef]
26. Senti, G.; Crameri, R.; Kuster, D.; Johansen, P.; Martinez-Gomez, J.M.; Graf, N.; Steiner, M.; Hothorn, L.A.; Gronlund, H.; Tivig, C.; et al. Intralymphatic immunotherapy for cat allergy induces tolerance after only 3 injections. *J. Allergy Clin. Immunol.* **2012**, *129*, 1290–1296. [CrossRef] [PubMed]
27. Senti, G.; Graf, N.; Haug, S.; Ruedi, N.; von Moos, S.; Sonderegger, T.; Johansen, P.; Kundig, T.M. Epicutaneous allergen administration as a novel method of allergen-specific immunotherapy. *J. Allergy Clin. Immunol.* **2009**, *124*, 997–1002. [CrossRef] [PubMed]
28. Senti, G.; Johansen, P.; Haug, S.; Bull, C.; Gottschaller, C.; Muller, P.; Pfister, T.; Maurer, P.; Bachmann, M.F.; Graf, N.; et al. Use of A-type CpG oligodeoxynucleotides as an adjuvant in allergen-specific immunotherapy in humans. A phase I/IIa clinical trial. *Clin. Exp. Allergy* **2009**, *39*, 562–570. [CrossRef]
29. Senti, G.; von Moos, S.; Tay, F.; Graf, N.; Sonderegger, T.; Johansen, P.; Kundig, T.M. Epicutaneous allergen-specific immunotherapy ameliorates grass pollen-induced rhinoconjunctivitis. A double-blind, placebo-controlled dose escalation study. *J. Allergy Clin. Immunol.* **2012**, *129*, 128–135. [CrossRef]

30. Basomba, A.; Tabar, A.I.; de Rojas, D.H.; Garcia, B.E.; Alamar, R.; Olaguibel, J.M.; del Prado, J.M.; Martin, S.; Rico, P. Allergen vaccination with a liposome-encapsulated extract of Dermatophagoides pteronyssinus. A randomized, double-blind, placebo-controlled trial in asthmatic patients. *J. Allergy Clin. Immunol.* **2002**, *109*, 943–948. [CrossRef]
31. Fonseca, D.E.; Kline, J.N. Use of CpG oligonucleotides in treatment of asthma and allergic disease. *Adv. Drug Deliv. Rev.* **2009**, *61*, 256–262. [CrossRef]
32. Patel, D.; Couroux, P.; Hickey, P.; Salapatek, A.M.; Laidler, P.; Larche, M.; Hafner, R.P. Fel d 1-derived peptide antigen desensitization shows a persistent treatment effect 1 year after the start of dosing. A randomized, placebo-controlled study. *J. Allergy Clin. Immunol.* **2013**, *131*, 103–109.e7. [CrossRef] [PubMed]
33. Orengo, J.M.; Radin, A.R.; Kamat, V.; Badithe, A.; Ben, L.H.; Bennett, B.L.; Zhong, S.; Birchard, D.; Limnander, A.; Rafique, A.; et al. Treating cat allergy with monoclonal IgG antibodies that bind allergen and prevent IgE engagement. *Nat. Commun.* **2018**, *9*, 1421. [CrossRef] [PubMed]
34. Satyaraj, E.; Li, Q.; Sun, P.; Sherrill, S. Anti-Fel d1 immunoglobulin Y antibody-containing egg ingredient lowers allergen levels in cat saliva. *J. Feline Med. Surg.* **2019**, 1098612X19861218. [CrossRef] [PubMed]
35. Satyaraj, E.; Gardner, C.; Filipi, I.; Cramer, K.; Sherrill, S. Reduction of active Fel d1 from cats using an antiFel d1 egg IgY antibody. *Immun. Inflamm. Dis.* **2019**, *7*, 68–73. [CrossRef] [PubMed]
36. Thoms, F.; Jennings, G.T.; Maudrich, M.; Vogel, M.; Haas, S.; Zeltins, A.; Hofmann-Lehmann, R.; Riond, B.; Grossmann, J.; Hunziker, P.; et al. Immunization of cats to induce neutralizing antibodies against Fel d 1, the major feline allergen in human subjects. *J. Allergy Clin. Immunol.* **2019**, *144*, 193–203. [CrossRef] [PubMed]
37. Zeltins, A.; West, J.; Zabel, F.; El Turabi, A.; Balke, I.; Haas, S.; Maudrich, M.; Storni, F.; Engeroff, P.; Jennings, G.T.; et al. Incorporation of tetanus-epitope into virus-like particles achieves vaccine responses even in older recipients in models of psoriasis, Alzheimer's and cat allergy. *NPJ Vaccines* **2017**, *2*, 30. [CrossRef]
38. Bachmann, M.F.; Rohrer, U.H.; Kundig, T.M.; Burki, K.; Hengartner, H.; Zinkernagel, R.M. The influence of antigen organization on B cell responsiveness. *Science* **1993**, *262*, 1448–1451. [CrossRef]
39. Bachmann, M.F.; Jennings, G.T. Vaccine delivery. A matter of size, geometry, kinetics and molecular patterns. *Nat. Rev. Immunol.* **2010**, *10*, 787–796. [CrossRef]
40. Pawankar, R. Allergic diseases and asthma. A global public health concern and a call to action. *World Allergy Organ. J.* **2014**, *7*, 1–3. [CrossRef]
41. Chan, S.K.; Leung, D.Y.M. Dog and Cat Allergies: Current State of Diagnostic Approaches and Challenges. *Allergy Asthma Immunol. Res.* **2018**, *10*, 97–105. [CrossRef]
42. Pfaar, O.; Demoly, P.; Gerth van Wijk, R.; Bonini, S.; Bousquet, J.; Canonica, G.W.; Durham, S.R.; Jacobsen, L.; Malling, H.J.; Mosges, R.; et al. Recommendations for the standardization of clinical outcomes used in allergen immunotherapy trials for allergic rhinoconjunctivitis: An EAACI Position Paper. *Allergy* **2014**, *69*, 854–867. [CrossRef] [PubMed]
43. Anonymous. *Guideline on the Clinical Development of Products for Specific Immunotherapy for the Treatment of Allergic Diseases*; European Medecine Agency: London, UK, 2008.
44. Pfaar, O.; Alvaro, M.; Cardona, V.; Hamelmann, E.; Mosges, R.; Kleine-Tebbe, J. Clinical trials in allergen immunotherapy: Current concepts and future needs. *Allergy* **2018**, *73*, 1775–1783. [CrossRef] [PubMed]
45. Macchia, D.; Melioli, G.; Pravettoni, V.; Nucera, E.; Piantanida, M.; Caminati, M.; Campochiaro, C.; Yacoub, M.-R.; Schiavino, D.; Paganelli, R.; et al. Guidelines for the use and interpretation of diagnostic methods in adult food allergy. *Clin. Mol. Allergy* **2015**, *13*, 27. [CrossRef] [PubMed]

Broad Protection of Pigs against Heterologous PRRSV Strains by a GP5-Mosaic DNA Vaccine Prime/GP5-Mosaic rVaccinia (VACV) Vaccine Boost

Junru Cui, Caitlin M. O'Connell, Connor Hagen, Kim Sawicki, Joan A. Smyth, Paulo H. Verardi, Herbert J. Van Kruiningen and Antonio E. Garmendia *

Department of Pathobiology and Veterinary Science, College of Agriculture, Health and Natural Resources, University of Connecticut, Storrs, CT 06269, USA; junru.cui@uconn.edu (J.C.); caitlin.o'connell@uconn.edu (C.M.O.); connor.hagen@uconn.edu (C.H.); kimitt@gmail.com (K.S.); joan.smyth@uconn.edu (J.A.S.); paulo.verardi@uconn.edu (P.H.V.); herbert.vankruiningen@uconn.edu (H.J.V.K.)

* Correspondence: antonio.garmendia@uconn.edu

Abstract: Background: Porcine reproductive and respiratory syndrome (PRRS) viruses are a major cause of disease and economic loss in pigs worldwide. High genetic diversity among PRRSV strains is problematic for successful disease control by vaccination. Mosaic DNA and vaccinia (VACV) vaccines were developed in order to improve protection against heterologous PRRSV strains. Methods: Piglets were primed and boosted with GP5-Mosaic DNA vaccine and recombinant GP5-Mosaic VACV (rGP5-Mosaic VACV), respectively. Pigs vaccinated with rGP5-WT (VR2332) DNA and rGP5-WT VACV, or empty vector DNA and empty VACV respectively, served as controls. Virus challenge was given to separate groups of vaccinated pigs with VR2332 or MN184C. Necropsies were performed 14 days after challenge. Results: Vaccination with the GP5-Mosaic-based vaccines resulted in cellular reactivity and higher levels of neutralizing antibodies to both VR2332 and MN184C PRRSV strains. In contrast, vaccination of animals with the GP5-WT vaccines induced responses only to VR2332. Furthermore, vaccination with the GP5-Mosaic based vaccines resulted in protection against challenge with two heterologous virus strains, as demonstrated by the significantly lower viral loads in serum, tissues, porcine alveolar macrophages (PAMs), and bronchoalveolar lavage (BAL) fluids, and less severe lung lesions after challenge with either MN184C or VR2332, which have only 85% identity. In contrast, significant protection by the GP5-WT based vaccines was only achieved against the VR2332 strain. Conclusions: GP5-Mosaic vaccines, using a DNA-prime/VACV boost regimen, conferred protection in pigs against heterologous viruses.

Keywords: PRRSV Mosaic T-cell DNA vaccine VACV; PRRS; cross protection; heterologous virus challenge

1. Introduction

Porcine reproductive and respiratory syndrome (PRRS) is a major disease in pigs that causes significant economic losses to industry across the world. In the United States alone, PRRS causes over $600 million in losses a year [1]. PRRS causes reproductive failure in pregnant sows and respiratory disease in young pigs. The causal virus, PRRSV, is a positive-sense, single-stranded RNA virus with a lipid envelope, and belongs to the Family *Arteriviridae,* Order *Nidovirales* [2–4]. The genome is approximately 15 Kb long and encodes at least 22 different viral proteins including fourteen non-structural and eight structural proteins [5]. PRRSV induces both humoral and cellular immune responses in pigs and some of the viral proteins inducing such responses have been identified; however, protection against reinfection is incomplete [6–9]. Killed virus (KV) vaccines and modified live virus (MLV) vaccines for PRRS have been licensed for more than two decades. These vaccines generally reduce the severity of clinical signs and the transmission of virus; however, they do not induce sterilizing immunity. In general, the efficacy of MLV vaccines is superior to that of KV vaccines [10–13]. Importantly, however, highly variable and generally sub-optimal levels of protection against heterologous PRRSV strains have been reported [10,14–18]. The potential for reversion to the virulence of MLV vaccines and subsequent transmission to susceptible pigs is a concern [19–21].

The major challenge for the development of efficacious, broadly protective PRRS vaccines is the extraordinary genetic variation among disease producing PRRSV strains. Currently, two major PRRSV genotypes are recognized, Genotype 1 (European) and Genotype 2 (North American), which exhibit nearly 40% sequence dissimilarity [22,23]. Genotype 1 and Genotype 2 PRRSVs can be further divided into four subgroups and nine different lineages, respectively, based on phylogenetic analysis of ORF5 [24]. The co-existence of multiple variants within one farm, or even within individual pigs, possibly indicates the occurrence of quasispecies variation of PRRSV [25]. Thus, the development of vaccines that can induce protection against different subgroups and lineages is highly desirable. Multi-subunit vaccines [26], consensus vaccines [27], molecular breeding of different viral structural proteins [28], Mosaic T-cell vaccines [29,30], a polyvalent vaccine containing five different live-attenuated PRRSV strains [31] and DNA prime-MLV boost [32] are just some of the vaccines that are or have been under evaluation recently.

Studies on potential vaccines against human immune deficiency virus type 1 (HIV-1), have shown that Mosaic sequences designed from naturally occurring HIV sequences could effectively address genetic diversity when used as vaccines [33,34]. Mosaic vaccines have been shown to elicit broader immune responses successfully and to confer cross protection in non-human primates and these Mosaic HIV vaccines have been trialed in humans [34–38]. We previously reported that a PRRSV Mosaic vaccine based on 748 GP5 sequences of the Genotype 2 PRRSV strain was immunogenic [29] and induced reactivity to four divergent Genotype-2 PRRSV strains that had at least 10% or more difference in their GP5 sequence—as shown by the expression of interferon gamma (IFN-γ) by peripheral blood mononuclear cells—and, further, that vaccinated pigs were protected against challenge with VR2332 [30]. The present study demonstrates further that vaccination of pigs with the GP5-Mosaic by using a DNA prime and rVaccinia boost approach protects them against strains that are more than 10% divergent in their sequences (VR2332 and MN184C).

2. Materials and Methods

2.1. Viruses and Cells

The viruses used in the study included the VR2332 NA reference strain (ATCC VR-2332) and the MN184C strain provided kindly by Drs. Kelly Lager and Kay Faaberg at U.S. Department of Agriculture-Agriculture Research Service (USDA-ARS). The viruses were propagated in MARC-145 cells [39] grown in Dulbecco's modified Eagle's medium (DMEM) containing 2 mM L-glutamine, 100 U penicillin/mL, 100 μg streptomycin/mL and 10% fetal bovine serum (FBS). The Reed–Muench formula was used to calculate virus titers [40]. Viruses were purified over continuous cesium chloride gradients, quantified using a NanoDrop 1000 spectrophotometer (Thermo Scientific, Waltham, MA, USA) and stored at −80 °C for later use. Titrated viruses were used for ex vivo recall immune response assay and challenge experiments.

2.2. Transfer Vector Construction

A combination of gene synthesis (DNA 2.0, Menlo Park, CA, USA) and standard sub-cloning was utilized to generate three transfer vectors. Each transfer vector contained a cassette with the tetR gene (based on GenBank: X00694), and either a natural or Mosaic version of Genotype 2 PRRSV ORF 5 [29,30], followed by the EMCV IRES (based on GenBank: NC_001479.1) and the EGFP gene (based on plasmid pEGFP-1, GenBank: U55761). The tetR gene and the ORF 5–IRES-EGFP genetic segment were placed under back-to-back synthetic VACV early/late promoters [41]. The tetO2 operator sequence was inserted after the putative VACV D6R promoter, as described in [42]. The cassettes were flanked by 600 bp of the VACV D5R gene to the left and 600 bp of the VACV D6R gene to the right (based on GenBank: NC_006998.1). Restriction endonuclease analysis was used to confirm plasmid identity.

2.3. Generation of Recombinant VACVs and Preparation of High-Titer Stocks

Standard homologous recombination was used to generate Tetracycline-inducible recombinant VACVs after the transfection of transfer vectors with FuGene HD Transfection Reagent (Promega, Madison, WI, USA) into BS-C-1 cells, infected 1 h before with an IPTG-inducible VACV strain (based on the WR clone 9.2.4.8.) in the presence of 0.1 mM IPTG and 1 μg/mL doxycycline. Recombinant EGFP-positive tetracycline-inducible VACVs were plaque purified in the absence of Isopropyl β-d-1-thiogalactopyranoside (IPTG) and in the presence of 1 μg/mL doxycycline. The elimination of the parental virus was confirmed by PCR analysis of viral DNA that was purified using a Nucleospin® Blood kit (Macherey-Nagel, Düren, Germany). High-titer stocks were generated by infecting HeLa S3 cells with recombinant virus at a multiplicity of infection (MOI)of 0.1 in the presence of 1 μg/mL doxycycline. Infected cells were harvested and homogenized 4 days post-infection. Homogenates were clarified by centrifugation at 750× *g* for 10 min, purified over a sucrose cushion [43], and resuspended in 1X PBS pH 7.3 (with no doxycycline).

2.4. Protein Sequence Alignment and Phylogenetic Analysis

MEGA 7 (Molecular Evolutionary Genetics Analysis) (www.megasoftware.net) (NIH, Bethesda, MD, USA) was utilized to evaluate protein sequence alignments between GP5 sequences of VR2332, MN184C, Mosaic 1 and Mosaic 2 and to create a phylogenetic tree.

2.5. Vaccination and Collection of Samples

Cross-bred three- to four-week-old male and female piglets, which were free of PRRSV and porcine circovirus-2, were used in this study. The experimental design is summarized in Table 1. GP5-Mosaic, GP5-WT and vector-control vaccines were administered by both intradermal and intramuscular injection. Briefly, 1 mL vaccine containing 500 μg DNA and 100 μg Quil-A® as adjuvant was injected intradermally (0.1 mL) on the back of ear and intramuscularly (0.9 mL) in the neck region at day 0 and again on day 14. The animals were further boosted at day 28 with a 1 mL suspension containing 10^8 PFU VACV expressing GP5-Mosaic, GP5-WT or VACV and 100 μg Quil-A® as adjuvant. Pigs were challenged at day 35 with VR2332 and at day 37 with MN184C to their respective groups. A total of 10^6 $TCID_{50}$ of each virus was administered by intranasal and intramuscular challenge to each animal. Blood was collected at days 0, 7, 14, 21, 28, the challenge day, and 4, 7, 10, and 14 days after challenge.

Table 1. Experimental design.

Group	Vaccination [a]	Challenge [b]
A (n = 8)	DNA/Vector-control/VACV	VR2332 (n = 4) MN184C (n = 4)
B (n = 8)	DNA GP5-WT/VACV GP5 WT	VR2332 (n = 4) MN184C (n = 4)
C (n = 8)	DNA GP5-Mosaic/VACV GP5-Mosaic	VR2332 (n = 4) MN184C (n = 4)

[a] One mL vaccine containing 500 μg DNA and 100 μg Quil-A® as adjuvant was injected intradermally (0.1 mL) on the back of ear and intramuscularly (0.9 mL) in the neck region at day 0 and again at day 14. VACV 10^8 PFU and 100 μg Quil-A® as adjuvant was administered at day 28. [b] Pigs were challenged at day 35 with $10^6 TCID_{50}$ VR2332 (n = 4/group) and day 37 with $10^6 TCID_{50}$ MN184C (n = 4/group) both intranasally and intramuscularly.

The pigs were euthanized at 14 days post-challenge. The lungs were evaluated macroscopically, weighed, and bronchoalveolar lavage (BAL) was then performed. Tissue samples were collected from each lung lobe, tracheobronchial lymph nodes (TBLN), spleen, inguinal lymph nodes (ILN) and tonsils: portions of each were either fixed in 10% neutral buffered formalin or kept frozen. Fixed tissues were routinely processed to paraffin, and 4–5 μm sections were stained with hematoxylin and eosin and evaluated histologically. Lung lesion scores were calculated as reported before [44]. All animal work was performed under a protocol approved by the University of Connecticut Institutional Animal Care and Use Committee, the animal protocol number under which the study was conducted is IACUC A17-003.

2.6. *Measurement of IFN-γ Immune Response to PRRSV*

Peripheral blood mononuclear cells harvested from blood collected at days 0 and on the challenge day, were seeded in 24-well flat-bottom plates (5×10^5 cells/well). They were then stimulated, in duplicate, by adding 200 $TCID_{50}$ VR2332 or MN184C/well, or mock treated for 48 h at 37 °C in a 5% CO_2 atmosphere. The cells were then collected and total RNA was extracted for quantitative real-time PCR analysis.

2.7. *Serum Neutralization Test*

Virus neutralization testing was carried out as previously reported [30]. Briefly, each serum was mixed with equal volumes of DMEM containing 100 $TCID_{50}$ of VR2332 or MN184C and the mixtures were incubated at 37 °C for 1 h. The serum–virus mixtures were then added to 96-well plates containing 80–90% confluent MARC-145 cells and incubated for 48 h at 37 °C in a 5% CO_2 atmosphere (final serum dilution 1:4). The VR2332 or MN184C virus, negative serum, and uninfected cells served as the virus control, negative serum control and cell control, respectively. The neutralizing capacity of serum was quantified by measuring the viral copy numbers by RT-qPCR in supernatants 48 h after the addition of pre-incubated serum–virus mixtures to the cells.

2.8. *Quantitative Real-Time PCR*

TRIzol LS Reagent or TRIzol Reagent (Invitrogen, Grand Island, NY, USA) was used to extract total RNA from serum/ culture supernatants or tissues, respectively. The extracted RNA was quantified in a NanoDrop 1000 spectrophotometer (Thermo Scientific, Waltham, MA, USA). The cDNA was synthesized from each sample RNA using a 20 μL reaction mixture and random primers (Invitrogen, Grand Island, NY, USA) and the following reaction conditions: 26 °C for 10 min, 42 °C for 45 min and 75 °C for 10 min. The cDNA was then amplified by SYBR Green real-time PCR. To this effect, SYBR qPCR Master Mix (Bimake, Huston, TX, USA), the cDNA template and 5′-ATG ATG RCC TGG CAT TCT-3′and 5′-ACA CGG TCG CCC TAA TTG-3′ were utilized as the forward and reverse primers for ORF7, respectively. Real time PCR was then performed as follows: 2 min at 95 °C, followed by 40 cycles at 95 °C for 15 s and 61 °C for 1 min using Bio-Rad CFX96 Touch System (Bio-Rad, Hercules, CA, USA). For use in quantification, a standard curve was generated using serial dilutions of viral RNA which contained 10^2–10^7 copies/μL. Both positive and negative reference samples were run concurrently with the test samples. Viral loads were determined by plotting the Ct values against the standard curve. Melting curves were analyzed to verify the specificity of the PCR.

To test for IFN-γ expression, total RNA was extracted by TRIzol Reagent from virus-stimulated or mock-treated PBMCs; this was then used as template for cDNA synthesis and this, in turn, was used for real-time PCR following the protocol described above. Glyceraldehyde 3-phosphate dehydrogenase (GAPDH) (forward primer: 5′-CGT CCC TGA GAC ACG ATG GT-3′and reverse primer: 5′-CCC GAT GCG GCC AAA T-3′) was used as internal control to calculate the fold changes in the expression of IFN-γ (forward primer: 5′-TGG TAG CTC TGG GAA ACT GAA TG-3′and reverse primer: 5′-GGC TTT GCG CTG GAT CTG-3′) by the delta–delta method [44].

2.9. Lung Lesion Scoring

The scoring of lung lesions was done systematically, as previously described [45], by a board-certified veterinary pathologist, blinded to the treatment groups. Nine sections, representing all six lung lobes, were scored, with one section from each division of the left cranial lung lobe and two sections from each diaphragmatic lobe.

2.10. Statistical Analysis

Two-way ANOVA or Student's t-test was used to evaluate the differences in measurements between the samples within or between groups. The data were analyzed using GraphPad Prism (version 7.0) (GraphPad Software, San Diego, CA, USA).

3. Results

3.1. Sequence Alignment and Analysis of GP5

The GP5 amino acid (aa) sequences in Mosaic 1, Mosaic 2, MN184C and VR2332 (the prototype of Genotype 2 PRRSV) were all the same size, with no deletions or insertions. Sequence alignments showed aa identity from 85% to 93%. To further investigate the antigenic relationship of these strains, a phylogenetic tree was constructed using the neighbor-joining method b. The four sequences clustered into two subgroups (Figure 1), with the two most distant being Mosaic 1 and MN184C. Mosaic 1 and Mosaic 2 were, relatively, more closely related to VR2332 and MN184C, respectively.

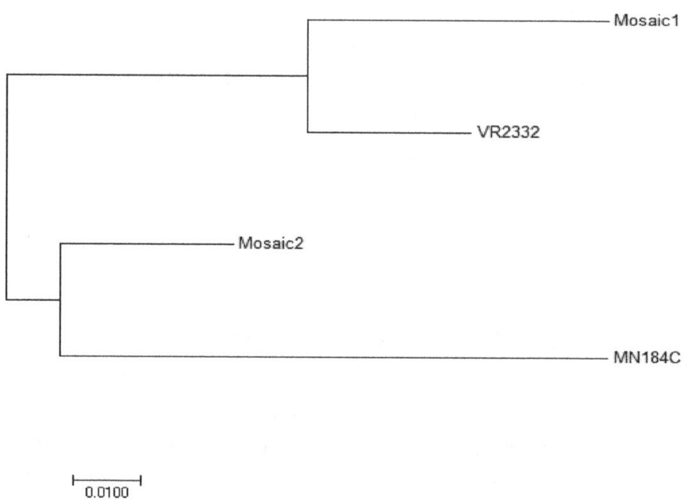

Figure 1. Phylogenetic analysis of the GP5 Amino acid sequence of the two Mosaic sequences, MN184C and VR2332. The analysis was done via the neighbor-joining method using MEGA7.0.

3.2. GP5-Mosaic Vaccines Induced Both Humoral and Cellular Response

GP5-Mosaic-vaccinated pigs had significantly higher levels of neutralizing antibodies in their serum compared to the vector-control animals, both to VR2332 ($p < 0.001$) and MN184C ($p < 0.05$) The virus neutralizing capability of serum from GP5-WT-vaccinated animals was greater against VR2332 ($p < 0.01$) and against MN184C ($p > 0.05$) when compared to serum from vector control animals (Figure 2A); vaccination with the GP5-Mosaic vaccine resulted in broader recall cellular responses than those induced with the GP5WT vaccine. Thus, a significantly higher ($p < 0.05$) relative fold-change in IFN-γ mRNA expression was detected upon stimulation of PBMCs derived from GP5-Mosaic-vaccinated pigs, with either VR2332 or MN184C strains, when compared to those in equally stimulated PMBCs from vector control pigs (Figure 2B). In contrast, the expression of IFN-γ mRNA in GP5-WT-vaccinated pigs was significantly higher only if their PBMCs were stimulated with

VR2332, when compared to those in the equally stimulated PBMCs of the control pigs at the same time points (Figure 2B). No changes were detected with the PBMCs of vector-control pigs with any type of stimulation.

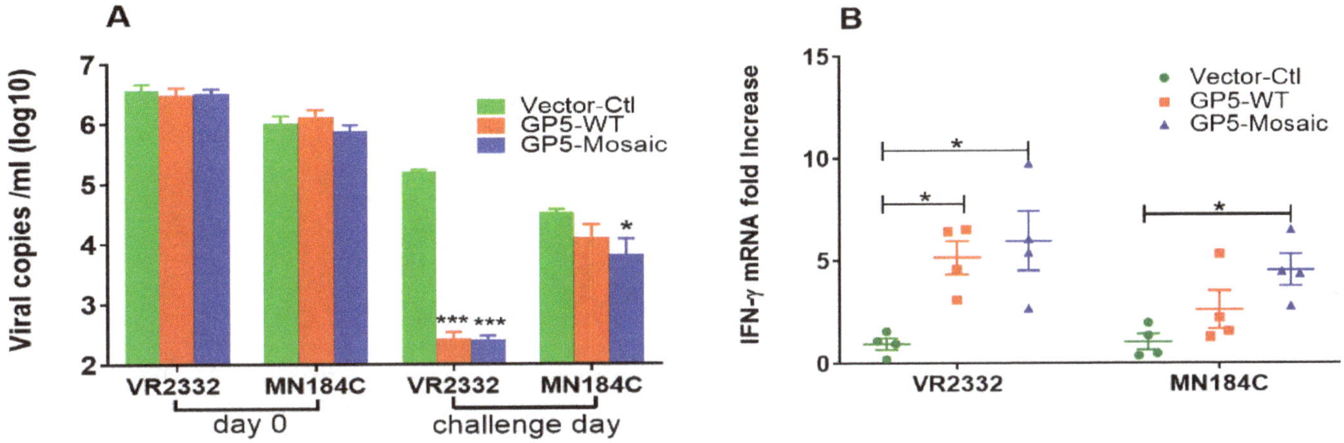

Figure 2. Vaccination-induced humoral and cellular responses. (**A**) The virus neutralization was expressed as viral copy numbers (log10 scale), as measured by RT-qPCR in cell supernatants after the infection of MARC-145 cells with pre-incubated serum–virus mixtures. (**B**) The expression of IFN-γ mRNA as fold changes, by either VR2332 or MN184C-stimulated PBMCs collected on the challenge day. Each dot represents the value of one animal. The variation is expressed as standard error of the means. There were three independent replications. Significant differences were calculated by a two-way ANOVA or Student's *t* test (* $p < 0.05$, *** $p < 0.0001$).

3.3. *GP5-Mosaic Vaccination Induced Cross-Protection in Pigs*

Viral loads in serum of both GP5-WT and GP5-Mosaic-vaccinated groups were significantly lower than those in the vector-control group at 7, 10 and 14 days after challenge with VR2332 (* $p < 0.05$, ** $p < 0.01$) (Figure 3A). Therefore, the capacity of reducing VR2332 virus loads in serum was relatively similar between the GP5-Mosaic and the GP5-WT vaccines. Furthermore, there was a steady decrease in viral loads from 4 days to 14 days after challenge in both GP5-WT and GP5-Mosaic vaccinated groups, while viral loads increased during the course of challenge and reached their peak at 10 days post-challenge (DPC), then declining slightly at 14 DPC in the vector-control group (Figure 3A). In contrast, the viral loads in serum of animals receiving the GP5-Mosaic-vaccine were significantly lower than those of animals receiving the GP5-WT vaccine or those of vector-control animals at 7 and 14 DPC with MN184C (* $p < 0.05$) (Figure 3B), which was different compared to VR2332-challenged groups. Viral load levels in GP5-WT vaccinated animals, increased during the infection with MN184C and reached their peak at 10DPC, which is comparable to the vector-control group. The viral loads in GP5-Mosaic vaccinated animals decreased steadily from 4 to 10 DPC and remained unchanged until 14 DPC (Figure 3B). Furthermore, the viral loads in lung, TBLN, spleen, ILN and tonsils were significantly lower in GP5-Mosaic-vaccinated animals than those in the vector-control group (* $p < 0.05$) after challenge with MN184C, while those of the GP5-WT group were similar or slightly lower compared to the vector-control group (Figure 3C). Viral loads in the lungs, TBLN, and tonsil were significantly lower in GP5-Mosaic-vaccinated animals than those in the vector-control group (* $p < 0.05$) after challenge with VR2332, while those of the GP5-WT group were significantly lower in the lungs, spleen and ILN compared to the vector-control group (* $p < 0.05$). There was no significant difference in VR2332 virus loads between the GP5-Mosaic and GP5-WT groups (Figure 3D).

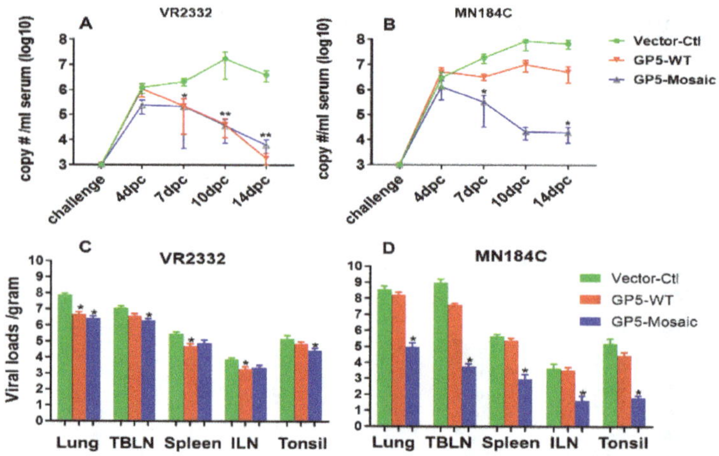

Figure 3. Virus clearance in sera and tissues. (**A**) Viral copy numbers in serum from 0 to 14 DPC upon VR2332 challenge. (**B**) The viral copy numbers in serum from 0 to 14 DPC upon MN184C challenge. Each dot represents the mean value of each group. The variation bars are expressed as the standard error of the mean. Three separate experiments were performed for each. A two-way ANOVA or Student's t test (* $p < 0.05$, ** $p < 0.01$, was used to calculate significant differences; days post-challenge (DPC). (**C**) The viral copy numbers in tissues at necropsy upon VR2332 challenge. (**D**) The viral copy numbers in tissues at necropsy upon MN184C challenge. Each bar represents the mean value of each group. The bars are the standard error of the mean. Three separate experiments were performed for each. Significant differences were calculated by Student's t test (* $p < 0.05$).

Tests in PAMs and BAL fluids showed a similar pattern in which the viral loads in both the GP5-Mosaic and GP5-WT groups were lower than those in the vector-control group after challenge with VR2332 (Figure 4A,C), meanwhile only the viral loads of GP5-Mosaic-vaccinated animals were significantly lower than those in the vector-control animals after challenge with MN184C (* $p < 0.05$ and ** $p < 0.01$, respectively), furthermore there was no apparent difference in MN184C viral loads between GP5-WT and vector-control animals (Figure 4B,D).

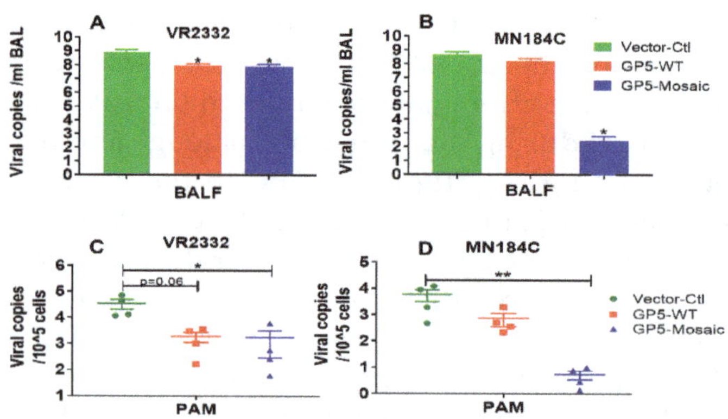

Figure 4. Virus clearance in bronchioalveolar lavage fluids (BAL) and PAMs. (**A**) The viral copy numbers in BAL fluids at necropsy upon challenge with VR2332. (**B**) The viral copy numbers in BAL fluids at necropsy upon challenge with MN184C. Each bar represents the mean value of each group. Bars represent the standard error of the mean. Three independent experiments were performed for each. Significant differences were calculated by Student's t test (* $p < 0.05$). (**C**) The viral copy numbers in PAMs at necropsy upon challenge with VR2332. (**D**) The viral copy numbers in PAMs at necropsy upon challenge with MN184C. Each dot represents the mean value of each animal. The bars represent the standard error of the mean. Three independent experiments were performed for each. Student's t test was used to calculate significant differences (* $p < 0.05$, ** $p < 0.01$).

3.4. Lower Lung Lesion Scores Detected in GP5-Mosaic-Vaccinated Animals

The lung lesion scores after challenge with MN184C were significantly lower in GP5-Mosaic-vaccinated animals than those in both GP5-WT and vector-control animals when evaluated using nine sections of lung (Figure 5 right panel, $p < 0.05$). In contrast, after VR2332 challenge, lung lesion scores were lower on average in both the GP5-Mosaic and GP5-WT groups than those in vector-control animals. There were no significant differences between the lung lesion scores of GP5-WT and GP5-Mosaic-vaccinated groups after challenge with VR2332 (Figure 5).

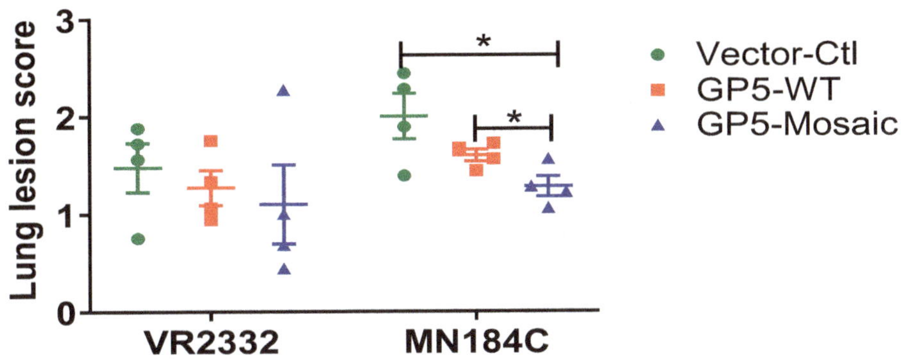

Figure 5. Lung lesion scores. The lung lesion scores of GP5-Mosaic-vaccinated animals were significantly lower ($p < 0.05$) than those of GP%-WT or vector-control animals after challenge with MN184C. Each figure represents the mean value of each individual. The bars represent the standard error of the mean. Three independent experiments were performed for each. Student's t test was utilized to calculate significant differences (days post-challenge (DPC)).

4. Discussion

There is extraordinary diversity among PRRSV strains. The diversity among PRRSV strains is as high as, or may even surpass that of, HIV. Recently, several vaccine candidates, including a synthetic consensus PRRSV strain [27], a chimeric PRRSV strain containing multiple ORFs DNA shuffled [46–48] and an intranasal live virus vaccine with adjuvant [49] induced various levels of heterologous protection in pigs. We have developed GP5-Mosaic vaccines that incorporate sequences derived from naturally circulating viruses. The data obtained from our GP5-Mosaic vaccinated pigs supports the Mosaic vaccine approach as an effective strategy to address PRRSV diversity. It has also been demonstrated that Mosaic T-cell vaccines have great potential for other viruses with extraordinary diversity, such as HIV [33–38]. In an earlier study, we demonstrated the immunogenicity of GP5-Mosaic vaccines in swine and their ability to induce cross-reactivity, as shown by their broad recall responses ex-vivo, and conferred the partial protection they provide in pigs [29,30]. The ability of the GP5-Mosaic vaccines to induce cross-protection in pigs against heterologous PRRSV strains was confirmed in the present study.

A sequence analysis of two GP5-Mosaic vaccines and the two Genotype 2 PRRSV strains utilized in the study, VR2332 and MN184C, that belong to lineage 5 and to lineage 1, respectively, revealed a 15% difference in the GP5 aa sequences. The aa sequences were used to generate a phylogenetic tree using the neighbor-joining method [24]. The GP5-Mosaic 1 was closer to VR2332 (93% aa identity), while GP5-Mosaic 2 was closer to MN184C (90% aa identity), which suggested that the two GP5-Mosaic sequences broaden the coverage to strains belonging to different lineages. Based on this analysis, a broader protection could be expected with GP5-Mosaic vaccines. The data of the present study supports clearly the capacity of the GP5-Mosaic vaccine to cross-protect pigs against VR2332 and MN184C that share only 85% aa identity.

VACV provides a very good platform for the development and testing of vaccines, including animal vaccines, human vaccines and cancer immunotherapy [50]. In our study, a GP5-Mosaic DNA vaccine prime/GP5-Mosaic rVaccinia (VACV) boost regime was used to immunize pigs. This type of prime-boost regime has previously been demonstrated to increase vaccination efficacy substantially [51,52]. In addition, Quil-A®, used as adjuvant for the priming of the GP5-Mosaic DNA vaccine, was previously shown to further increase the immune responses [53–55]. Therefore, the prime-boost vaccination regime used here for testing GP5-Mosaic vaccine efficacy, in terms of broad protection, proved appropriate for testing the hypothesis.

PBMCs collected on the challenge day from GP5-Mosaic-vaccinated pigs responded to a broader range of virus strains, as measured by IFN-γ mRNA expression, than those from GP5-WT vaccinates. Thus, PBMC from GP5-Mosaic-vaccinated pigs expressed higher levels of IFN-γ mRNA in response to stimulation with VR2332 or MN184C strains, respectively, compared to those of the vector-control pigs. In contrast, PBMC from GP5-WT vaccinated pigs expressed higher levels of IFN-γ mRNA only when stimulated with VR2332. These data were consistent with those of our previous study where the GP5-Mosaic vaccine induced broad recall cellular responses, as measured by significantly higher levels of IFN-γ mRNA expression in response to the four diverse Genotype 2 PRRSV strains tested, including VR2332, NADC9, NADC30 and SDSU73 [30]. The significant induction of IFN-γ is an important asset of a PRRSV vaccine, as IFN-γ reportedly plays a critical role in the control of and protection from PRRSV infection [56]. In addition, both the GP5-Mosaic and the GP5-WT vaccines induced relatively high levels of neutralizing antibodies in VR2332-challenged pigs. These data indicate that the GP5-Mosaic vaccine preserves virus-neutralizing epitopes that appear to contribute to the overall efficacy of this vaccine.

In terms of vaccine-induced protection, both GP5-Mosaic and GP5-WT-vaccinated pigs had significantly lower serum viral loads at 7, 10 and 14 DPC than the vector-control group after the VR2332 challenge. In contrast, only the GP5-Mosaic-vaccinated group showed significantly lower viral loads in sera at 7 and 14 DPC than the vector-control group after the MN184C challenge. These data demonstrate that the GP5-Mosaic vaccine is capable of cross-protecting pigs against two divergent PRRSV strains (15% difference) while the GP5-WT vaccine only provided protection in pigs against the homologous strain. Furthermore, a similar pattern was found with respect to viral loads in tissues, where the GP5-Mosaic-vaccinated pigs had significantly lower viral loads in their lungs, TBLN, spleen, ILN and tonsils compared to the vector-control group after challenge with MN184C, while the GP5-WT group only showed slightly lower (numerically, but not significant) viral loads. In the VR2332 challenge experiment, both the GP5-Mosaic and GP5-WT vaccinates had significantly lower viral loads in tissues generally—the viral loads in the GP5-Mosaic vaccinates were significantly lower in their lungs, TBLN and tonsils, while viral loads in the GP5-WT group were significantly lower in their lungs, ILN and spleen, compared to the vector-control group. Similar protective effects were also demonstrated in the GP5-Mosaic vaccine vaccinates, where lower viral loads were detected in the BAL fluids or PAMs after MN184C challenge, further confirming the cross-protective capability of the GP5-Mosaic vaccine. Indeed, this is finding may be particularly relevant since PAMs are the primary target of PRRSV infection. Lung lesion scoring is an essential and crucial method to evaluate vaccine efficacy, as infection by PRRSV tends to increase susceptibility to coinfection with other virus or bacterial pathogens [57–59] which may result in more severe lesions and mortality. Pigs vaccinated with the GP5-Mosaic vaccine had significantly lower lung lesion scores than both the GP5-WT and vector-control groups after challenge with MN184C, while both the GP5-Mosaic and GP5-WT groups had lower lung lesion scores compared to the vector-control group in the VR2332 challenge experiment.

5. Conclusions

Taken altogether, our results clearly demonstrate that the GP5-Mosaic vaccine provided cross-protection against two heterologous PRRSV strains, VR2332, the prototype Genotype 2 strain, and MN184C, a highly virulent strain, while the GP5-WT vaccine provided only homologous protection against VR2332. In summary, our results demonstrate that our GP5-Mosaic vaccine is able to induce broader protection against PRRS and warrants further research for field applications.

Author Contributions: Conceptualization, P.H.V. and A.E.G.; Methodology, J.C., C.M.O., J.A.S., P.H.V. and A.E.G.; Formal analysis, J.C. and A.E.G.; Investigation, J.C., C.M.O., C.H., K.S., J.A.S., P.H.V., H.J.V.K., and A.E.G.; Data curation, J.C. and A.E.G.; Writing—original draft preparation, J.C.; Writing—review and editing, J.C., C.M.O., J.A.S., P.H.V. and A.E.G.; Supervision, A.E.G.; Project administration, A.E.G.; Funding acquisition, J.A.S., P.H.V. and A.E.G. All authors have read and agreed to the published version of the manuscript.

Acknowledgments: The authors thank Kay Faaberg and Kelly Lager kindly providing the PRRSV strains.

References

1. Holtkamp, D.J.; Kliebenstein, J.B.; Neumann, E.J.; Zimmerman, J.J.; Rotto, H.F.; Yoder, T.K.; Wang, C.; Yeske, P.E.; Mowrer, C.L.; Haley, C.A. Assessment of the economic impact of porcine reproductive and respiratory syndrome virus on United States pork producers. *J. Swine Health Prod.* **2013**, *21*, 72–84.
2. Collins, J.; Benfield, D.; Christianson, W.T.; Harris, L.; Hennings, J.C.; Shaw, D.P.; Goyal, S.M.; McCullough, S.; Morrison, R.B.; Joo, H.S.; et al. Isolation of Swine Infertility and Respiratory Syndrome Virus (Isolate ATCC VR-2332) in North America and Experimental Reproduction of the Disease in Gnotobiotic Pigs. *J. Veter Diagn. Investig.* **1992**, *4*, 117–126. [CrossRef] [PubMed]
3. Wensvoort, G.; Terpstra, C.; Pol, J.M.; Ter Laak, E.A.; Bloemraad, M.; de Kluyver, E.P.; Kragten, C.; van Buiten, L.; den Besten, A.; Wagenaar, F. Mystery swine disease in The Netherlands: The isolation of Lelystad virus. *Veter Q.* **1991**, *13*, 121–130. [CrossRef] [PubMed]
4. Cavanagh, D. Nidovirales: A new order comprising Coronaviridae and Arteriviridae. *Arch. Virol.* **1997**, *142*, 629–633. [PubMed]
5. Lunney, J.K.; Fang, Y.; Ladinig, A.; Chen, N.; Li, Y.; Rowland, B.; Renukaradhya, G. Porcine Reproductive and Respiratory Syndrome Virus (PRRSV): Pathogenesis and Interaction with the Immune System. *Annu. Rev. Anim. Biosci.* **2016**, *4*, 129–154. [CrossRef]
6. Mokhtar, H.; Eck, M.; Morgan, S.B.; Essler, S.E.; Frossard, J.-P.; Ruggli, N.; Graham, S. Proteome-wide screening of the European porcine reproductive and respiratory syndrome virus reveals a broad range of T cell antigen reactivity. *Vaccine* **2014**, *32*, 6828–6837. [CrossRef]
7. Parida, R.; Choi, I.-S.; Peterson, D.A.; Pattnaik, A.K.; Laegreid, W.; Zuckermann, F.A.; Osorio, F. Location of T-cell epitopes in nonstructural proteins 9 and 10 of type-II porcine reproductive and respiratory syndrome virus. *Virus Res.* **2012**, *169*, 13–21. [CrossRef]
8. Brown, E.; Lawson, S.; Welbon, C.; Gnanandarajah, J.; Li, J.; Murtaugh, M.P.; Nelson, E.; Molina, R.; Zimmerman, J.; Rowland, R.; et al. Antibody response to porcine reproductive and respiratory syndrome virus (PRRSV) nonstructural proteins and implications for diagnostic detection and differentiation of PRRSV types I and II. *Clin. Vaccine Immunol.* **2009**, *16*, 628–635. [CrossRef]
9. Vanhee, M.; Van Breedam, W.; Costers, S.; Geldhof, M.; Noppe, Y.; Nauwynck, H. Characterization of antigenic regions in the porcine reproductive and respiratory syndrome virus by the use of peptide-specific serum antibodies. *Vaccine* **2011**, *29*, 4794–4804. [CrossRef]
10. Zuckermann, F.A.; Garcia, E.A.; Luque, I.D.; Christopher-Hennings, J.; Doster, A.; Brito, M.; Osorio, F. Assessment of the efficacy of commercial porcine reproductive and respiratory syndrome virus (PRRSV) vaccines based on measurement of serologic response, frequency of gamma-IFN-producing cells and virological parameters of protection upon challenge. *Veter Microbiol.* **2007**, *123*, 69–85. [CrossRef]
11. Osorio, F.A.; Galeota, J.A.; Nelson, E.; Brodersen, B.; Doster, A.; Wills, R.; Zuckermann, F.; Laegreid, W.W. PRRSV: Comparison of commercial vaccines in their ability to induce protection against current PRRSV strains of high virulence. In Proceedings of the Allen D Leman Swine Conference, St. Paul, MN, USA, 14–17 September 2019; 1998; pp. 176–182.
12. Scortti, M.; Prieto, C.; Alvarez, E.; Simarro, I.; Castro, J.M. Failure of an inactivated vaccine against porcine reproductive and respiratory syndrome to protect gilts against a heterologous challenge with PRRSV. *Veter Rec.* **2007**, *161*, 809–813.
13. Geldhof, M.F.; Vanhee, M.; Van Breedam, W.; Van Doorsselaere, J.; Karniychuk, U.U.; Nauwynck, H.J. Comparison of the efficacy of autogenous inactivated Porcine Reproductive and Respiratory Syndrome Virus (PRRSV) vaccines with that of commercial vaccines against homologous and heterologous challenges. *BMC Veter Res.* **2012**, *8*, 182. [CrossRef] [PubMed]

14. Labarque, G.; Reeth KVan Nauwynck, H.; Drexler, C.; Gucht SVan Pensaert, M. Impact of genetic diversity of European-type porcine reproductive and respiratory syndrome virus strains on vaccine efficacy. *Vaccine* **2004**, *22*, 4183–4190. [CrossRef] [PubMed]
15. Okuda, Y.; Kuroda, M.; Ono, M.; Chikata, S.; Shibata, I. Efficacy of Vaccination with Porcine Reproductive and Respiratory Syndrome Virus Following Challenges with Field Isolates in Japan. *J. Veter Med. Sci.* **2008**, *70*, 1017–1025. [CrossRef]
16. Han, K.; Seo, H.W.; Park, C.; Chae, C. Vaccination of sows against type 2 Porcine Reproductive and Respiratory Syndrome Virus (PRRSV) before artificial insemination protects against type 2 PRRSV challenge but does not protect against type 1 PRRSV challenge in late gestation. *Veter Res.* **2014**, *45*, 12. [CrossRef]
17. Kim, T.; Park, C.; Choi, K.; Jeong, J.; Kang, I.; Park, S.-J.; Chae, C. Comparison of Two Commercial Type 1 Porcine Reproductive and Respiratory Syndrome Virus (PRRSV) Modified Live Vaccines against Heterologous Type 1 and Type 2 PRRSV Challenge in Growing Pigs. *Clin. Vaccine Immunol.* **2015**, *22*, 631–640. [CrossRef]
18. Trus, I.; Bonckaert, C.; van der Meulen, K.; Nauwynck, H.J. Efficacy of an attenuated European subtype 1 porcine reproductive and respiratory syndrome virus (PRRSV) vaccine in pigs upon challenge with the East European subtype 3 PRRSV strain Lena. *Vaccine* **2014**, *32*, 2995–3003. [CrossRef]
19. Bøtner, A.; Strandbygaard, B.; Sørensen, K.J.; Have, P.; Madsen, K.G.; Madsen, E.S.; Alexandersen, S. Appearance of acute PRRS-like symptoms in sow herds after vaccination with a modified live PRRS vaccine. *Veter Rec.* **1997**, *141*, 497–499. [CrossRef]
20. Madsen, K.G.; Hansen, C.M.; Madsen, E.S.; Strandbygaard, B.; Bøtner, A.; Sørensen, K.J. Sequence analysis of porcine reproductive and respiratory syndrome virus of the American type collected from Danish swine herds. *Arch. Virol.* **1998**, *143*, 1683–1700. [CrossRef]
21. Nielsen, H.S.; Stadejek, T.; Bøtner, A.; Oleksiewicz, M.B.; Forsberg, R. Reversion of a live porcine reproductive and respiratory syndrome virus vaccine investigated by parallel mutations. *J. Gen. Virol.* **2015**, *82*, 1263–1272. [CrossRef]
22. Nelsen, C.J.; Murtaugh, M.P.; Faaberg, K.S. Porcine reproductive and respiratory syndrome virus comparison: Divergent evolution on two continents. *J. Virol.* **1999**, *73*, 270–280. [CrossRef] [PubMed]
23. Kim, H.K.; Yang, J.S.; Moon, H.J.; Park, S.J.; Luo, Y.; Lee, C.S.; Song, D.; Kang, B.; Ann, S.; Jun, C.; et al. Genetic analysis of ORF5 of recent Korean porcine reproductive and respiratory syndrome viruses (PRRSVs) in viremic sera collected from MLV-vaccinating or non-vaccinating farms. *J. Veter Sci.* **2009**, *10*, 121–130. [CrossRef] [PubMed]
24. Shi, M.; Lam, T.T.-Y.; Hon, C.-C.; Murtaugh, M.P.; Davies, P.R.; Hui, R.K.-H.; Li, J.; Wong, L.; Yip, C.; Jiang, J.; et al. Phylogeny-Based Evolutionary, Demographical, and Geographical Dissection of North American Type 2 Porcine Reproductive and Respiratory Syndrome Viruses. *J. Virol.* **2010**, *84*, 8700–8711. [CrossRef] [PubMed]
25. Goldberg, T.L.; Lowe, J.F.; Milburn, S.M.; Firkins, L.D. Quasispecies variation of porcine reproductive and respiratory syndrome virus during natural infection. *Virology* **2003**, *317*, 197–207. [CrossRef]
26. Jiang, Y.; Xiao, S.; Fang, L.; Yu, X.; Song, Y.; Niu, C.; Chen, H. DNA vaccines co-expressing GP5 and M proteins of porcine reproductive and respiratory syndrome virus (PRRSV) display enhanced immunogenicity. *Vaccine* **2006**, *24*, 2869–2879. [CrossRef]
27. Vu, H.L.; Ma, F.; Laegreid, W.W.; Pattnaik, A.K.; Steffen, D.; Doster, A.R.; Osorio, F. A Synthetic Porcine Reproductive and Respiratory Syndrome Virus Strain Confers Unprecedented Levels of Heterologous Protection. *J. Virol.* **2015**, *89*, 12070–12083. [CrossRef]
28. Zhou, L.; Ni, Y.Y.; Pineyro, P.; Sanford, B.J.; Cossaboom, C.M.; Dryman, B.A.; Huang, Y.; Cao, D.; Meng, X. DNA shuffling of the GP3 genes of porcine reproductive and respiratory syndrome virus (PRRSV) produces a chimeric virus with an improved cross-neutralizing ability against a heterologous PRRSV strain. *Virology* **2012**, *434*, 96–109. [CrossRef]
29. Cui, J.; O'Connell, C.M.; Smith, J.D.; Pan, Y.; Smyth, J.A.; Verardi, P.H.; Garmendia, A.E. A GP5 Mosaic T-cell vaccine for porcine reproductive and respiratory syndrome virus is immunogenic and confers partial protection to pigs. *Vaccine Rep.* **2016**, *6*, 77–85. [CrossRef]

30. Cui, J.; O'Connell, C.M.; Costa, A.; Pan, Y.; Smyth, J.A.; Verardi, P.H.; Burgess, D.; Van Kruiningen, H.; Garmendia, A.E. A PRRSV GP5-Mosaic vaccine: Protection of pigs from challenge and ex vivo detection of IFNγ responses against several genotype 2 strains. *PLoS ONE* **2019**, *14*, e0208801. [CrossRef]
31. Mengeling, W.L.; Lager, K.M.; Vorwald, A.C.; Clouser, D.F. Comparative safety and efficacy of attenuated single-strain and multi-strain vaccines for porcine reproductive and respiratory syndrome. *Veter Microbiol.* **2003**, *93*, 25–38. [CrossRef]
32. Bernelin-Cottet, C.; Urien, C.; Fretaud, M.; Langevin, C.; Trus, I.; Jouneau, L.; Blanc, F.; Leplat, J.; Barc, C.; Boulesteix, O.; et al. A DNA Prime Immuno-Potentiates a Modified Live *Vaccine* against the Porcine Reproductive and Respiratory Syndrome Virus but Does Not Improve Heterologous Protection. *Viruses* **2019**, *11*, 576. [CrossRef] [PubMed]
33. Fischer, W.; Perkins, S.; Theiler, J.; Bhattacharya, T.; Yusim, K.; Funkhouser, R.; Kuiken, C.; Haynes, B.; Letvin, N.; Walker, B.; et al. Polyvalent vaccines for optimal coverage of potential T-cell epitopes in global HIV-1 variants. *Nat. Med.* **2007**, *13*, 100–106. [CrossRef] [PubMed]
34. Thurmond, J.; Yoon, H.; Kuiken, C.; Yusim, K.; Perkins, S.; Theiler, J.; Bhattacharya, T.; Korber, B.; Fisher, W. Web-based design and evaluation of T-cell vaccine candidates. *Bioinformatics* **2008**, *24*, 1639–1640. [CrossRef] [PubMed]
35. Kong, W.P.; Wu, L.; Wallstrom, T.C.; Fischer, W.; Yang, Z.Y.; Ko, S.Y.; Letvin, N.; Haynes, B.; Hahn, B.; Korber, B.; et al. Expanded breadth of the T-cell response to mosaic human immunodeficiency virus type 1 envelope DNA vaccination. *J. Virol.* **2009**, *83*, 2201–2215. [CrossRef]
36. Barouch, D.H.; O'Brien, K.L.; Simmons, N.L.; King, S.L.; Abbink, P.; Maxfield, L.F.; Sun, Y.; La Port, A.; Riggs, A.; Lynch, D.; et al. Mosaic HIV-1 vaccines expand the breadth and depth of cellular immune responses in rhesus monkeys. *Nat. Med.* **2010**, *16*, 319–323. [CrossRef]
37. Santra, S.; Liao, H.X.; Zhang, R.; Muldoon, M.; Watson, S.; Fischer, W.; Theiler, J.; Szinger, J.; Balachandran, H.; Buzby, A.; et al. Mosaic vaccines elicit CD8+ T lymphocyte responses that confer enhanced immune coverage of diverse HIV strains in monkeys. *Nat. Med.* **2010**, *16*, 324–328. [CrossRef]
38. Barouch, D.H.; Tomaka, F.L.; Wegmann, F.; Stieh, D.J.; Alter, G.; Robb, M.L.; Nelson, L.; Michael, N.L.; Peter, L.; Nkolola, J.P.; et al. Evaluation of a mosaic HIV-1 vaccine in a multicentre, randomised, double-blind, placebo-controlled, phase 1/2a clinical trial (APPROACH) and in rhesus monkeys (NHP 13–19). *Lancet* **2018**, *392*, 232–243. [CrossRef]
39. Kim, H.S.; Kwang, J.; Yoon, I.J.; Joo, H.S.; Frey, M.L. Enhanced replication of porcine reproductive and respiratory syndrome (PRRS) virus in a homogeneous subpopulation of MA-104 cell line. *Arch. Virol.* **1993**, *133*, 477–483. [CrossRef]
40. Reed, L.J.; Muench, H. A simple method of estimating fifty percent endpoints. *Am. J. Hyg.* **1938**, *27*, 493–497.
41. Chakrabarti, S.; Sisler, J.R.; Moss, B. Compact, synthetic, vaccinia virus early/late promoter for protein expression. *Biotechniques* **1997**, *23*, 1094–1097. [CrossRef]
42. Hagen, C.J.; Titong, A.; Sarnoski, E.A.; Verardi, P.H. Antibiotic-dependent expression of early transcription factor subunits leads to stringent control of vaccinia virus replication. *Virus Res.* **2014**, *181*, 43–52. [CrossRef] [PubMed]
43. Cotter, C.A.; Earl, P.L.; Wyatt, L.S.; Moss, B. Preparation of Cell Cultures and Vaccinia Virus Stocks. *Curr. Protoc. Protein Sci.* **2017**, *89*, 5121–5128. [CrossRef]
44. Livak, K.J.; Schmittgen, T.D. Analysis of Relative Gene Expression Data Using Real-Time Quantitative PCR and the $2-\Delta\Delta CT$ Method. *Methods* **2001**, *25*, 402–408. [CrossRef] [PubMed]
45. Halbur, P.G.; Paul, P.S.; Meng, X.J.; Lum, M.A.; Andrews, J.J.; Rathje, J.A. Comparative pathogenicity of nine US porcine reproductive and respiratory syndrome virus (PRRSV) isolates in a five-week-old cesarean-derived, colostrum-deprived pig model. *J. Veter Diagn. Investig.* **1996**, *8*, 11–20. [CrossRef]
46. Ni, Y.Y.; Opriessnig, T.; Zhou, L.; Cao, D.; Huang, Y.W.; Halbur, P.G.; Meng, X. Attenuation of porcine reproductive and respiratory syndrome virus by molecular breeding of virus envelope genes from genetically divergent strains. *J. Virol.* **2013**, *87*, 304–313. [CrossRef]
47. Zhou, L.; Ni, Y.-Y.; Piñeyro, P.; Cossaboom, C.M.; Subramaniam, S.; Sanford, B.J.; Dryman, B.; Huang, Y.; Meng, X. Broadening the heterologous cross-neutralizing antibody inducing ability of porcine reproductive and respiratory syndrome virus by breeding the GP4 or M genes. *PLoS ONE* **2013**, *8*, e66645. [CrossRef]

48. Tian, D.; Ni, Y.-Y.; Zhou, L.; Opriessnig, T.; Cao, D.; Piñeyro, P.; Yugo, D.; Overend, C.; Cao, Q.; Lynn Heffron, C.; et al. Chimeric porcine reproductive and respiratory syndrome virus containing shuffled multiple envelope genes confers cross-protection in pigs. *Virology* **2015**, *485*, 402–413. [CrossRef]
49. Dwivedi, V.; Manickam, C.; Patterson, R.; Dodson, K.; Murtaugh, M.; Torrelles, J.B.; Schlesinger, L.; Renukaradhya, G. Cross-protective immunity to porcine reproductive and respiratory syndrome virus by intranasal delivery of a live virus vaccine with a potent adjuvant. *Vaccine* **2011**, *29*, 4058–4066. [CrossRef]
50. Verardi, P.H.; Titong, A.; Hagen, C.J. A vaccinia virus renaissance. *Hum. Vaccines Immunother.* **2012**, *8*, 961–970. [CrossRef]
51. Chapman, R.; Jongwe, T.I.; Douglass, N.; Chege, G.; Williamson, A.L. Heterologous prime-boost vaccination with DNA and MVA vaccines, expressing HIV-1 subtype C mosaic Gag virus-like particles, is highly immunogenic in mice. *PLoS ONE* **2017**, *12*, e0173352. [CrossRef]
52. Deng, Y.; Chuai, X.; Chen, P.; Chen, H.; Wang, W.; Ruan, L.; Li, W.; Tan, W. Recombinant vaccinia vector-based vaccine (Tiantan) boosting a novel HBV subunit vaccine induced more robust and lasting immunity in rhesus macaques. *Vaccine* **2017**, *35*, 3347–3353. [CrossRef] [PubMed]
53. Lampe, K.; Gottstein, B.; Becker, T.; Stahl-Hennig, C.; Kaup, F.J.; Mätz-Rensing, K. Immunization of rhesus macaques with Echinococcus multilocularis recombinant 14-3-3 antigen leads to specific antibody response. *Parasitol. Res.* **2017**, *116*, 435–439. [CrossRef] [PubMed]
54. Tahoun, A.; Jensen, K.; Corripio-Miyar, Y.; McAteer, S.P.; Corbishley, A.; Mahajan, A.; Brown, H.; Frew, D.; Aumeunier, A.; Smith, D.G.; et al. Functional analysis of bovine TLR5 and association with IgA responses of cattle following systemic immunisation with H7 flagella. *Veter Res.* **2015**, *46*, 9. [CrossRef] [PubMed]
55. Gómez-Gascón, L.; Cardoso-Toset, F.; Tarradas, C.; Gómez-Laguna, J.; Maldonado, A.; Nielsen, J.; Olaya-Abril, A.; Rodriguez-Ortega, M.; Luque, I. Characterization of the immune response and evaluation of the protective capacity of rSsnA against Streptococcus suis infection in pigs. *Comp. Immunol. Microbiol. Infect. Dis.* **2016**, *47*, 52–59. [CrossRef] [PubMed]
56. Morgan, S.B.; Graham, S.P.; Salguero, F.J.; Sánchez Cordón, P.J.; Mokhtar, H.; Rebel, J.M.J.; Weesendorp, E.; Bodman-Smith, K.; Steinbach, F.; Frossard, J. Increased pathogenicity of European porcine reproductive and respiratory syndrome virus is associated with enhanced adaptive responses and viral clearance. *Veter Microbiol.* **2013**, *163*, 13–22. [CrossRef] [PubMed]
57. Thanawongnuwech, R.; Brown, G.B.; Halbur, P.G.; Roth, J.A.; Royer, R.L.; Thacker, B.J. Pathogenesis of Porcine Reproductive and Respiratory Syndrome Virus-induced Increase in Susceptibility to Streptococcus suis Infection. *Veter Pathol.* **2000**, *37*, 143–152. [CrossRef] [PubMed]
58. Van Reeth, K.; Nauwynck, H.; Pensaert, M. Dual infections of feeder pigs with porcine reproductive and respiratory syndrome virus followed by porcine respiratory coronavirus or swine influenza virus: A clinical and virological study. *Veter Microbiol.* **1996**, *48*, 325–335. [CrossRef]
59. Tsai, Y.C.; Chang, H.W.; Jeng, C.R.; Lin, T.L.; Lin, C.M.; Wan, C.H.; Pang, V. The effect of infection order of porcine circovirus type 2 and porcine reproductive and respiratory syndrome virus on dually infected swine alveolar macrophages. *BMC Veter Res.* **2012**, *8*, 174. [CrossRef]

10

Influenza Virus Like Particles (VLPs): Opportunities for H7N9 Vaccine Development

Peter Pushko * **and Irina Tretyakova**

Medigen, Inc., 8420 Gas House Pike, Suite S, Frederick, MD 21701, USA; itretyakova@medigen-usa.com
* Correspondence: ppushko@medigen-usa.com

Abstract: In the midst of the ongoing COVID-19 coronavirus pandemic, influenza virus remains a major threat to public health due to its potential to cause epidemics and pandemics with significant human mortality. Cases of H7N9 human infections emerged in eastern China in 2013 and immediately raised pandemic concerns as historically, pandemics were caused by the introduction of new subtypes into immunologically naïve human populations. Highly pathogenic H7N9 cases with severe disease were reported recently, indicating the continuing public health threat and the need for a prophylactic vaccine. Here we review the development of recombinant influenza virus-like particles (VLPs) as vaccines against H7N9 virus. Several approaches to vaccine development are reviewed including the expression of VLPs in mammalian, plant and insect cell expression systems. Although considerable progress has been achieved, including demonstration of safety and immunogenicity of H7N9 VLPs in the human clinical trials, the remaining challenges need to be addressed. These challenges include improvements to the manufacturing processes, as well as enhancements to immunogenicity in order to elicit protective immunity to multiple variants and subtypes of influenza virus.

Keywords: H7N9, pandemic influenza A; avian flu; IAV; VLP vaccine

---

1. Introduction

In addition to pandemic COVID-19 virus infections, influenza virus remains a major threat to public health and causes significant morbidity and mortality worldwide from annual seasonal epidemics and periodic pandemics [1,2]. According to WHO, seasonal influenza affects 5–10% of the global population annually and results in 3-5 million hospitalizations and about half a million deaths per year. Pandemic influenza A virus (IAV) represents an even greater concern. Due to the rapid mutation rate of human IAVs, antigenically novel viruses are emerging periodically, which are difficult to predict, prevent, or treat [3]. Zoonotic influenza viruses of H5N1, H9N2 and recently, H7N9 and H10N8 subtypes have been identified as potentially pandemic [4,5].

Influenza viruses belong to the *Orthomyxoviridae* family and comprise negative-sense, single stranded, segmented RNA genome. The RNA genome segments are loosely encapsidated by the nucleoprotein into virus particle. There are four types of influenza virus—types A, B, C, and D. Influenza A viruses (IAV) and type B viruses are clinically relevant for humans.

IAV are further sub-divided based on the antigenic properties of surface glycoproteins into 18 hemagglutinin (HA) and 11 neuraminidase (NA) subtypes. Only a few IAV subtypes have been known to infect humans, while the majority of them are harbored in their natural hosts such as waterfowl, shorebirds, and other species [6]. Cases of H7N9 human infections caused by an avian-origin H7N9 virus emerged in eastern China in March 2013 [7,8]. This novel virus has immediately raised pandemic concerns as historically, pandemics were caused by the introduction of new subtypes into immunologically naïve human populations [9]. Phylogenetic results indicate that novel H7N9 virus was a triple reassortant derived from avian influenza viruses [7]. Since 2013, surveillance of live poultry markets routinely detected H7N9 virus [10]. Human infections with H7N9 virus were associated mainly with the exposure to infected poultry [11] and were identified in many cities in China [12]. Both low pathogenicity avian influenza (LPAI) and high pathogenicity avian influenza (HPAI) H7N9 viruses have been recorded. The first wave of H7N9 was associated with LPAI virus and lasted from March until September 2013. The following four waves occurred annually until 2017 (Figure 1). During the fifth wave in the 2016/17 season, the emergence of HPAI H7N9 viruses was detected. After no reported human cases of HPAI H7N9 for over a year, another HPAI H7N9 case with severe disease was reported in mainland China in late March 2019, indicating the continuing public health threat from the H7N9 subtype [13]. HPAI subtype H5 and H7 proteins contain multiple basic amino acid cleavage sites between HA1 and HA2 domains within HA proteins, which can be cleaved by furin-like proteases [14] in many host cells and organs that can lead to the efficient spread of the virus and severe disease in humans. In contrast, HA of LPAI viruses does not have the furin cleavage site.

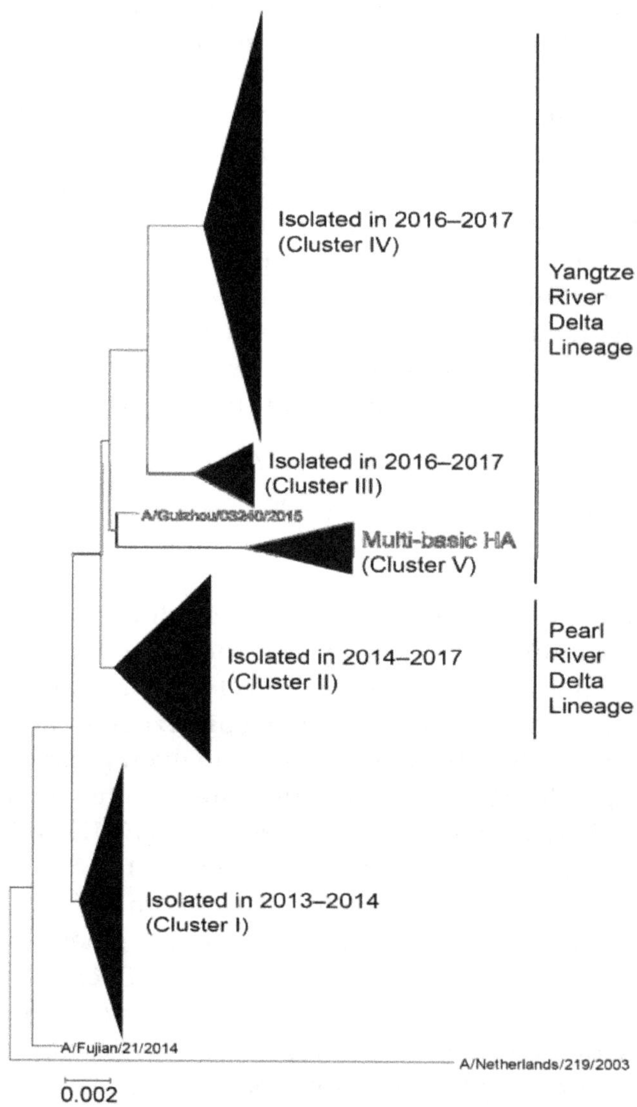

Figure 1. Phylogenetic tree of hemagglutinin (HA) sequences derived from human H7N9 viruses [15]. The evolutionary history was inferred using the neighbor-joining method with Kimura distances. Five major clusters are shown as a collapsed branch. A/Netherlands/219/2003 is defined as an outgroup. The Yangtze River Delta and Pearl River Delta lineages are circulating in China. HPAI H7N9 viruses, which harbor multiple basic amino acids in the HA cleave site, are included in the Yangtze River Delta lineage. Permission: Viruses https://doi.org/10.3390/v11020149.

A fatality rate of up to 38% was reported for H7N9 viruses [16], which highlights the need for a safe and effective vaccine [17]. Several candidate H7N9 vaccine viruses have been prepared and listed by WHO (Table 1). These candidate vaccine viruses are available to vaccine developers for the preparation of H7N9 vaccine in the case of a pandemic. The majority of current vaccine manufacturers prepare vaccines either as split subvirions or live-attenuated viruses, and they are mostly dependent on fertilized chicken eggs as production "bioreactors". This technology is unlikely to meet the vaccine production demand during the rapid pandemic spread [18]. Scalability issues (one vaccine dose/egg), the relatively long 6-month time period from strain isolation to final dose formulation and the requirement of biosecurity facilities for HPAI are the major obstacles for egg-based production [19]. In addition, IAV can acquire adaptive mutations when grown in eggs, which can interfere with the vaccine performance and efficacy. According to the action plan published by WHO in 2006, more than 2.34 billion monovalent vaccine doses will be needed in the case of a global pandemic, which justifies the development of novel technologies capable of supporting surge demand for pandemic influenza vaccine within a short period of time [20].

Table 1. WHO-recommended vaccine strains for H7N9 virus (adapted from [21]).

Vaccine Prototype Strain	Vaccine Candidate	Examples
A/Guangdong/17SF003/2016		*Wild Type Virus*
	Reverse genetics	CBER-RG7C, IDCDC-RG56N, CBER-RG7D, NIBRG-375
A/Hong Kong/125/2017		*Wild type virus*
	Reverse genetics	IDCDC-RG56B
A/Shanghai/2/2013		*Wild type virus*
	Reverse genetics	IDCDC-RG32A, IDCDC-RG32A.3, NIBRG-267, CBER-RG4A
A/Anhui/1/2013		*Wild type virus*
	Reverse genetics	NIBRG-268, NIIDRG-10.1, IDCDC-RG33A, SJ005

2. Recombinant Influenza Virus-Like Particles (VLPs) as Vaccines

Recently, several new platform technologies including recombinant VLPs have been developed in order to facilitate the scale-up of vaccine production including overcoming the drawbacks of the egg-based vaccine production method. The first recombinant influenza vaccine FluBlok based on HA antigen has received FDA approval [22]. The surface envelope glycoproteins such as influenza HA and NA generally are viewed as the primary targets for vaccine development. HA currently represents the major target for vaccine development including approved and experimental vaccines [22]. Recombinant HA-based vaccines have been shown to be efficacious against influenza including H7N9 [17,23–31]. Experimental NA-based vaccines have been reported [32,33]. The induction of immune responses against the surface envelope proteins has advantages, because virus-neutralizing antibody response to the viral envelope proteins can prevent early steps of viral infection. Human monoclonal antibodies targeting the HA glycoprotein can neutralize H7N9 influenza virus [34]. Importantly, the neutralizing antibodies protected against A/Shanghai/2/2013 (H7N9) virus challenge [35].

The novel recombinant VLP vaccine platforms included VLPs prepared in mammalian, insect, and plant expression systems. Recombinant VLPs are morphologically and biochemically similar to the wild type influenza virus (Figure 2); however, they lack viral genetic material and are unable to replicate and cause infection. Table 2 shows examples of various VLPs prepared from H7N9 virus antigens. Cell culture-based production of VLPs can potentially overcome limitations of classic influenza vaccines [36].

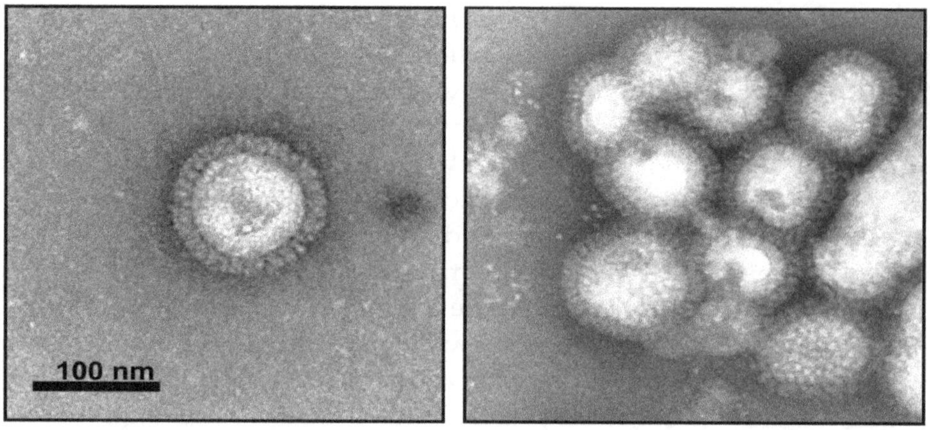

Figure 2. Electron microscopy images of influenza VLPs prepared in Sf9 cells using baculovirus expression system. Recombinant VLPs contain three subtypes (H5, H7, H9), morphologically and biochemically are similar to the wild type influenza virus, and can be found as individual particles (left) or groups of particles (right). Characterization of triple-subtype VLPs was done by negative staining transmission electron microscopy. (Adapted from [50].

Table 2. Examples of virus-like particle (VLP) vaccines against H7N9 influenza.

VLP Antigen	Expression System	Vaccination			Protection from Intranasal Challenge	References
		Animals	Dose	Route		
HA	High Five insect cells	mice	10 μg protein plus 10 μg poly(I·C) in PBS	IM	100 mLD_{50}	[37]
HA	Insect Sf9	mice ferrets	5 μg 15 μg	IN IM	10 mLD_{50} 10^6 PFU	[38]
HA	Insect Sf9	ferrets	15 μg	SC	10^7 PFU	[31]
HA	Plants	mice ferrets	3 μg 15 μg	IM IM	100 mLD_{50} 10^6 $TCID_{50}$	[39]
HA, M1	Insect *Trichoplusia ni* cell line High Five (BTI-TN-5B1-4)	mice	0.03, 0.3, 3 μg	IM	fully protected against 100 mLD_{50}	[40]
HA, M1	Insect Sf9	mice	1.5 μg	IN	10 mLD_{50}	[41]
HA, NA, M1	Insect Sf9	mice	6 μg	IM	4.4X10^3 $TCID_{50}$ PFU	[42]
HA, NA, M1	HEK293T	mice	40 μg total protein	IM	NA	[43]
HA, NA, M1	Insect Sf9	mice	3 μg	SC	10^6 $TCID_{50}$	[44]
HA, NA, M1	Insect Sf9	mice chickens	10 μg	IM	NA	[45]
HA, NA, M1	Insect Sf9	mice	40 μg	IM, IN		[46]
HA, NA, BIV Gag	Insect Sf9	chickens	1536 HA units per dose of VLPs	SC	10^6 EID_{50}	[47]
HA/M1, M2/NA, BAFF-HA_{tm}/M1, APRILHA_{tm}/M1	Insect Sf9	mice	0.5 μg HA content	IM	10 mLD_{50} of NIBRG-14 vaccine strain	[48]
Combined HA and M2e5x (Universal)	Insect Sf9	mice	5 μg HA + 10 μg M2e5x VLPs	IM	7.5 x 10^2 PFU = 5 mLD_{50}	[49]

mLD_{50}, mouse median lethal dose.

As VLPs closely resemble viruses, they contain immunological epitopes in the natural conformation, are highly immunogenic, but they are non-infectious because they are prepared in the absence of viral genomic RNA segments. Each VLP represents a repetitive and highly organized molecular array of antigens displayed on the VLP surface. VLPs have been shown to be better immunogens than subunit vaccines because of their self-adjuvant properties [51]. The antigens present in VLP bind pattern recognition receptors on innate immune effector cells and trigger the innate immunity of host cells [52,53]. The molecular arrays displayed on VLP's surface are also potent inducers of Type 2 T-independent B-cell response [54]. Cryo-electron microscopy of VLPs from 1918 pandemic influenza virus demonstrated a uniform distribution of HA molecules on the surface of VLPs along with prefusion state confirmation [55]. Two types of spike on the surface of virus are formed by trimers of HA and tetramers of NA. It has been estimated that a spherical influenza virion of average diameter 120 nm has ~375 spikes [56].

3. Recombinant Platforms for Expression of H7N9 VLPs

The recombinant platforms using either mammalian, insect, or plant cells have many potential advantages including scalability and intrinsic safety, especially for HPAI viruses such as H7N9 (Table 2). Mammalian cells, such as MDCK, Vero and PERC.C6 cell lines have been extensively studied and applied to influenza vaccine production. The use of VLPs expressed from mammalian cell platform has advantages for VLP production such as flexibility and a similar glycosylation pattern to the human virus. In some reports, VLPs expressed from HEK293T cells containing HA and NA proteins on their surface with a HA:NA ratio of 1:1, which is higher than natural influenza viruses, where the HA:NA ratio is 4:1 [57]. VLPs isolated from HEK293SF cells were also characterized by nano-LC-MS/MS analysis to identify the protein cargo. Nucleolin was the most abundant cellular protein present in VLPs, in addition to the recombinant influenza VLP proteins [58]. However, production of VLPs in mammalian cell expression system is difficult to scale up to the commercial scale, especially when using the transient transfection method. This limitation can be addressed by preparing stable cell line of corresponding genes. For example, a stable cell line expressing H1 and N1 genes under the cumate inducible promoter was generated to create 293HA-NA cells. Plasmid with either Gag or M1 gene was transiently transfected in 293HA-NA cells and VLP yield was compared with Gag or M1 protein. 293HA-NA cells produced seven times more HA and NA with Gag plasmid transfected cells than its counterpart matrix M1-encoding plasmid [59]. Gag VLPs produced by this approach elicited strong antibody response and provided complete protection against the homologous virus strain. Optimization of cell density at the time of induction in inducible stable HEK293 cell lines also increased VLP yield by five-fold [60].

Insect cells such as Sf9 can be maintained in serum-free suspension cultures and have been often used to prepare recombinant VLPs including H7N9. When influenza VLPs were compared between insect Sf9 cells and mammalian HEK293 suspension cells, Thompson et al. found that Sf9 cells produce approximately 35 times more VLP than HEK293 cells [61]. VLPs produced from Sf9 cells also showed higher HA titer and more homogenous VLPs than HEK293 cells derived VLPs [61]. As expected, the high titer of baculovirus vector was also present in VLPs prepared in Sf9 cells. However, VLPs generated in HEK293 cells contained extracellular vesicles, such as exosomes and microvesicles. VLPs produced from Sf9 insect cells may have a safety advantage over other expression system because insect cells are unlikely to contain human pathogens, and baculovirus vector cannot replicate in human cells. VLPs produced from insect cells show higher yields as compared to mammalian cell-produced VLPs, which is beneficial for commercial production. In the above study, Sf9 cells produced up to 35 times higher yield than the HEK293 cells' expression system [61]. In addition, VLPs had higher HA activity and they were more homogenous in morphology and size than mammalian cells produced VLPs [61]. Sf9 cells are usually maintained in a serum free, animal product-free medium. Some of the chemical compounds known as M2 inhibitors, such as amantadine-enhanced expression of HA protein in VLPs by seven-fold in Sf9 expression system [62]. However, the challenge for VLPs expressed using baculovirus expression system is that it is difficult to separate VLPs from the baculovirus expression vector during vaccine manufacturing.

H7N9 VLPs have been prepared from the full-length HA, NA, and matrix M1 genes in Sf9 cells. The H7 HA was derived from A/Shanghai/2/2013 (H7N9) virus, while both NA and M1 proteins were derived from A/Puerto Rico/8/1934 (H1N1) virus, a standard donor virus that is often used for preparation of influenza reassortant viruses used in human influenza vaccine production [63]. VLPs have been isolated from Sf9 cells and their morphology resembling native H7N9 virus envelope was confirmed.

In another study, recombinant H7N9 VLP vaccine was prepared from HA and NA derived from the A/Anhui/1/2013 (H7N9) virus and the matrix M1 protein derived from the H5N1 virus (A/Indonesia/05/2005) [42]. As control vaccines, VLPs were prepared from A/chicken/Jalisco/CPA1/2012 (H7N3) and A/Indonesia/05/2005 (H5N1) viruses. The H7N9 VLPs elicited hemagglutination-inhibition (HAI) antibody response against the homologous H7N9 virus, cross-reactive HAI against the heterologous H7N3 virus, and three- to four-fold higher HAI response if VLPs were administered with ISCOMATRIX™ saponin-based adjuvant. Similarly, all doses of H7N9 VLP elicited anti-NA antibody, with three- to four-fold higher responses measured in the corresponding ISCOMATRIX subgroups. A lethal murine wild-type A/Anhui/1/2013 (H7N9) challenge demonstrated 100% survival of all animals receiving H7N9 or H7N3 VLP vaccines, versus 0% survival in A(H5N1) vaccine and placebo groups [42].

Another study reported a VLP from Sf9 cells that consisted of HA, NA and M1 proteins derived from the human isolate A/Taiwan/S02076/2013(H7N9) as a potential vaccine. In animal experiments, BALB/c mice and specific-pathogen-free chickens receiving the VLP immunization developed HAI serum titer and antibodies against NA and M1 proteins [45].

The immunogenicity and protective efficacy of a H7N9 VLP vaccine were evaluated in the ferret challenge model considered the most appropriate animal model for influenza [31]. Purified recombinant H7N9 VLPs morphologically resembled influenza virions and elicited high-titer serum HAI and neutralizing antibodies to A/Anhui/1/2013 (H7N9) virus. H7N9 VLP-immunized ferrets were challenged with homologous virus. After challenge, VLP-vaccinated animals displayed reductions in fever, weight loss, and virus shedding as compared to the same parameters in the unimmunized control ferrets. H7N9 VLP was also effective in protecting against lung and tracheal infection. The addition of either ISCOMATRIX or Matrix-M1 adjuvant further improved immunogenicity and protection of the VLP vaccine against H7N9 virus [31].

Another recombinant influenza vaccine was developed by expressing H7 from H7N9 (A/Shanghai/2/2013) on the surface of recombinant baculovirus. Although this approach would not result in a typical influenza VLP morphology, the spatial conformation of H7 in the resulting vaccine is expected to be similar to that in an influenza virion or in a cognate VLP. Mice were immunized twice, either intranasally or subcutaneously, with the vaccine. The immunogenicity and cross-protective efficacy of the vaccine were evaluated against H7N9 or H7N7 subtype challenges. The authors concluded that intranasal administration of H7 protein expressed on the baculovirus envelope can be an alternative way to prime the immune system against influenza infection during a pandemic situation [64]. Recently, a baculovirus vaccine expressing the HA of H7N9 strain A/Chicken/Jiaxing/148/2014 was prepared [65]. The recombinant baculovirus-HA generated in this study showed favorable growth characteristics in insect cells, good safety profile, and induced high-level hemagglutination inhibition antibody titer. Moreover, this vaccine demonstrated better efficacy than inactivated whole-virus vaccine JX148, provided complete protection of chickens against challenge with HPAI H7N9 virus, and effectively inhibited viral shedding.

Plant-based VLP vaccines can be produced from *Agrobacterium*-mediated transient expression of influenza HA proteins in *Nicotiana benthamiana*. Plant-made H1 or H5 VLPs mimicked the structure of influenza virions to some extent, they are immunogenic and elicit both humoral and cellular responses [66,67]. Each HA-only particle contains 30–50 homo-trimer HA incorporated into lipid bilayer envelope of plant cell origin [68]. Plant-based recombinant VLP vaccines elicited humoral and cellular responses and protected against challenges. For example, a plant-derived VLP vaccine based on the HA of influenza H7N9 A/Hangzhou/1/2013 was prepared, with no other influenza proteins included in the vaccine. The immunogenicity of such H7-only VLP vaccine was assessed in mice and ferrets after one or two intramuscular dose(s) with, and without, adjuvant (alum or GLA-SE™). In ferrets, H7-specific cell-mediated immunity was also evaluated. The mice and ferrets were challenged with H7N9 A/Anhui/1/2013 influenza virus. A single immunization with the adjuvanted vaccine elicited a strong humoral response and protected mice against an otherwise lethal challenge. Two doses of unadjuvanted vaccine significantly increased humoral response and resulted in 100% protection with significant reduction in clinical signs, leading to nearly asymptomatic infections. In ferrets, a single immunization with the alum-adjuvanted H7 VLP vaccine induced strong humoral and CMI responses with antigen-specific activation of CD3(+) T cells. This plant-made H7 vaccine therefore induced protective responses after either one adjuvanted or two unadjuvanted doses [39]. Potentially, the plant-based transient expression system can allow the production of VLP structures, which contain HA only, without other influenza proteins.

The recombinant HA-only H7 vaccine against H7N9 virus has been also prepared in insect cells [30]. The study has shown that purified HA formed rosette-shaped nanoparticles of approximately 30–50 nm in diameter [69]. Similarly, subviral particles containing the full-length H7 rHA (A/Anhui/1/2013 (H7N9) were isolated from Sf9 cells treated with mild detergent [38]. Similarly to a previous study [30], purified rHA formed particulate structures; the particles were approximately 20 nm in diameter, exhibited hemagglutination activity, and consisted of approximately 3–4 trimers of the full-length HA molecules.

4. Considerations for Immune Responses and Protection

As noted above, immunization with VLPs have shown promising results in protecting from influenza infections with H7N9 [27,70,71] (Table 2). Potentially, antibody induced by VLPs can be more effective than those of subunit vaccines containing recombinant protein antigens [72]. In addition, experimental VLP vaccines generally show higher protective rates to high-risk groups such as children and the elderly [26]. However, the full spectrum of factors affecting immunogenicity of VLPs requires additional studies. For example, it has been shown that amino acid residues of HA that are related to receptor specificity can affect the protective efficacy of H5N1 and H7N9 vaccines in mice [44]. H7N9 VLP vaccine that contained L226 (mammalian specificity) and G228 (avian specificity) in HA showed better immunogenicity and protection efficacy than VLP containing HA with either L226 + S228 or Q226 + S228. This observation indicated that specific HA residues could enhance a vaccine's protection efficacy and HA glycoproteins with both avian-type and human-type receptor specificities may produce better pandemic influenza vaccines for humans [44].

While inactivated vaccines have been shown to induce predominantly systemic humoral response, VLP vaccines stimulate both humoral and cellular immune responses. H7N9 VLPs secreted from 293T cells triggered both humoral and cellular immune responses in mice. This vaccine produced higher levels and antibody and isotypes of IgG, as well as cross-reactive HAI titer against heterologous H1N1 and H1N3 subtypes [43].

The presence of NA and potentially other IAV proteins in VLP could be beneficial. The NA was demonstrated to protect host from influenza infection [73]. Mice immunized with NA VLPs (without HA) were protected against lethal challenge of homologous A/PR/8/34 virus without any weight loss [74].

Furthermore, both the exterior and interior of VLPs can be altered to enhance their stability and immunogenicity. Various adjuvants such as alum, CpG DNA, monophosphoryl lipid A (MPL), poly IC, gardiquimod, cholera toxin (CT) can be encapsulated into VLPs by exogenous and endogenous methods [75,76]. These adjuvanted VLPs show higher levels of antibodies in both sera and mucosa. In another study, adjuvants that stimulate TLR3 or NLPR3 pathways showed higher efficiency of influenza VLP vaccine in aged group of mice [77]. The CpG-adjuvanted intranasal immunization with an egg-derived split H7N9 vaccine offered a high level of protection against H7N9 infection in mice [78].

5. Human Clinical Trials with H7N9 VLP Vaccines

Two phase I clinical trials of experimental H7N9 VLP vaccines with, and without, adjuvant have been completed, NCT01897701 and NCT02078674. The first study enrolled 284 adults (≥18 years of age) in a randomized, observer-blinded, placebo-controlled clinical trial [79]. Interestingly enough, significant increases in N9 neuraminidase-inhibiting antibodies occurred in up to 71.9% of recipients of the vaccine without adjuvant, 92.0% of recipients of vaccine with 30 units of adjuvant, and 97.2% of recipients of vaccine with 60 units of adjuvant. Remarkably, the vaccines that were studied were released for human use within 3 months after the availability of the HA and NA sequences. This illustrates the possibility of rapid response to the public health emergency situations, such as in the case of pandemic influenza outbreaks, as well as other health emergencies such as the ongoing COVID-19 coronavirus pandemic.

In another previously reported phase I clinical trial, subjects vaccinated with two doses of an unadjuvanted H7N9 VLP vaccine responded poorly (15.6% seroconversion rates with 45 μg HA dose). In contrast, 80.6% of subjects receiving H7N9 VLP vaccine (5μg HA) with ISCOMATRIX adjuvant developed HAI responses [80]. The results suggest that adjuvants can be important component for the development of safe and effective H7N9 human vaccines [81].

Plant-derived quadrivalent seasonal VLP vaccine has been evaluated and elicited cross-reactive antibody and T cell response in healthy adults [82]. Although H7N9 antigens have not been included in this study, the confirmed safety profile of VLP in humans suggests an attractive alternative manufacturing method for producing effective and HA-strain matching influenza vaccines.

6. Broadly Protective Influenza VLP Vaccines

Current annual vaccines (inactivated, live attenuated, and recombinant subunit) protect from circulating, antigenically matching IAV and influenza B virus strains. Broad protection is difficult to achieve because of the frequent emergence of new strains [83]. Therefore, current approved and experimental vaccines have limited protection against antigenically mismatched variants and newly emerging viral strains. For new strains, antigenically matching new vaccines have to be developed within short periods of time. Therefore, vaccines are needed that can protect from an antigenically divergent strain, especially from potentially pandemic viruses with a new HA subtype. In addition to H7N9 virus described above, multiple other viruses with pandemic potential, including H5N1, H9N2, and H10N8 subtypes, that have caused human infections in the past, continue to circulate in birds and other animals. Therefore, vaccines capable of protecting against multiple potentially pandemic influenza strains would be advantageous for pandemic preparedness and public health.

One way to achieve protection against multiple strains and increase the breadth of immune response afforded by VLPs can be a blended formulation of monovalent vaccines. A vaccine was prepared by mixing VLPs that display H1, H3, H5 or H7 HA molecules. Mice vaccinated with these VLPs intranasally showed significant protection (94% aggregate survival following vaccination) against 1918 H1, 1957 H2, and avian H5, H6, H7, H10 and H11 HA subtypes [41]. These experiments suggest a promising and practical strategy for developing a broadly protective influenza vaccine.

Potentially, HA molecules from different subtypes can be co-localized within recombinant VLP envelope for broader immune coverage. A multi-subtype, mosaic VLP design containing three or four subtypes of the full-length rHA within the envelope has also been described [50,71]. A triple-subtype VLP contained HA proteins from the potentially pandemic H5N1, H7N2, and H9N2 subtypes [50]. A recombinant baculovirus vector was prepared to co-express the H5, H7, and H9 genes from A/Viet Nam/1203/2004 (H5N1), A/New York/107/2003 (H7N2) and A/Hong Kong/33982/2009 (H9N2) viruses, respectively, as well as NA and M1 genes from A/Puerto Rico/8/1934 (H1N1) virus. VLPs were prepared in Sf9 cells, and the immunogenicity and efficacy of the resulting H5/H7/H9 VLPs were evaluated in a ferret animal model following intranasal (i.n.) vaccination. We showed that i.n. vaccination with the H5/H7/H9 triple-subtype VLP induced immune responses and protected ferrets from experimental challenges with three subtypes of avian influenza viruses [50]. We also prepared triple-HA mosaic VLPs that co-localized A/Vietnam/1203/2004 (H5N1), A/Hong Kong/33982/2009 (H9N2) and A/Shanghai/2/2013 (H7N9) rHA proteins, as well as quadri-HA VLPs (Figure 3).

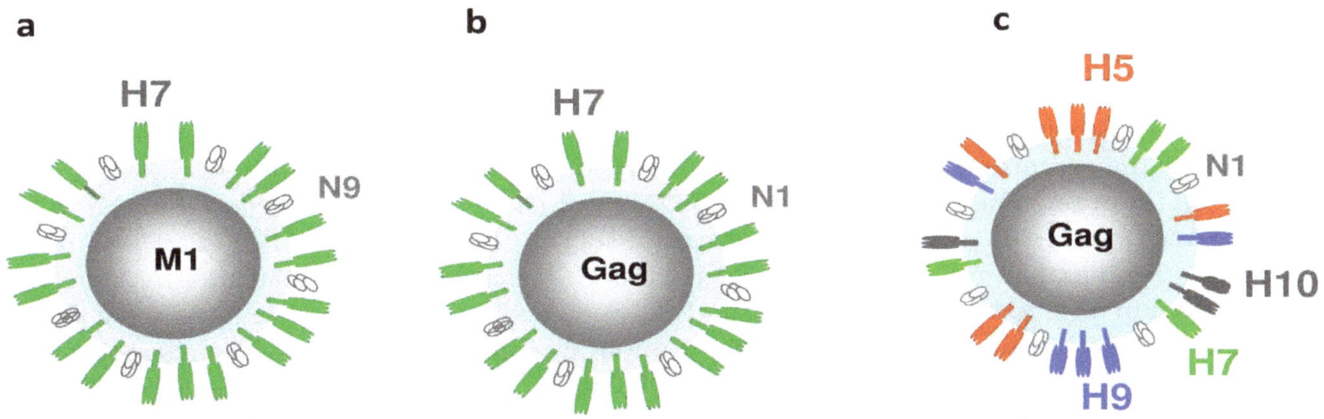

Figure 3. Structural proteins in mono- and quadri-subtype VLPs. (**a**) Mono-subtype H7N9 VLP with H7, N9 and M1 genes; (**b**) Mono-subtype chimeric H7N1 VLP with H7, N1, and Gag genes; (**c**) Quadri-subtype VLPs co-localizing H5, H7, H9 and H10 subtypes along with N1 and Gag within a VLP.

By using Group antigen (Gag) derived from bovine retrovirus as a VLP core in place of M1 protein, quadri-subtype VLPs were prepared, which co-expressed within the VLP the four HA subtypes derived from avian-origin H5N1, H7N9, H9N2 and H10N8 viruses. VLPs showed hemagglutination and neuraminidase activities and reacted with specific antisera [84]. Quadri-subtype vaccine elicited serum antibody in ferrets to the homologous H5, H7, H9, and H10 antigens. Antiserum was also evaluated for cross-reaction with multiple clades of H5N1 virus, and cross-reactivity has been confirmed. The level of immune response suggests protection against multiple influenza subtypes, which was experimentally confirmed by challenge with H10 IAV. Ferrets were protected from challenge with H10 virus [85]. Overall, such multi-subtype, mosaic VLPs that co-localize distinct HA subtypes in the envelope showed broader protection range against different influenza viruses [47,85,86]. Multi-subtype mosaic VLPs combine advantages of conserved HA epitope and blended VLPs, as VLPs contain both subtype-specific head epitopes and the conserved stem epitopes.

Recently, a VLP preparation consisting of retroviral Gag-VLPs pseudo-typed with the HA was expressed using the novel *Trichoplusia ni* (*T.ni*)-derived insect cell line *Tnms*42 and tested successfully to assess the sole contribution of anti-HA immunity in limiting post-influenza secondary *Staphylococcus aureus* bacterial infection, morbidity and mortality in a situation of a vaccine match and mismatch [87]. The results demonstrate that matched anti-HA immunity elicited by a VLP preparation may suffice to prevent morbidity and mortality caused by lethal secondary bacterial infection.

It should also be noted that cross-reactive antibodies to the H7N9 virus were also induced by recombinant viral vectors, such as Newcastle disease virus (NDV) [88–90] and parainfluenza virus PIV5 [91].

7. Expression of H7N9 Influenza Epitopes Using VLP Carriers

The emerging strains potentially can be also targeted by "universal" vaccines consisting of conserved viral proteins or epitopes, such as stem region of HA, or extracellular domain M2e of the ion channel protein M2, which are both considered capable of inducing cross-reactive immune responses. Targeting the stem region of HA for antibody production could be a promising approach to generate a broadly protective influenza vaccine. The immune response can be elicited against both the head and stem region of HA protein. However, because of the constantly changing nature of the head region due to the antigenic drift, new vaccine candidates need to be updated frequently. Since the stem region is evolutionally more stable and more conserved among different influenza strains, vaccine candidates targeting the stem region might not need to be updated every year and could induce a broad range of protective immunity against different influenza strains [92,93]. However, the stem region is less immunogenic in the virus. Therefore, chimeric VLP approaches have been used to elicit antibodies to the stem region of HA. The long alpha-helix (LAH) region located in influenza virus hemagglutinin (HA) shows conservation among different influenza A strains, and could be used as a candidate target for influenza vaccines. The hepatitis B virus core protein (HBc) was used as a carrier for heterologous LAH epitopes to elicit effective immune responses [94]. The spatial conformation of LAH epitope cloned in the major immunodominant region (MIR) of the HBc molecule and expressed in yeast is shown on Figure 4. The LAH region of the H7N9 influenza virus was inserted into the HBc to prepare chimeric LAH-HBc protein, which was capable of self-assembly into VLPs in *E. coli* expression system [95]. Intranasal immunization of the LAH-HBc VLP in combination with chitosan adjuvant or CTB* adjuvant in mice induced both humoral and cellular immune responses effectively and conferred complete protection against lethal challenge with homologous H7N9 virus or heterologous H3N2 virus, as well as partial protection against lethal challenge of heterologous H1N1 virus. These results provide a proof of concept for LAH-HBc VLP vaccine that can be rapidly produced and potentially can serve as an antigen against a future influenza pandemic [95].

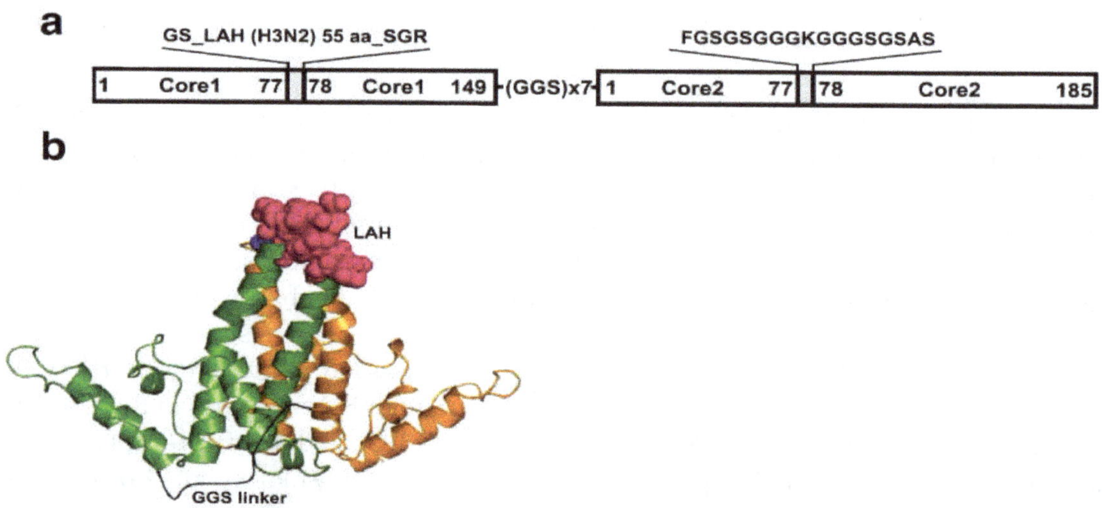

Figure 4. An example of expression of influenza epitope using chimeric VLP based on recombinant LAH3-HBc gene. Design (**a**) and cartoon (**b**) of the LAH3-HBc dimer. Individual hepatitis B virus core protein (HBc) monomers are shown in green and orange. The first major immunodominant region (MIR) contains the LAH domain (the 55 amino acid long influenza H3N2 virus (A/Hong Kong/1/1968, Accession No. AAK51718) HA stalk domain, corresponding to HA amino acids 420–474, shown as pink spheres) while the second MIR contains lysine linker (blue spheres)). The model was created using PyMOL version 1.7rc1. The tandem core dimer is based on the structure from PDB-1QGT, with the linker shown in black.

In another study, the globular head domain (HA1-2, aa 62–284) of the protective H7 HA was fused to the potent TLR5 ligand, *Salmonella typhimurium* flagellin (FliC) [96]. The resulting fusion protein, HA1-2-fliC, which apparently did not form VLPs, was efficiently expressed in *E. coli*, retained the native HA and fliC conformations, and was highly immunogenic in mice by intraperitoneal vaccination. Furthermore, highly immunogenic influenza VLPs have been prepared via the overexpression of four viral proteins, HA, NA, M1, and M2, using M2 fusion with the FliC [97]. The chimeric H5N1 VLPs were further combined with the molecular adjuvant, granulocyte-macrophage colony-stimulating factor (GM-CSF), FliC, or a GM-CSF/FliC [98]. All three forms of the chimeric H5N1 VLPs elicited protective immunity against live virus. Next, the GM-CSF/FliC H5N1 VLPs were obtained to include H7 or H1H7 antigens for developing multi-subtype influenza vaccines [98].

The chimeric norovirus VLPs, P particles, were used to express the trivalent HA2:90-105 epitopes derived from H1, H3 and B subtypes, with 24 copies in total, on the surface loops [99].

Finally, trimeric H7 transiently expressed in *N. benthamiana* was conjugated successfully onto the surface of nanodiamond particles [100]. After two or three immunizations in mice, the mixture of trimeric H7 protein and nanodiamond elicited statistically significant stronger H7-specific-IgG response demonstrated by higher amounts of H7N9-specific IgG.

Other universal influenza vaccine approaches applicable to H7N9 were based on ion channel protein M2. Extracellular part of M2 protein, ~23 aa residues, is highly conserved among human IAV strains, suggesting its potential utility as a broadly protective immunogen for the development of broadly protective influenza vaccines. Tandem repeats of heterologous M2e sequences (M2e5x) derived from human, swine, and avian origin influenza A viruses were expressed on influenza VLPs in a membrane-anchored form. Immunization of mice with M2e5x VLPs induced antibodies that were cross-reactive to antigenically distinct influenza A viruses and conferred cross-protection [101]. Furthermore, the M2e5x VLPs demonstrated a clear advantage in inducing IgG2a isotype antibodies, T cell responses, plasma cells and germinal center B cells as well as in conferring cross protection [102]. These studies paved the way to a novel vaccination strategy by enhancing the cross protective efficacy of live attenuated influenza virus vaccines by supplemented vaccination with M2e5x VLPs [103].

High immunogenicity in mice, even in the absence of adjuvants, was demonstrated by the M2e displayed on VLPs of *Macrobrachium rosenbergii* nodavirus [104,105]. This novel vaccine candidate was tested by the H1N1 and H3N2 challenge in mice, and potentially, it can be universal and applicable to H7N9 virus. In another example, the M2e proteins, as well as NA, were expressed on recombinant *Lactococcus lactis*, which conferred effective mucosal and systemic immune responses [106].

8. Challenges for Recombinant VLPs as Influenza Vaccines

Heterogenous composition is one of the challenges associated with the use of influenza VLPs as a vaccine candidate. VLPs produced by using baculovirus expression system contain live baculovirus vector as impurity. Moreover, considerable fraction of HA protein is bound to viral envelope of baculovirus [107]. Therefore, it is difficult to distinguish whether the HA activity is associated with influenza VLP or with baculovirus-displayed HA in the unpurified samples during vaccine manufacturing, which also causes difficulty for HA quantification. VLPs produced from mammalian expression system do not contain baculovirus contamination but they contain extracellular particles and produce low yields, with VLPs needing to be concentrated up to 200 times to reach measurable titers [72]. The current methods that are used for quantification are mostly applicable to concentrated and purified VLPs; however, better methods need to be developed to characterize the materials at the different stage of bioprocessing during the manufacturing process. Other potential challenges include the presence of endogenous rhabdovirus in standard Sf9 cell lines [108]. Although insect rhabdovirus is not associated with any human disease, the development of rhabdovirus-free cell line can resolve this potential safety concern [108,109].

To overcome manufacturing challenges, technological improvements to production of H7N9 VLPs in baculovirus-Sf9 insect cell cultures have been reported [110–112]. The yield and quality of influenza VLPs produced in insect cells could be improved by inhibiting cytopathic effects of the protein M2 [62]. The ion channel activity of M2 induces significant cytopathic effects in Sf9 insect cells. These effects include altered Sf9 cell morphology and reduced baculovirus replication, resulting in impaired influenza protein expression and thus VLP production. The use of the M2 inhibitor amantadine indeed improved Sf9 cellular expression not only of M2 (~three-fold), but also of HA (~seven-fold) and of matrix protein M1 (~three-fold) when co-expressed to produce influenza VLPs. This increased cellular expression of all three influenza proteins further led to ~two-fold greater VLP yield. The quality of the resulting influenza VLPs was significantly improved, as demonstrated by the ~two-fold, ~50-fold, and ~two-fold increase in the antigen density to approximately 53 HA, 48 M1, and 156 M2 per influenza VLP, respectively [62].

For purification of influenza VLPs, a nitrocellulose membrane-based filtration system [113] and a cascade of ultrafiltration and diafiltration steps, followed by a sterile filtration step [109,114] were used successfully. The bioprocessing of influenza VLPs was recently reviewed [115]. Recently, a fast chromatography step purification method was developed for chimeric HIV-1 Gag influenza-HA VLPs produced in *Tnms*42 insect cells using the baculovirus insect cell expression vector system [116]. The absence of the baculovirus capsid protein p39 in the product fraction was confirmed by HPLC-MS. The process is simple and includes only a few handling steps, which has promising characteristics to become a platform for purification of these types of VLPs [116].

Regarding the detection and quality assessment of influenza vaccines, several methodologies are being used. These include development of standards for potency determination [117]. A high-resolution LC-MS method allows the quantitation of both HA and NA protein concentrations in influenza VLP vaccine candidates [118].

9. Conclusions

Recombinant VLPs were developed with the purpose of rapidly preparing influenza vaccines including against pandemic threat viruses such as H7N9 virus. Multiple designs of VLPs have been evaluated including the use of multivalent VLPs, multi-subtype mosaic VLP, and rationally designed VLPs containing conserved influenza virus epitopes. The use of highly conserved epitopes remains a promising approach for the improved design of highly immunogenic VLPs. Blended VLPs have been used as a classic approach to broaden immune coverage. Multi-subtype mosaic VLPs potentially combine the conserved epitope and blended approaches, as VLPs contain both subtype-specific head epitopes and the conserved stem epitopes. In addition to VLPs, other novel technologies have been used to develop improved influenza vaccines including DNA vaccines, viral vectors, advanced adjuvants, and other approaches. Potentially, the combination of various technologies can prove beneficial for the development of next-generation influenza vaccines including H7N9.

Acknowledgments: We thank Tek Lamichhane and Paul Pumpens for their valuable contributions. This works was supported by the NIH NIAID grant R43AI136220. The views and conclusions in this report are those of the authors and do not necessarily reflect the views of the funding agency.

References

1. Gostin, L.O.; Phelan, A.; Stoto, M.A.; Kraemer, J.D.; Reddy, K.S. Virus sharing, genetic sequencing, and global health security. *Science* **2014**, *345*, 1295–1296. [CrossRef] [PubMed]
2. Dormitzer, P.R.; Suphaphiphat, P.; Gibson, D.G.; Wentworth, D.E.; Stockwell, T.B.; Algire, M.A.; Alperovich, N.; Barro, M.; Brown, D.M.; Craig, S.; et al. Synthetic generation of influenza vaccine viruses for rapid response to pandemics. *Sci. Transl. Med.* **2013**, *5*, 185ra68. [CrossRef] [PubMed]
3. Mostafa, A.; Abdelwhab, E.M.; Mettenleiter, T.C.; Pleschka, S. Zoonotic Potential of Influenza A Viruses: A Comprehensive Overview. *Viruses* **2018**, *10*, 497. [CrossRef] [PubMed]
4. Philippon, D.A.M.; Wu, P.; Cowling, B.J.; Lau, E.H.Y. Avian influenza human infections at the human-animal interface. *J. Infect. Dis.* **2020**. [CrossRef]
5. Wu, X.; Xiao, L.; Li, L. Research progress on human infection with avian influenza H7N9. *Front. Med.* **2020**, *14*, 8–20. [CrossRef]
6. Yoon, S.W.; Webby, R.J.; Webster, R.G. Evolution and ecology of influenza A viruses. *Curr. Top. Microbiol. Immunol.* **2014**, *385*, 359–375.
7. Gao, R.; Cao, B.; Hu, Y.; Feng, Z.; Wang, D.; Hu, W.; Chen, J.; Jie, Z.; Qiu, H.; Xu, K.; et al. Human infection with a novel avian-origin influenza A (H7N9) virus. *N. Engl. J. Med.* **2013**, *368*, 1888–1897. [CrossRef]
8. Chen, F.; Li, J.; Sun, B.; Zhang, H.; Zhang, R.; Yuan, J.; Ou, X.; Ye, W.; Chen, J.; Liu, Y.; et al. Isolation and characteristic analysis of a novel strain H7N9 of avian influenza virus A from a patient with influenza-like symptoms in China. *Int. J. Infect. Dis.* **2015**, *33*, 130–131. [CrossRef]

9. Pu, J.; Wang, S.; Yin, Y.; Zhang, G.; Carter, R.A.; Wang, J.; Xu, G.; Sun, H.; Wang, M.; Wen, C.; et al. Evolution of the H9N2 influenza genotype that facilitated the genesis of the novel H7N9 virus. *Proc. Natl. Acad. Sci. USA* **2015**, *112*, 548–553. [CrossRef]
10. Jones, J.C.; Sonnberg, S.; Webby, R.J.; Webster, R.G. Influenza A(H7N9) Virus Transmission between Finches and Poultry. *Emerg. Infect. Dis.* **2015**, *21*, 619–628. [CrossRef]
11. Zaraket, H.; Baranovich, T.; Kaplan, B.S.; Carter, R.; Song, M.S.; Paulson, J.C.; Rehg, J.E.; Bahl, J.; Crumpton, J.C.; Seiler, J.; et al. Mammalian adaptation of influenza A(H7N9) virus is limited by a narrow genetic bottleneck. *Nat. Commun.* **2015**, *6*, 6553. [CrossRef] [PubMed]
12. Yang, J.R.; Kuo, C.Y.; Huang, H.Y.; Wu, F.T.; Huang, Y.L.; Cheng, C.Y.; Su, Y.T.; Wu, H.S.; Liu, M.T. Characterization of Influenza A (H7N9) Viruses Isolated from Human Cases Imported into Taiwan. *PLoS ONE* **2015**, *10*, e0119792. [CrossRef] [PubMed]
13. Yu, D.; Xiang, G.; Zhu, W.; Lei, X.; Li, B.; Meng, Y.; Yang, L.; Jiao, H.; Li, X.; Huang, W.; et al. The re-emergence of highly pathogenic avian influenza H7N9 viruses in humans in mainland China, 2019. *Eurosurveillance* **2019**, *24*, 1900273. [CrossRef] [PubMed]
14. Horimoto, T.; Nakayama, K.; Smeekens, S.P.; Kawaoka, Y. Proprotein-processing endoproteases PC6 and furin both activate hemagglutinin of virulent avian influenza viruses. *J. Virol.* **1994**, *68*, 6074–6078. [CrossRef] [PubMed]
15. Ito, M.; Yamayoshi, S.; Murakami, K.; Saito, K.; Motojima, A.; Nakaishi, K.; Kawaoka, Y. Characterization of Mouse Monoclonal Antibodies Against the HA of A(H7N9) Influenza Virus. *Viruses* **2019**, *11*, 149. [CrossRef]
16. Guo, Z.; Xiao, D.; Li, D.; Wang, Y.; Yan, T.; Dai, B. The temporal distribution of new H7N9 avian influenza infections based on laboratory-confirmed cases in Mainland China, 2013–2017. *Sci. Rep.* **2018**, *8*, 4051. [CrossRef]
17. Isakova-Sivak, I.; Rudenko, L. Tackling a novel lethal virus: A focus on H7N9 vaccine development. *Expert Rev. Vaccines* **2017**, *16*, 1–13. [CrossRef]
18. Trombetta, C.M.; Marchi, S.; Manini, I.; Lazzeri, G.; Montomoli, E. Challenges in the development of egg-independent vaccines for influenza. *Expert Rev. Vaccines* **2019**, *18*, 737–750. [CrossRef]
19. Gerdil, C. The annual production cycle for influenza vaccine. *Vaccine* **2003**, *21*, 1776–1779. [CrossRef]
20. WHO. *Department of Immunization, Vaccines and Biologicals. Geneva: Global Pandemic Influenza Action Plan to Increase Vaccine Supply 2006*; WHO: Geneva, Switzerland, 2006.
21. WHO. *Summary of Status of Development and Availability of Avian Influenza A(H7N9) Candidate Vaccine Viruses and Potency Testing Reagents*; WHO: Geneva, Switzerland, 2020.
22. Woo, E.J.; Moro, P.L.; Cano, M.; Jankosky, C. Postmarketing safety surveillance of trivalent recombinant influenza vaccine: Reports to the Vaccine Adverse Event Reporting System. *Vaccine* **2017**, *35*, 5618–5621. [CrossRef]
23. Galarza, J.M.; Latham, T.; Cupo, A. Virus-like particle (VLP) vaccine conferred complete protection against a lethal influenza virus challenge. *Viral Immunol.* **2005**, *18*, 244–251. [CrossRef] [PubMed]
24. Kang, S.M.; Pushko, P.; Bright, R.A.; Smith, G.; Compans, R.W. Influenza virus-like particles as pandemic vaccines. *Curr. Top. Microbiol. Immunol.* **2009**, *333*, 269–289. [PubMed]
25. Perrone, L.A.; Ahmad, A.; Veguilla, V.; Lu, X.; Smith, G.; Katz, J.M.; Pushko, P.; Tumpey, T.M. Intranasal vaccination with 1918 influenza virus-like particles protects mice and ferrets from lethal 1918 and H5N1 influenza virus challenge. *J. Virol.* **2009**, *83*, 5726–5734. [CrossRef] [PubMed]
26. Bright, R.A.; Carter, D.M.; Daniluk, S.; Toapanta, F.R.; Ahmad, A.; Gavrilov, V.; Massare, M.; Pushko, P.; Mytle, N.; Roweet, T.; et al. Influenza virus-like particles elicit broader immune responses than whole virion inactivated influenza virus or recombinant hemagglutinin. *Vaccine* **2007**, *25*, 3871–3878. [CrossRef] [PubMed]
27. Pushko, P.; Tumpey, T.M.; Bu, F.; Knell, J.; Robinson, R.; Smith, G. Influenza virus-like particles comprised of the, H.A.; NA, and M1 proteins of H9N2 influenza virus induce protective immune responses in BALB/c mice. *Vaccine* **2005**, *23*, 5751–5759. [CrossRef] [PubMed]
28. Quan, F.S.; Vunnava, A.; Compans, R.W.; Kang, S.M. Virus-like particle vaccine protects against 2009 H1N1 pandemic influenza virus in mice. *PLoS ONE* **2010**, *5*, e9161. [CrossRef]
29. Ross, T.M.; Mahmood, K.; Crevar, C.J.; Schneider-Ohrum, K.; Heaton, P.M.; Bright, R.A. A trivalent virus-like particle vaccine elicits protective immune responses against seasonal influenza strains in mice and ferrets. *PLoS ONE* **2009**, *4*, e6032. [CrossRef]

30. Buckland, B.; Boulanger, R.; Fino, M.; Srivastava, I.; Holtz, K.; Khramtsov, N.; McPherson, C.; Meghrous, J.; Kubera, P.; Cox, M.M. Technology transfer and scale-up of the Flublok recombinant hemagglutinin (HA) influenza vaccine manufacturing process. *Vaccine* **2014**, *32*, 5496–5502. [CrossRef]
31. Liu, Y.V.; Massare, M.J.; Pearce, M.B.; Sun, X.; Belser, J.A.; Maines, T.R.; Creager, H.M.; Glenn, G.M.; Pushko, P.; Smith, G.E.; et al. Recombinant virus-like particles elicit protective immunity against avian influenza A(H7N9) virus infection in ferrets. *Vaccine* **2015**, *33*, 2152–2158. [CrossRef] [PubMed]
32. Smith, G.E.; Sun, X.; Bai, Y.; Liu, Y.V.; Massare, M.J.; Pearce, M.B.; Belser, J.A.; Maines, T.R.; Creager, H.M.; Glenn, G.M.; et al. Neuraminidase-based recombinant virus-like particles protect against lethal avian influenza A(H5N1) virus infection in ferrets. *Virology* **2017**, *509*, 90–97. [CrossRef]
33. Kingstad-Bakke, B.; Kamlangdee, A.; Osorio, J.E. Mucosal administration of raccoonpox virus expressing highly pathogenic avian H5N1 influenza neuraminidase is highly protective against H5N1 and seasonal influenza virus challenge. *Vaccine* **2015**, *33*, 5155–5162. [CrossRef] [PubMed]
34. Chen, Z.; Wang, J.; Bao, L.; Guo, L.; Zhang, W.; Xue, Y.; Zhou, H.; Xiao, Y.; Wang, J.; Wu, F.; et al. Human monoclonal antibodies targeting the haemagglutinin glycoprotein can neutralize H7N9 influenza virus. *Nat. Commun.* **2015**, *6*, 6714. [CrossRef] [PubMed]
35. Schmeisser, F.; Vasudevan, A.; Verma, S.; Wang, W.; Alvarado, E.; Weiss, C.; Atukorale, V.; Meseda, C.; Weir, J.P. Antibodies to antigenic site A of influenza H7 hemagglutinin provide protection against H7N9 challenge. *PLoS ONE* **2015**, *10*, e0117108. [CrossRef] [PubMed]
36. Perez Rubio, A.; Eiros, J.M. Cell culture-derived flu vaccine: Present and future. *Hum. Vaccines Immunother.* **2018**, *14*, 1874–1882. [CrossRef]
37. Krammer, F.; Albrecht, R.A.; Tan, G.S.; Margine, I.; Hai, R.; Schmolke, M.; Runstadler, J.; Andrews, S.F.; Wilson, P.C.; Cox, R.J.; et al. Divergent H7 immunogens offer protection from H7N9 virus challenge. *J. Virol.* **2014**, *88*, 3976–3985. [CrossRef]
38. Pushko, P.; Pujanauski, L.M.; Sun, X.; Pearce, M.; Hidajat, R.; Kort, T.; Schwartzman, L.M.; Tretyakova, I.; Chunqing, L.; Taubenberger, J.K.; et al. Recombinant H7 Hemagglutinin Forms Subviral Particles that Protect Mice and Ferrets from Challenge with H7N9 Influenza Virus submitted for publication. *Vaccine* **2015**, *33*, 4975–4982. [CrossRef]
39. Pillet, S.; Racine, T.; Nfon, C.; Di Lenardo, T.Z.; Babiuk, S.; Ward, B.J.; Kobinger, G.P.; Landry, N. Plant-derived H7 VLP vaccine elicits protective immune response against H7N9 influenza virus in mice and ferrets. *Vaccine* **2015**, *33*, 6282–6289. [CrossRef]
40. Klausberger, M.; Wilde, M.; Palmberger, D.; Hai, R.; Albrecht, R.A.; Margine, I.; Hirsh, A.; Garcia-Sastre, A.; Grabherr, R.; Krammer, F. One-shot vaccination with an insect cell-derived low-dose influenza A H7 virus-like particle preparation protects mice against H7N9 challenge. *Vaccine* **2014**, *32*, 355–362. [CrossRef]
41. Schwartzman, L.M.; Cathcart, A.L.; Pujanauski, L.M.; Qi, L.; Kash, J.C.; Taubenberger, J.K. An Intranasal Virus-Like Particle Vaccine Broadly Protects Mice from Multiple Subtypes of Influenza A Virus. *MBio* **2015**, *6*, e01044. [CrossRef]
42. Smith, G.E.; Flyer, D.C.; Raghunandan, R.; Liu, Y.; Wei, Z.; Wu, Y.; Kpamegan, E.; Courbron, D.; Fries, L.F., 3rd; Glenn, G.M. Development of influenza H7N9 virus like particle (VLP) vaccine: Homologous A/Anhui/1/2013 (H7N9) protection and heterologous A/chicken/Jalisco/CPA1/2012 (H7N3) cross-protection in vaccinated mice challenged with H7N9 virus. *Vaccine* **2013**, *31*, 4305–4313. [CrossRef]
43. Zhang, L.; Lu, J.; Chen, Y.; Shi, F.; Yu, H.; Huang, C.; Cui, L.; Shi, Z.; Jiao, Y.; Hu, Y. Characterization of Humoral Responses Induced by an H7N9 Influenza Virus-Like Particle Vaccine in BALB/C Mice. *Viruses* **2015**, *7*, 4369–4384. [CrossRef] [PubMed]
44. Xu, L.; Bao, L.; Lau, S.Y.; Wu, W.L.; Yuan, J.; Gu, S.; Li, F.; Lv, Q.; Xu, Y.; Pushko, P.; et al. Hemagglutinin amino acids related to receptor specificity could affect the protection efficacy of H5N1 and H7N9 avian influenza virus vaccines in mice. *Vaccine* **2016**, *34*, 2627–2633. [CrossRef] [PubMed]
45. Hu, C.J.; Chien, C.Y.; Liu, M.T.; Fang, Z.S.; Chang, S.Y.; Juang, R.H.; Chang, S.C.; Chen, H.W. Multi-antigen avian influenza a (H7N9) virus-like particles: Particulate characterizations and immunogenicity evaluation in murine and avian models. *BMC Biotechnol.* **2017**, *17*, 2. [CrossRef] [PubMed]
46. Ren, Z.; Zhao, Y.; Liu, J.; Ji, X.; Meng, L.; Wang, T.; Sun, W.; Zhang, K.; Sang, X.; Yu, Z.; et al. Intramuscular and intranasal immunization with an H7N9 influenza virus-like particle vaccine protects mice against lethal influenza virus challenge. *Int. Immunopharmacol.* **2018**, *58*, 109–116. [CrossRef]

47. Pushko, P.; Tretyakova, I.; Hidajat, R.; Zsak, A.; Chrzastek, K.; Tumpey, T.M.; Kapczynski, D.R. Virus-like particles displaying H5, H7, H9 hemagglutinins and N1 neuraminidase elicit protective immunity to heterologous avian influenza viruses in chickens. *Virology* **2017**, *501*, 176–182. [CrossRef]
48. Hong, J.Y.; Chen, T.H.; Chen, Y.J.; Liu, C.C.; Jan, J.T.; Wu, S.C. Highly immunogenic influenza virus-like particles containing B-cell-activating factor (BAFF) for multi-subtype vaccine development. *Antivir. Res.* **2019**, *164*, 12–22. [CrossRef]
49. Kang, H.J.; Chu, K.B.; Lee, D.H.; Lee, S.H.; Park, B.R.; Kim, M.C.; Kang, S.M.; Quan, F.S. Influenza M2 virus-like particle vaccination enhances protection in combination with avian influenza HA VLPs. *PLoS ONE* **2019**, *14*, e0216871. [CrossRef]
50. Tretyakova, I.; Pearce, M.B.; Florese, R.; Tumpey, T.M.; Pushko, P. Intranasal vaccination with H5, H7 and H9 hemagglutinins co-localized in a virus-like particle protects ferrets from multiple avian influenza viruses. *Virology* **2013**, *442*, 67–73. [CrossRef]
51. Hervas-Stubbs, S.; Rueda, P.; Lopez, L.; Leclerc, C. Insect baculoviruses strongly potentiate adaptive immune responses by inducing type I IFN. *J. Immunol.* **2007**, *178*, 2361–2369. [CrossRef]
52. Buonaguro, L.; Tornesello, M.L.; Tagliamonte, M.; Gallo, R.C.; Wang, L.X.; Kamin-Lewis, R.; Abdelwahab, S.; Lewis, G.K.; Buonaguro, F.M. Baculovirus-derived human immunodeficiency virus type 1 virus-like particles activate dendritic cells and induce ex vivo T-cell responses. *J. Virol.* **2006**, *80*, 9134–9143. [CrossRef]
53. Sailaja, G.; Skountzou, I.; Quan, F.S.; Compans, R.W.; Kang, S.M. Human immunodeficiency virus-like particles activate multiple types of immune cells. *Virology* **2007**, *362*, 331–341. [CrossRef] [PubMed]
54. Bachmann, M.F.; Rohrer, U.H.; Kundig, T.M.; Burki, K.; Hengartner, H.; Zinkernagel, R.M. The influence of antigen organization on B cell responsiveness. *Science* **1993**, *262*, 1448–1451. [CrossRef] [PubMed]
55. McCraw, D.M.; Gallagher, J.R.; Torian, U.; Myers, M.L.; Conlon, M.T.; Gulati, N.M.; Harris, A.K. Structural analysis of influenza vaccine virus-like particles reveals a multicomponent organization. *Sci. Rep.* **2018**, *8*, 10342. [CrossRef] [PubMed]
56. Harris, A.; Cardone, G.; Winkler, D.C.; Heymann, J.B.; Brecher, M.; White, J.M. Influenza virus pleiomorphy characterized by cryoelectron tomography. *Proc. Natl. Acad. Sci. USA* **2006**, *103*, 19123–19127. [CrossRef]
57. Buffin, S.; Peubez, I.; Barriere, F.; Nicolai, M.C.; Tapia, T.; Dhir, V.; Forma, E.; Seve, N.; Legastelois, I. Influenza A and B virus-like particles produced in mammalian cells are highly immunogenic and induce functional antibodies. *Vaccine* 2019. [CrossRef]
58. Venereo-Sanchez, A.; Fulton, K.; Koczka, K.; Twine, S.; Chahal, P.; Ansorge, S.; Gilbert, R.; Henry, O.; Kamen, A. Characterization of influenza H1N1 Gag virus-like particles and extracellular vesicles co-produced in HEK-293SF. *Vaccine* **2019**, *37*, 7100–7107. [CrossRef] [PubMed]
59. Venereo-Sanchez, A.; Gilbert, R.; Simoneau, M.; Caron, A.; Chahal, P.; Chen, W.; Ansorge, S.; Li, X.; Henry, O.; Kamen, A. Hemagglutinin and neuraminidase containing virus-like particles produced in HEK-293 suspension culture: An effective influenza vaccine candidate. *Vaccine* **2016**, *34*, 3371–3380. [CrossRef]
60. Venereo-Sanchez, A.; Simoneau, M.; Lanthier, S.; Chahal, P.; Bourget, L.; Ansorge, S.; Gilbert, R.; Henry, O.; Kamen, A. Process intensification for high yield production of influenza H1N1 Gag virus-like particles using an inducible HEK-293 stable cell line. *Vaccine* **2017**, *35*, 4220–4228. [CrossRef]
61. Thompson, C.M.; Petiot, E.; Mullick, A.; Aucoin, M.G.; Henry, O.; Kamen, A.A. Critical assessment of influenza VLP production in Sf9 and HEK293 expression systems. *BMC Biotechnol.* **2015**, *15*, 31. [CrossRef]
62. Zak, A.J.; Hill, B.D.; Rizvi, S.M.; Smith, M.R.; Yang, M.; Wen, F. Enhancing the Yield and Quality of Influenza Virus-like Particles (VLPs) Produced in Insect Cells by Inhibiting Cytopathic Effects of Matrix Protein M2. *ACS Synth. Biol.* **2019**, *8*, 2303–2314. [CrossRef]
63. Li, X.; Pushko, P.; Tretyakova, I. Recombinant Hemagglutinin and Virus-Like Particle Vaccines for H7N9 Influenza Virus. *J. Vaccines Vaccin.* **2015**, *6*, 287. [PubMed]
64. Prabakaran, M.; Kumar, S.R.; Raj, K.V.; Wu, X.; He, F.; Zhou, J.; Kwang, J. Cross-protective efficacy of baculovirus displayed hemagglutinin against highly pathogenic influenza H7 subtypes. *Antivir. Res.* **2014**, *109*, 149–159. [CrossRef] [PubMed]
65. Hu, J.; Liang, Y.; Hu, Z.; Wang, X.; Gu, M.; Li, R.; Ma, C.; Liu, X.; Hu, S.; Chen, S.; et al. Recombinant baculovirus vaccine expressing hemagglutinin of H7N9 avian influenza virus confers full protection against lethal highly pathogenic H7N9 virus infection in chickens. *Arch. Virol.* **2019**, *164*, 807–817. [CrossRef] [PubMed]

66. Makarkov, A.I.; Chierzi, S.; Pillet, S.; Murai, K.K.; Landry, N.; Ward, B.J. Plant-made virus-like particles bearing influenza hemagglutinin (HA) recapitulate early interactions of native influenza virions with human monocytes/macrophages. *Vaccine* **2017**, *35*, 4629–4636. [CrossRef] [PubMed]
67. Lindsay, B.J.; Bonar, M.M.; Costas-Cancelas, I.N.; Hunt, K.; Makarkov, A.I.; Chierzi, S.; Krawczyk, C.M.; Landry, N.; Ward, B.J.; Rouiller, I. Morphological characterization of a plant-made virus-like particle vaccine bearing influenza virus hemagglutinins by electron microscopy. *Vaccine* **2018**, *36*, 2147–2154. [CrossRef]
68. Le Mauff, F.; Mercier, G.; Chan, P.; Burel, C.; Vaudry, D.; Bardor, M.; Vezina, L.P.; Couture, M.; Lerouge, P.; Landry, N. Biochemical composition of haemagglutinin-based influenza virus-like particle vaccine produced by transient expression in tobacco plants. *Plant Biotechnol. J.* **2015**, *13*, 717–725. [CrossRef]
69. Holtz, K.M.; Robinson, P.S.; Matthews, E.E.; Hashimoto, Y.; McPherson, C.E.; Khramtsov, N.; Reifler, M.J.; Meghrous, J.; Rhodes, D.G.; Cox, M.M.; et al. Modifications of cysteine residues in the transmembrane and cytoplasmic domains of a recombinant hemagglutinin protein prevents cross-linked multimer formation and potency loss. *BMC Biotechnol.* **2014**, *14*, 1. [CrossRef]
70. Latham, T.; Galarza, J.M. Formation of wild-type and chimeric influenza virus-like particles following simultaneous expression of only four structural proteins. *J. Virol.* **2001**, *75*, 6154–6165. [CrossRef]
71. Pushko, P.; Pearce, M.B.; Ahmad, A.; Tretyakova, I.; Smith, G.; Belser, J.A.; Tumpey, T.M. Influenza virus-like particle can accommodate multiple subtypes of hemagglutinin and protect from multiple influenza types and subtypes. *Vaccine* **2011**, *29*, 5911–5918. [CrossRef]
72. Thompson, C.M.; Petiot, E.; Lennaertz, A.; Henry, O.; Kamen, A.A. Analytical technologies for influenza virus-like particle candidate vaccines: Challenges and emerging approaches. *Virol. J.* **2013**, *10*, 141. [CrossRef]
73. Marcelin, G.; DuBois, R.; Rubrum, A.; Russell, C.J.; McElhaney, J.E.; Webby, R.J. A contributing role for anti-neuraminidase antibodies on immunity to pandemic H1N1 2009 influenza A virus. *PLoS ONE* **2011**, *6*, e26335. [CrossRef] [PubMed]
74. Quan, F.S.; Kim, M.C.; Lee, B.J.; Song, J.M.; Compans, R.W.; Kang, S.M. Influenza M1 VLPs containing neuraminidase induce heterosubtypic cross-protection. *Virology* **2012**, *430*, 127–135. [CrossRef] [PubMed]
75. Gomes, A.C.; Flace, A.; Saudan, P.; Zabel, F.; Cabral-Miranda, G.; Turabi, A.E.; Manolova, V.; Bachmann, M.F. Adjusted Particle Size Eliminates the Need of Linkage of Antigen and Adjuvants for Appropriated T Cell Responses in Virus-Like Particle-Based Vaccines. *Front. Immunol.* **2017**, *8*, 226. [CrossRef] [PubMed]
76. Quan, F.S.; Ko, E.J.; Kwon, Y.M.; Joo, K.H.; Compans, R.W.; Kang, S.M. Mucosal adjuvants for influenza virus-like particle vaccine. *Viral Immunol.* **2013**, *26*, 385–395. [CrossRef] [PubMed]
77. Schneider-Ohrum, K.; Giles, B.M.; Weirback, H.K.; Williams, B.L.; DeAlmeida, D.R.; Ross, T.M. Adjuvants that stimulate TLR3 or NLPR3 pathways enhance the efficiency of influenza virus-like particle vaccines in aged mice. *Vaccine* **2011**, *29*, 9081–9092. [CrossRef] [PubMed]
78. Zhou, Y.; Li, S.; Bi, S.; Li, N.; Bi, Y.; Liu, W.; Wang, B. Long-lasting protective immunity against H7N9 infection is induced by intramuscular or CpG-adjuvanted intranasal immunization with the split H7N9 vaccine. *Int. Immunopharmacol.* **2020**, *78*, 106013. [CrossRef]
79. Fries, L.F.; Smith, G.E.; Glenn, G.M. A recombinant viruslike particle influenza A (H7N9) vaccine. *N. Engl. J. Med.* **2013**, *369*, 2564–2566. [CrossRef]
80. Chung, K.Y.; Coyle, E.M.; Jani, D.; King, L.R.; Bhardwaj, R.; Fries, L.; Smith, G.; Glenn, G.; Golding, H.; Khurana, S. ISCOMATRIX adjuvant promotes epitope spreading and antibody affinity maturation of influenza A H7N9 virus like particle vaccine that correlate with virus neutralization in humans. *Vaccine* **2015**, *33*, 3953–3962. [CrossRef]
81. Zheng, D.; Gao, F.; Zhao, C.; Ding, Y.; Cao, Y.; Yang, T.; Xu, X.; Chen, Z. Comparative effectiveness of H7N9 vaccines in healthy individuals. *Hum. Vaccin. Immunother.* **2019**, *15*, 80–90. [CrossRef]
82. Pillet, S.; Aubin, E.; Trepanier, S.; Bussiere, D.; Dargis, M.; Poulin, J.F.; Yassine-Diab, B.; Ward, B.J.; Landry, N. A plant-derived quadrivalent virus like particle influenza vaccine induces cross-reactive antibody and T cell response in healthy adults. *Clin. Immunol.* **2016**, *168*, 72–87. [CrossRef]
83. Osterholm, M.T.; Kelley, N.S.; Sommer, A.; Belongia, E.A. Efficacy and effectiveness of influenza vaccines: A systematic review and meta-analysis. *Lancet Infect. Dis.* **2012**, *12*, 36–44. [CrossRef]
84. Tretyakova, I.; Hidajat, R.; Hamilton, G.; Horn, N.; Nickols, B.; Prather, R.O.; Tumpey, T.M.; Pushko, P. Preparation of quadri-subtype influenza virus-like particles using bovine immunodeficiency virus gag protein. *Virology* **2016**, *487*, 163–171. [CrossRef] [PubMed]

85. Pushko, P.; Sun, X.; Tretyakova, I.; Hidajat, R.; Pulit-Penaloza, J.A.; Belser, J.A.; Maines, T.R.; Tumpey, T.M. Mono- and quadri-subtype virus-like particles (VLPs) containing H10 subtype elicit protective immunity to H10 influenza in a ferret challenge model. *Vaccine* **2016**, *34*, 5235–5242. [CrossRef] [PubMed]
86. Pushko, P.; Tretyakova, I.; Hidajat, R.; Sun, X.; Belser, J.A.; Tumpey, T.M. Multi-clade H5N1 virus-like particles: Immunogenicity and protection against H5N1 virus and effects of beta-propiolactone. *Vaccine* **2018**, *36*, 4346–4353. [CrossRef] [PubMed]
87. Klausberger, M.; Leneva, I.A.; Egorov, A.; Strobl, F.; Ghorbanpour, S.M.; Falynskova, I.N.; Poddubikov, A.V.; Makhmudova, N.R.; Krokhin, A.; Svitich, O.A.; et al. Off-target effects of an insect cell-expressed influenza HA-pseudotyped Gag-VLP preparation in limiting postinfluenza Staphylococcus aureus infections. *Vaccine* **2020**, *38*, 859–867. [CrossRef] [PubMed]
88. Goff, P.H.; Krammer, F.; Hai, R.; Seibert, C.W.; Margine, I.; Garcia-Sastre, A.; Palese, P. Induction of cross-reactive antibodies to novel H7N9 influenza virus by recombinant Newcastle disease virus expressing a North American lineage H7 subtype hemagglutinin. *J. Virol.* **2013**, *87*, 8235–8240. [CrossRef] [PubMed]
89. Liu, Q.; Mena, I.; Ma, J.; Bawa, B.; Krammer, F.; Lyoo, Y.S.; Lang, Y.; Morozov, I.; Mahardika, G.N.; Ma, W.; et al. Newcastle Disease Virus-Vectored H7 and H5 Live Vaccines Protect Chickens from Challenge with H7N9 or H5N1 Avian Influenza Viruses. *J. Virol.* **2015**, *89*, 7401–7408. [CrossRef]
90. Hu, Z.; Liu, X.; Jiao, X.; Liu, X. Newcastle disease virus (NDV) recombinant expressing the hemagglutinin of H7N9 avian influenza virus protects chickens against NDV and highly pathogenic avian influenza A (H7N9) virus challenges. *Vaccine* **2017**, *35*, 6585–6590. [CrossRef]
91. Li, Z.; Gabbard, J.D.; Johnson, S.; Dlugolenski, D.; Phan, S.; Tompkins, S.M.; He, B. Efficacy of a parainfluenza virus 5 (PIV5)-based H7N9 vaccine in mice and guinea pigs: Antibody titer towards HA was not a good indicator for protection. *PLoS ONE* **2015**, *10*, e0120355. [CrossRef] [PubMed]
92. Mallajosyula, V.V.; Citron, M.; Ferrara, F.; Temperton, N.J.; Liang, X.; Flynn, J.A.; Varadarajan, R. Hemagglutinin Sequence Conservation Guided Stem Immunogen Design from Influenza A H3 Subtype. *Front. Immunol.* **2015**, *6*, 329. [CrossRef]
93. Ellebedy, A.H.; Krammer, F.; Li, G.M.; Miller, M.S.; Chiu, C.; Wrammert, J.; Chang, C.Y.; Davis, C.W.; McCausland, M.; Elbein, R.; et al. Induction of broadly cross-reactive antibody responses to the influenza HA stem region following H5N1 vaccination in humans. *Proc. Natl. Acad. Sci. USA* **2014**, *111*, 13133–13138. [CrossRef] [PubMed]
94. Kazaks, A.; Lu, I.N.; Farinelle, S.; Ramirez, A.; Crescente, V.; Blaha, B.; Ogonah, O.; Mukhopadhyay, T.; de Obanos, M.P.; Krimer, A.; et al. Production and purification of chimeric HBc virus-like particles carrying influenza virus LAH domain as vaccine candidates. *BMC Biotechnol.* **2017**, *17*, 79. [CrossRef] [PubMed]
95. Zheng, D.; Chen, S.; Qu, D.; Chen, J.; Wang, F.; Zhang, R.; Chen, Z. Influenza H7N9 LAH-HBc virus-like particle vaccine with adjuvant protects mice against homologous and heterologous influenza viruses. *Vaccine* **2016**, *34*, 6464–6471. [CrossRef] [PubMed]
96. Song, L.; Xiong, D.; Kang, X.; Yang, Y.; Wang, J.; Guo, Y.; Xu, H.; Chen, S.; Peng, D.; Pan, Z.; et al. An avian influenza A (H7N9) virus vaccine candidate based on the fusion protein of hemagglutinin globular head and Salmonella typhimurium flagellin. *BMC Biotechnol.* **2015**, *15*, 79. [CrossRef] [PubMed]
97. Wei, H.J.; Chang, W.; Lin, S.C.; Liu, W.C.; Chang, D.K.; Chong, P.; Wu, S.C. Fabrication of influenza virus-like particles using M2 fusion proteins for imaging single viruses and designing vaccines. *Vaccine* **2011**, *29*, 7163–7172. [CrossRef]
98. Liu, W.C.; Liu, Y.Y.; Chen, T.H.; Liu, C.C.; Jan, J.T.; Wu, S.C. Multi-subtype influenza virus-like particles incorporated with flagellin and granulocyte-macrophage colony-stimulating factor for vaccine design. *Antivir. Res.* **2016**, *133*, 110–118. [CrossRef]
99. Gong, X.; Yin, H.; Shi, Y.; He, X.; Yu, Y.; Guan, S.; Kuai, Z.; Haji, N.M.; Haji, N.M.; Kong, W.; et al. Evaluation of the immunogenicity and protective effects of a trivalent chimeric norovirus P particle immunogen displaying influenza HA2 from subtypes H1, H3 and, B. *Emerg. Microbes Infect.* **2016**, *5*, e51. [CrossRef]
100. Pham, N.B.; Ho, T.T.; Nguyen, G.T.; Le, T.T.; Le, N.T.; Chang, H.C.; Pham, M.D.; Conrad, U.; Chu, H.H. Nanodiamond enhances immune responses in mice against recombinant HA/H7N9 protein. *J. Nanobiotechnol.* **2017**, *15*, 69. [CrossRef]
101. Kim, M.C.; Lee, J.S.; Kwon, Y.M.; O, E.; Lee, Y.J.; Choi, J.G.; Wang, B.Z.; Compans, R.W.; Kang, S.M. Multiple heterologous M2 extracellular domains presented on virus-like particles confer broader and stronger M2 immunity than live influenza A virus infection. *Antivir. Res.* **2013**, *99*, 328–335. [CrossRef]

102. Kim, K.H.; Kwon, Y.M.; Lee, Y.T.; Kim, M.C.; Hwang, H.S.; Ko, E.J.; Lee, Y.; Choi, H.J.; Kang, S.M. Virus-Like Particles Are a Superior Platform for Presenting M2e Epitopes to Prime Humoral and Cellular Immunity against Influenza Virus. *Vaccines* **2018**, *6*, 66. [CrossRef]
103. Lee, Y.T.; Kim, K.H.; Ko, E.J.; Kim, M.C.; Lee, Y.N.; Hwang, H.S.; Lee, Y.; Jung, Y.J.; Kim, Y.J.; Santos, J.; et al. Enhancing the cross protective efficacy of live attenuated influenza virus vaccine by supplemented vaccination with M2 ectodomain virus-like particles. *Virology* **2019**, *529*, 111–121. [CrossRef] [PubMed]
104. Yong, C.Y.; Yeap, S.K.; Ho, K.L.; Omar, A.R.; Tan, W.S. Potential recombinant vaccine against influenza A virus based on M2e displayed on nodaviral capsid nanoparticles. *Int. J. Nanomed.* **2015**, *10*, 2751–2763.
105. Ong, H.K.; Yong, C.Y.; Tan, W.S.; Yeap, S.K.; Omar, A.R.; Razak, M.A.; Ho, K.L. An Influenza A Vaccine Based on the Extracellular Domain of Matrix 2 Protein Protects BALB/C Mice Against H1N1 and H3N2. *Vaccines* **2019**, *7*, 91. [CrossRef] [PubMed]
106. Lahiri, A.; Sharif, S.; Mallick, A.I. Intragastric delivery of recombinant Lactococcus lactis displaying ectodomain of influenza matrix protein 2 (M2e) and neuraminidase (NA) induced focused mucosal and systemic immune responses in chickens. *Mol. Immunol.* **2019**, *114*, 497–512. [CrossRef] [PubMed]
107. Tang, X.C.; Lu, H.R.; Ross, T.M. Hemagglutinin displayed baculovirus protects against highly pathogenic influenza. *Vaccine* **2010**, *28*, 6821–6831. [CrossRef]
108. Ma, H.; Nandakumar, S.; Bae, E.H.; Chin, P.J.; Khan, A.S. The Spodoptera frugiperda Sf9 cell line is a heterogeneous population of rhabdovirus-infected and virus-negative cells: Isolation and characterization of cell clones containing rhabdovirus X-gene variants and virus-negative cell clones. *Virology* **2019**, *536*, 125–133. [CrossRef]
109. Geisler, C.; Jarvis, D.L. Adventitious viruses in insect cell lines used for recombinant protein expression. *Protein Expr. Purif.* **2018**, *144*, 25–32. [CrossRef]
110. Margine, I.; Palese, P.; Krammer, F. Expression of functional recombinant hemagglutinin and neuraminidase proteins from the novel H7N9 influenza virus using the baculovirus expression system. *J. Vis. Exp.* **2013**, *81*, e51112. [CrossRef]
111. Lai, C.C.; Cheng, Y.C.; Chen, P.W.; Lin, T.H.; Tzeng, T.T.; Lu, C.C.; Lee, M.S.; Hu, A.Y. Process development for pandemic influenza VLP vaccine production using a baculovirus expression system. *J. Biol. Eng.* **2019**, *13*, 78. [CrossRef]
112. Effio, C.L.; Hubbuch, J. Next generation vaccines and vectors: Designing downstream processes for recombinant protein-based virus-like particles. *Biotechnol. J.* **2015**, *10*, 715–727. [CrossRef]
113. Park, Y.C.; Song, J.M. Preparation and immunogenicity of influenza virus-like particles using nitrocellulose membrane filtration. *Clin. Exp. Vaccine Res.* **2017**, *6*, 61–66. [CrossRef] [PubMed]
114. Carvalho, S.B.; Silva, R.J.S.; Moleirinho, M.G.; Cunha, B.; Moreira, A.S.; Xenopoulos, A.; Alves, P.M.; Carrondo, M.J.T.; Peixoto, C. Membrane-Based Approach for the Downstream Processing of Influenza Virus-Like Particles. *Biotechnol. J.* **2019**, *14*, e1800570. [CrossRef] [PubMed]
115. Durous, L.; Rosa-Calatrava, M.; Petiot, E. Advances in influenza virus-like particles bioprocesses. *Expert Rev. Vaccines* **2019**, *18*, 1285–1300. [CrossRef] [PubMed]
116. Reiter, K.; Aguilar, P.P.; Grammelhofer, D.; Joseph, J.; Steppert, P.; Jungbauer, A. Separation of influenza virus-like particles from baculovirus by polymer grafted anion-exchanger. *J. Sep. Sci.* **2020**. [CrossRef]
117. Li, C.; Xu, K.; Hashem, A.; Shao, M.; Liu, S.; Zou, Y.; Gao, Q.; Zhang, Y.; Yuan, L.; Xu, M.; et al. Collaborative studies on the development of national reference standards for potency determination of H7N9 influenza vaccine. *Hum. Vaccin Immunother.* **2015**, *11*, 1351–1356. [CrossRef]
118. Guo, J.; Lu, Y.; Zhang, Y.; Mugabe, S.; Wei, Z.; Borisov, O.V. Development and fit-for-purpose verification of an LC-MS method for quantitation of hemagglutinin and neuraminidase proteins in influenza virus-like particle vaccine candidates. *Anal. Biochem.* **2020**, *592*, 113577. [CrossRef]

11

Quality Assessment of Virus-Like Particles at Single Particle Level: A Comparative Study

Irene González-Domínguez *,†, Eduard Puente-Massaguer *,†, Laura Cervera and Francesc Gòdia

Departament d'Enginyeria Química Biològica i Ambiental, Universitat Autònoma de Barcelona, Cerdanyola del Vallès, 08193 Barcelona, Spain; laura.cervera@uab.cat (L.C.); francesc.godia@uab.cat (F.G.)

* Correspondence: irene.gonzalez@uab.cat (I.G.-D.); eduard.puente.massaguer@gmail.com (E.P.-M.)

† These authors contributed equally to the work.

Abstract: Virus-like particles (VLPs) have emerged as a powerful scaffold for antigen presentation and delivery strategies. Compared to single protein-based therapeutics, quality assessment requires a higher degree of refinement due to the structure of VLPs and their similar properties to extracellular vesicles (EVs). Advances in the field of nanotechnology with single particle and high-resolution analysis techniques provide appealing approaches to VLP characterization. In this study, six different biophysical methods have been assessed for the characterization of HIV-1-based VLPs produced in mammalian and insect cell platforms. Sample preparation and equipment set-up were optimized for the six strategies evaluated. Electron Microscopy (EM) disclosed the presence of several types of EVs within VLP preparations and cryogenic transmission electron microscopy (cryo-TEM) resulted in the best technique to resolve the VLP ultrastructure. The use of super-resolution fluorescence microscopy (SRFM), nanoparticle tracking analysis (NTA) and flow virometry enabled the high throughput quantification of VLPs. Interestingly, differences in the determination of nanoparticle concentration were observed between techniques. Moreover, NTA and flow virometry allowed the quantification of both EVs and VLPs within the same experiment while analyzing particle size distribution (PSD), simultaneously. These results provide new insights into the use of different analytical tools to monitor the production of nanoparticle-based biologicals and their associated contaminants.

Keywords: VLP; viral quantification; NTA; flow virometry; SRFM; cryo-TEM; SEM

1. Introduction

Virus-like particles (VLPs) are considered a promising platform in the field of vaccine development. Nowadays, there are several licensed VLP-based vaccines, such as Cervarix®, Gardasil®, Hecolin® or Porcilis PCV® and more than 100 candidates are undergoing clinical trials [1]. Their success as immunogens lies on their ability to mimic native viruses without containing a viral genome. Their highly organized and repetitive antigen structure has shown effective cellular and humoral immune responses [2]. Furthermore, advances in the field of bioengineering have widened their possible applications; VLP technology accepts several modifications including encapsulation, chemical conjugation or genetic engineering. By doing so, VLPs can be pseudotyped or used either as DNA or drug nanocarriers [1,3].

VLP quality assessment is of major importance since both, the physicochemical and biological properties, are responsible of their clinical efficacy. The preservation of their structural integrity during all the stages of vaccine manufacturing, storage and administration is critical to ensure their success [4]. The study of particle size distribution (PSD) or particle concentration are some of the critical quality attributes (CQA) that could be monitored in this regard [5]. Overall, the specific detection and quantification of VLPs entails several difficulties, especially for enveloped VLPs, which are composed of a protein capsid surrounded by the host-cell lipid membrane. VLPs must be distinguished from other similar nanovesicle structures; extracellular vesicles (EVs), including exosomes and microvesicles [6], adventitious viruses, or baculoviruses (BV) in insect cell systems [7], are important process-related impurities. In this sense, traditional quantification methods such as $TCID_{50}$ or PCR have a limited applicability due to the non-infective nature of VLPs.

Comprehensive studies on VLP-based vaccine candidates have been conducted by multiple approaches, including biochemical, biological and biophysical methods [3]. Biochemical protein gels, biological enzyme-linked immunosorbent assay (ELISA) or immunoblot are normally used [8–11]. Nonetheless, these assays cannot distinguish assembled from non-assembled structures [12]. Among biophysical methods, analytical ultracentrifugation, dynamic light scattering (DLS) and transmission electron microscopy (TEM) are the reference methods used to assess VLP physical properties [3]. Recently, technical progress in the field of microscopy, as well as the application of nanotechnology to virology, have given rise to several single nanoparticle analytical technologies. These techniques represent the most advanced methods to evaluate VLP size, polydispersity, purity and even nanoparticle composition simultaneously [3,12].

Among them, electron microscopy (EM) has traditionally been the preferred technique since resolution at the nanometric or even atomic level is achieved [13]. Within EM methods, transmission (TEM), scanning (SEM) and cryogenic (cryo-TEM) methodologies are frequently used. TEM is the gold standard technique for the characterization of virus-like structures as reported in a myriad of studies [3,14]. This methodology requires a contrast medium for sample visualization, typically a heavy metal solution containing a cationic or anionic salt, being negative staining the most extended strategy [15]. In TEM-Negative staining, a thin layer of biological material is covered by a dried non-crystalline amorphous layer of a heavy metal salt, typically uranyl acetate. Differential electron scattering between the biological material and the surrounding staining layer enables the visualization of the specimen. The application of SEM in the characterization of different materials has been demonstrated in several works [16]. However, few studies address its use as a tool for VLP characterization. The addition of Alcian Blue solution to the grid before sample deposition results in the activation of the grid with a net positive charge, with successful results reported for the visualization of other negatively charged specimens such as nucleic acids [17]. Since viral structures and EVs are known to have an overall negative charge at physiological pH [18,19], this strategy could improve their adsorption and reduce nanoparticle loss during the sample preparation process. Cryo-TEM has also gained increasing interest as a tool for nanoparticle visualization over the last years [13]. Essentially, this technique enables the visualization of viruses and VLPs in their native conformation at nanometric and even atomic scale [3], and the addition of a contrast solution is not required. A key point of this technique is the rapid freezing process which reduces sample damage. Therefore, the selection of an adequate grid and support film is of upmost importance since the correct formation of a thin ice film is pivotal for an adequate sample visualization. Perforated carbon films are generally the preferred option since they allow the biological material to be imaged in the ice generated between holes in the carbon support film [20,21].

The study of viral vectors and nanoparticles by confocal microscopy has been traditionally restricted by the Abbe diffraction limit. However, the appearance of super-resolution fluorescence microscopy (SRFM) enabling to surpass this constraint has opened a breadth of opportunities to apply confocal microscopy to the nanoscale [22]. Despite SRFM has been mainly used to study cellular processes, its application to appraise individual viral structures is becoming more popular [23]. In previous works, a method for VLP quantification by HyVolution2 SRFM has been described by González-Domínguez and co-workers [24,25]. This method combines sub-Airy confocal microscopy with mathematical deconvolution, which has been described to achieve resolutions up to 140 nm [26]. Finally, light scatter-based technologies, such as nanoparticle tracking analysis (NTA) and flow virometry are also gaining attention for viral particle and EV quantification [5,12,27,28]. NTA is a method to characterize and quantify nanoparticles in solution that relates the rate of Brownian motion to nanoparticle size. Its use in the assessment of nanoparticles has been reported for viruses, VLPs and other nanoparticles [5,29–31]. This technique is theoretically able to detect nanoparticles with a size comprised between 30 and 1000 nm, but the nanoparticle concentration has to be maintained around 10^8 particles/mL and 20–60 particles/frame [29]. The latter indicates that the range of possible nanoparticle concentrations is narrow, and it is often required to dilute the sample to meet this criterion, which is generally based on trial-and-error. Flow virometry has recently emerged as a technique to specifically detect viruses similarly to conventional cell-based flow cytometry [27]. Labeling studies at single particle level, particle quantification or virus sorting are some of the applications that can be performed with this technology [27]. Considering the high difference in volume between a cell and a nanoparticle, which can be one million-fold [32], the acquisition settings need to be adjusted to detect the scattered or fluorescence signal from nanoparticles. Still, a significant loss of scattered light that fall in the range of the background noise of the instrument and different sensitivities between equipments are a general concern [33]. To address this issue, the implementation of the violet (405 nm) side scatter (V-SSC) has been reported to improve the sensitivity but also the resolution of the technique [34]. Owing to the specific features of each analytical method, characterization results such as particle concentration obtained by different techniques are often difficult to compare.

The aim of this work is the characterization of VLPs using several advanced nanoparticle analytical methods, and to discuss the technological limitations that may affect their use, including sample preparation or equipment set-up. The study of PSD, particle ultrastructural analysis, VLP quantification and differentiation from other nanoparticle subpopulations has been performed. The VLPs analyzed in this work are HIV-1 Gag VLPs, which are a promising platform for the development of a vaccine candidate against HIV, but also as a scaffold for chimeric or multivalent vaccine development [2,35]. Upon expression in the host cell, the Gag polyprotein travels to the cell membrane and after an oligomerization process, HIV-1 Gag VLPs are released from the cell through a budding process [36,37]. Thus, the final nanoparticles are enveloped by the host cell lipid membrane [38], with sizes comprised between 100–200 nm. In previous works, the Gag polyprotein has been fused to GFP to track the VLP production process [36]. By doing so, VLPs could be easily quantified and distinguished from other contaminant particles. Besides, product characteristics are known to be affected by the expression system selected for VLP production [39]. Here, the two most relevant systems for the generation of HIV-1 Gag-based VLPs have been used [40]. VLPs obtained by transient gene expression in HEK 293 cells and baculovirus (BV) infection in Sf9 cells have been characterized in parallel. This study provides relevant data on the use of different analytical methods to evaluate the production of VLPs and their associated contaminants in animal cell-based bioprocesses.

2. Materials and Methods

2.1. HEK 293 Mammalian Cell Line, Culture Conditions and Transient Transfection

The mammalian cell line used in this work is a serum-free suspension-adapted HEK 293 cell line (HEK 293SF-3F6 from NRC, Montreal, QC, Canada) kindly provided by Dr. Amine Kamen from McGill University (Montreal, QC, Canada). Cells were cultured as previously described [36]. HIV-1 Gag-eGFP VLP production was achieved by transient transfection. Briefly, the pGag-eGFP plasmid encoding for the Gag-eGFP polyprotein, is diluted with FreeStyle 293 medium (Invitrogen, Carlsbad, CA, USA) and vortexed for 10 s, then polyethylenimine (PEI) is added at 1:2 DNA:PEI ratio (*w/w*) and vortexed three times, the mixture is incubated for 15 min at RT and is added to the cell culture, where a medium exchange has been already performed. HIV-1 Gag-eGFP VLPs were harvested at 72 h post transfection (hpt) by centrifugation at 1000× *g* during 15 min. Supernatants were stored at 4 °C until analysis. Non-transfected negative controls reproducing cell growth conditions were also produced, for comparison.

2.2. *Sf9 Insect Cell Line, Culture Conditions and Baculovirus Infection*

The suspension-adapted lepidopteran insect cell line used in this work is the *Spodoptera frugiperda* (Sf9, cat. num. 71104, Merck, Darmstadt, Germany) gently provided by Dr. Berrow (Institute of Biomedical Research, Barcelona, Spain). Sf9 cells were cultured in Sf900III medium (Thermo Fisher Scientific, Grand Island, NY, USA) in 125-mL disposable polycarbonate Erlenmeyer flasks [25]. Cell cultures were shaken at 130 rpm using an orbital shaker (Stuart, Stone, United Kingdom) and maintained at 27 °C. HIV-1 Gag-eGFP VLP production was achieved through infection with the recombinant baculovirus *Autographa californica* multiple nucleopolyhedrovirus (*Ac*MNPV) (BD Biosciences, San José, CA, USA) enconding for the Gag-eGFP protein. Shortly, Sf9 cells were grown to 2–3 × 10^6 cells/mL and were infected at a multiplicity of infection (MOI) of 1. HIV-1 Gag-eGFP VLPs were harvested at 40 or 72 h post infection (hpi) by centrifugation at 1000× *g* during 15 min, and supernatants were kept at 4 °C until analysis. Non-infected negative controls reproducing cell growth conditions were also produced, for comparison.

Biophysical analyses were performed on HIV-1 Gag-eGFP VLP supernatants obtained as previously described. FreeStyle and Sf900III cell culture media and conditioned cell culture media obtained from HEK 293 and Sf9 non-transfected/infected conditions were also assessed in each analysis as negative controls.

2.3. *Electron Microscopy (EM)*

EM analyses were performed at Servei de Microscòpia at Universitat Autònoma de Barcelona (UAB, Barcelona, Spain). Particle size distribution (PSD) analyses were performed with ImageJ Fiji (ImageJ, NIH, WI, USA) and SigmaPlot 12.0 (Systat Software Inc., San Jose, CA, USA).

2.3.1. Transmission Electron Microscopy (TEM)-Negative Staining

Prior to negative staining, HIV-1 Gag-eGFP VLPs were concentrated by double sucrose cushion 25–45% (w:v) at 31.000 rpm and centrifuged for 2.5 h at 4 °C in a Beckman Optima L100XP centrifuge using a SW32 Ti rotor (Beckman Coulter, Brea, CA, USA). The 25–45% interphase was recovered and stored at 4 °C until analysis [41]. TEM micrographs were analyzed after air-dried negative staining. The protocol used is summarized in Figure 1A. Briefly, VLP samples were deposited onto carbon-coated copper or Holey carbon 200 mesh grids (Micro to Nano, Wateringweg, the Netherlands). Grids were glow discharged in a PELCO easiGlow glow discharge unit (PELCO, Fresno, CA, USA). Thereafter, 8 µL of sample were loaded onto the grid and incubated at RT for 1 min. Excess sample was carefully drained off the grid with the aid of filter paper. Samples were negatively stained with 8 µL of 2% w:v uranyl acetate by incubation at RT for 1 min. Excess stain was drained off as previously indicated and grids were dried at RT until analysis. TEM examinations were performed with a Jeol JEM-1400 (JEOL USA, Pleasanton, CA, USA) transmission electron microscope equipped with an ES1000W Erlangshen charge-coupled device camera (CCD) (Model No. 785; Gatan, Pleasanton, CA, USA).

2.3.2. Scanning Electron Microscopy (SEM)-Alcian Blue Staining

HIV-1 Gag-eGFP VLP visualization by SEM was performed by staining VLP-containing supernatants with Alcian Blue solution, adapted from Gállego [17]. The protocol used is shown in Figure 2A. Briefly, Alcian Blue solution 1% w:v in 3% v:v acetic acid (Sigma Aldrich, St Louis, MO, USA) was diluted in ultrapure water achieving a final concentration of 1 µg/mL. Carbon-coated copper or Holey carbon 200 mesh grids were placed in this solution for 5 min, then the excess of Alcian Blue solution was removed by washing the grid in ultrapure water. Grids were dried with filter paper. Thereafter, 8 µL of the sample were placed on the grid and incubated at RT for 5 min. Excess sample was carefully drained off the grid with the aid of filter paper. Negative staining was applied to the samples when required, using the protocol described in Section 2.3.1. SEM micrographs were performed in a FE-SEM Merlin scanning electron microscope (Zeiss, Jena, Germany). Micrographs were taken with the lens mode and secondary electron detector, with an electron high tension (EHT) comprised between 1–2 eV and 2.9–7.5 mm of working distance using a protocol adapted from González-Domínguez et al. [31].

2.3.3. Cryogenic Transmission Electron Microscopy (cryo-TEM)

Cryo-TEM analyses of HIV-1 Gag-eGFP VLPs were conducted from harvested supernatants. In Figure 3A, the sample preparation procedure for VLP visualization is presented. 2–3 μL of sample were blotted onto 200 or 400 mesh Holey carbon grids (Micro to Nano, Wateringweg, the Netherlands) previously glow discharged in a PELCO easiGlow glow discharge unit. Samples were subsequently plunged into liquid ethane at −180 °C using a Leica EM GP cryo workstation and observed in a Jeol JEM-2011 TEM electron microscope operating at 200 kV. During imaging, samples were maintained at −173 °C, and pictures were taken using a CCD multiscan camera (Model No. 895, Gatan).

2.4. Super-Resolution Fluorescence Microscopy (SRFM)

SRFM was performed with a TCS SP8 confocal microscope equipped with Huygens deconvolution suite embedded via a direct interface with LAS X software and GPU arrays (Leica Microsystems, Wetzlar, Germany) at Servei d'Anatomia Patològica from Hospital Sant Joan de Déu (Esplugues de Llobregat, Barcelona, Spain), as previously described [24]. A summary of the protocol is depicted in Figure 4A. Briefly, harvested VLPs were directly loaded onto the microscope slide and adsorbed to the surface of the cover glass after an incubation time of 30 min at RT (Figure 4A). HIV-1 Gag-eGFP VLP preparations were analyzed with 100 X magnification (zoom 5), a line average of 3 and 496 x 496 pixels with HC PL APO CS2 100 X/1.40 OIL objective with the HyVolution2 mode (Leica). Five fields of 13 sections per each biological triplicate were studied in harvested HIV-1 Gag-eGFP VLPs. Deconvolution was performed with the SVI Huygens Professional program and the best resolution strategy (Scientific Volume Imaging B.V., Hilversum, the Netherlands). HIV-1 Gag-eGFP VLP concentration was calculated based on the division of particle number by 3D image volume as previously described [24]. Briefly, direct quantification was performed on deposited HIV-1 Gag-eGFP VLP samples with 23 × 23 × 3 μm in *xyz* from a total loaded volume of 50 μL distributed in 24 × 60 mm under the cover glass and a total height of 34 μm. Assuming complete sample deposition, minimum concentration of Gag-eGFP VLPs was also calculated. PSD analyses were performed using SigmaPlot 12.0 software.

2.5. Nanoparticle Tracking Analysis (NTA)

HIV-1 Gag-eGFP VLPs and total particle content were analyzed by NTA. A NanoSight® NS300 device (Malvern Panalytical, Malvern, United Kingdom) equipped with a blue filter module (488 nm) and a neutral filter was used to quantify GFP-fluorescent nanoparticles and total particle by light diffraction, respectively. The measurements were performed at Service of Preparation and Characterization of Soft Materials located at Institut de Ciència de Materials de Barcelona (ICMAB, CSIC, Campus UAB). The workflow used for HIV-1 Gag-eGFP VLP quantification is summarized in Figure 5A. Prior to injection into the device chamber, each sample was diluted to obtain 1 mL sample with a concentration of around 10^8 particles/mL. Sample injection into the chamber was continuously added using a pump to improve the robustness of the measurement and minimize the photobleaching effect due to fluorescence depletion over time (Figure 5B) [42]. The videos recorded were then analyzed with the NTA 3.2 software (Malvern Panalytical) by tracking the individual particle movement, where camera level and detection threshold were adjusted manually for each sample (Table 1). Three independent analyses were carried out and videos of 60 s were recorded at RT, with particles identified and tracked by their Brownian motion. HIV-1 Gag-eGFP VLP concentrations were calculated as the total fluorescent particles and the concentration of EVs was calculated as the difference between light scattering particles and fluorescent particles. PSD analyses were performed with NTA 3.2 software and SigmaPlot 12.0 software.

Table 1. NTA analysis settings.

	VLPs		Total Nanoparticles	
2-5	**Camera Level**	**Threshold**	**Camera Level**	**Threshold**
1-5 HEK 293 supernatants	16	4	10	4
Sf9 supernatants	16	3	8	3
HEK 293 conditioned medium	-	-	10	4
Sf9 conditioned medium	-	-	14	3
FreeStyle culture medium	-	-	13	5
Sf900III culture medium	-	-	13	4

2.6. *Flow Virometry*

Flow virometry experiments were performed with a CytoFLEX LX (Beckman Coulter) with violet side scatter (V-SSC) 405 nm filter configuration at Servei de Cultius Cel·lulars, Producció d'Anticossos i Citometria (UAB, Barcelona, Spain). The different steps required in the analysis are described in Figure 6A. Measurements from different experiments were standardized using a mixture of Megamix-Plus Side Scatter and Forward Scatter (FSC) fluorescent polystyrene beads (100, 160, 200, 240, 300, 500 and 900 nm; Biocytex, Marseille, France). The threshold of height trigger signal in Violet Side Scatter (V-SSC) was manually adjusted to 1200 and laser gains were set as 72, 9 and 106 for FSC, V-SSC and B525-FITC, respectively. Samples were diluted with 1 X Dulbecco's phosphate-buffered saline (DPBS, Thermo Fisher Scientific) until the abort rate value was below the 2%. Three-hundred thousand events were analyzed per sample at a flow rate of 10 μL/min. V-SSC vs B525-FITC density plots were used to gate the different EVs and VLPs populations. Gating was manually adjusted for each channel. Results were analyzed with the CytExpert v.2.3 software (Beckman Coulter). Nanoparticle concentrations were calculated with Equation (1):

$$Particle\ concentration\left(\frac{Events}{mL}\right) = (Events)\cdot\frac{\mu L}{mL}\cdot Dilution \quad (1)$$

Particle size diameters based on the median violet side scatter were calculated by Mie correlation [43] using FCM_{PASS} software [33]. Megamix-Plus SSC and FSC fluorescent polystyrene beads were used as the reference material with a refractive index (RI) of 1.633 with a 405 nm illumination wavelength [43]. The following RI were used for Mie correlation: 1.374 (vesicle cytosol), 1.394 (vesicle upper cytosol), 1.354 (vesicle lower cytosol), 1.474 (vesicle membrane) and 1.345 (vesicle surrounding medium) considering 405 nm as the illumination wavelength. The vesicle membrane thickness was defined as 10 nm [43]. The half angle parameter was set as circular aperture geometry. The maximum diameter was fixed as 3000 nm, the triggering threshold as 60 arbitrary units (a.u.) and the log decade number parameter comprised between 0–6. Thereafter, HIV-1 Gag-eGFP VLP and EV mean sizes were exported with the FlowJo v.10 software (BD Biosciences).

3. Results

3.1. *Transmission Electron Microscopy (TEM)-Negative Staining*

Virus-like particle (VLP) characterization by TEM with uranyl acetate as the negative staining solution is shown in Figure 1. VLPs were concentrated by ultracentrifugation according to previous studies [36]. VLPs produced in HEK 293 (Figure 1B,D) and Sf9 cells (Figure 1C,E) were examined in order to identify differences arising from the expression of these nanoparticles in each specific cell platform. Uranium strongly reacts with phosphate and amino groups and typically stains proteins, nucleic acids and lipid membranes [44]. Thus, VLPs were observed as spherical electrodense structures surrounded by a bright corona (white arrows) that might correspond to structured Gag-eGFP monomers surrounded by the lipid membrane [36,45]. As expected, the presence of baculoviruses (BV) (black arrows) was detected along with VLPs (white arrows) in infected Sf9 samples. EVs were observed as less electrodense nanoparticles (dashed grey arrows) and that could also be identified in conditioned medium samples (Supplementary materials S1) [46]. Interestingly, differences between VLPs and EVs were less evident in Sf9 micrographs compared to HEK 293 ones. A mean population diameter of 165 ± 54 nm (n = 71) and 146 ± 33 nm (n = 69) was quantified in HEK 293 and Sf9 samples, respectively (Figure 1F,G). Moreover, TEM characterizations revealed that only the 52 ± 6% and 55 ± 14% of the nanoparticles analyzed were VLPs in HEK 293 and Sf9 concentrated samples. The use of negative staining for sample visualization hindered a more detailed characterization of the structure of the different specimens due to the presence of artifacts and background noise in all samples (Figure 1B,E) [1].

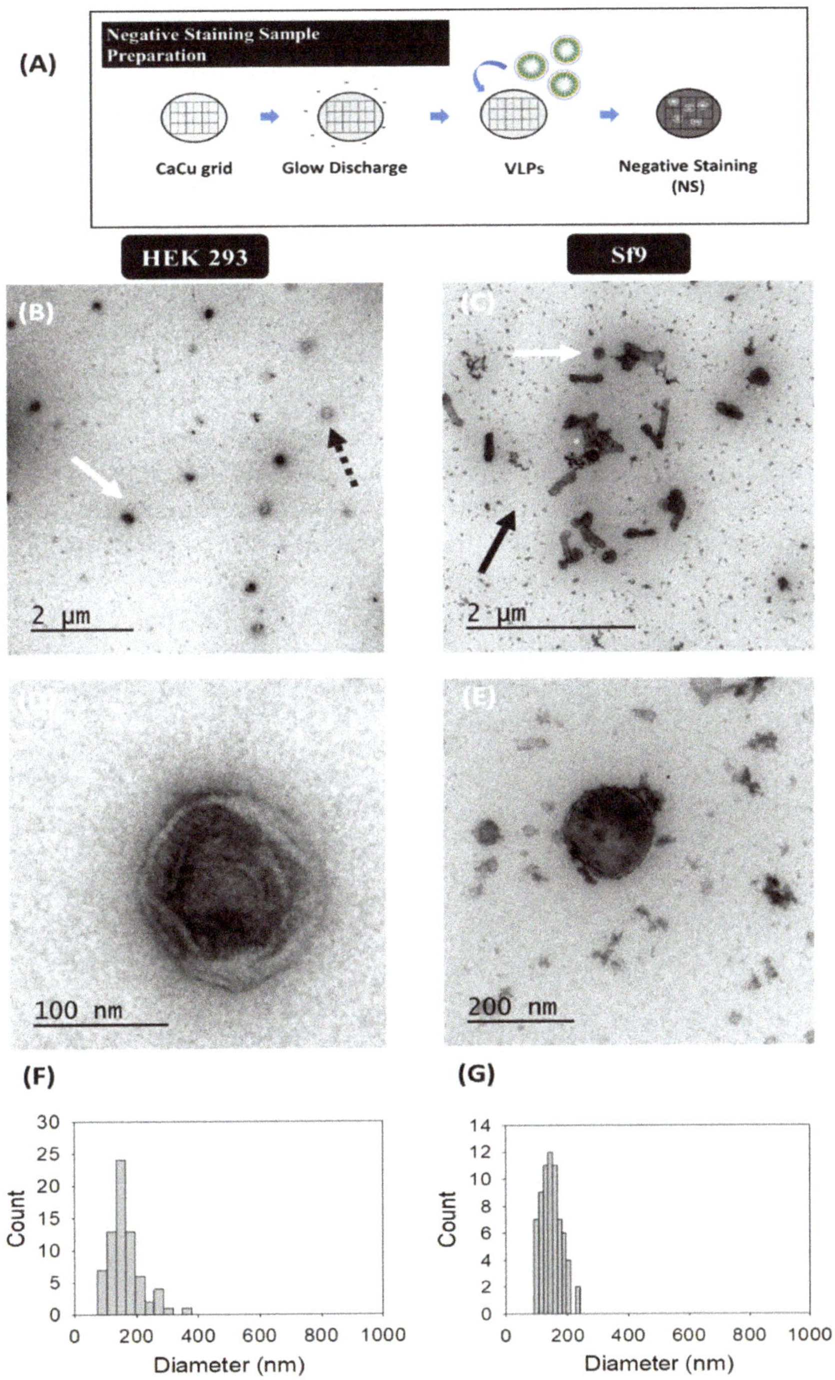

Figure 1. Transmission electron microscopy with negative staining analysis of HIV-1 Gag-eGFP VLPs produced in HEK 293 and Sf9 cells harvested at 72 hpt and 72 hpi, respectively. (**A**) Sample preparation

protocol; (**B–E**) samples corresponding to the 25–45% ultracentrifugation fraction from HEK 293 supernatants (**B**,**D**) and Sf9 supernatants (**C**,**E**). All samples were stained with uranyl acetate in Ca-Cu grids. (**F**,**G**) PSD analysis of HEK 293 and Sf9 concentrated samples, respectively. White and grey dashed arrows indicate the presence of VLPs and EVs in HEK 293 and Sf9 productions, respectively, and black arrows indicate the presence of BVs in Sf9 samples. Negative controls were assessed using the same conditions as in VLP samples (Supplementary materials S1).

3.2. Scanning Electron Microscopy (SEM)-Alcian Blue Staining

SEM analyses were directly performed on harvested VLP supernatants from transfected HEK 293 (Figure 2B,D,F) and BV infected Sf9 cells (Figure 2E,G). Initial analyses using standard sample preparation protocols resulted in the loss of a high portion of the nanoparticles prior to visualization [47]. Thus, the combination of SEM with Alcian Blue solution was investigated (Figure 2) and compared to uranyl acetate staining as the reference methodology. The comparison between negative staining, Alcian Blue grid pre-treatment followed by negative staining, and only Alcian Blue grid pre-treatment is shown in Figure 2B–E, respectively.

Samples stained with uranyl acetate presented an important background regardless the grid treatment or not with Alcian Blue solution (Figure 2B,C and Figure S1). Indeed, large and irregular salt stacks deposited on the sample grid were detected probably related to the interaction of uranium with phosphate salts and amino acids from cell culture media, with similar results as observed in TEM micrographs (Figure 1). A decrease in the load of background signal was achieved by Alcian Blue grid pre-treatment without negative staining (white arrows) and nanoparticles could be individually resolved as 3D sphere-like structures. Despite the improvement in nanoparticle resolution achieved by the Alcian Blue grid pre-treatment, VLPs and EVs could not be distinguished in these analyses. Thus, the calculation of particle size distribution (PSD) was performed considering all nanoparticles as a single population, resulting in 296 ± 88 nm (n = 94) for HEK 293 and 162 ± 60 nm (n = 57) for Sf9 supernatants. The presence of EVs in conditioned supernatants could also be observed by SEM-Alcian Blue staining (Supplementary Materials S1), as well as the typical rod-shaped capsids of BVs (black arrows) in infected Sf9 supernatants (Figure 2E).

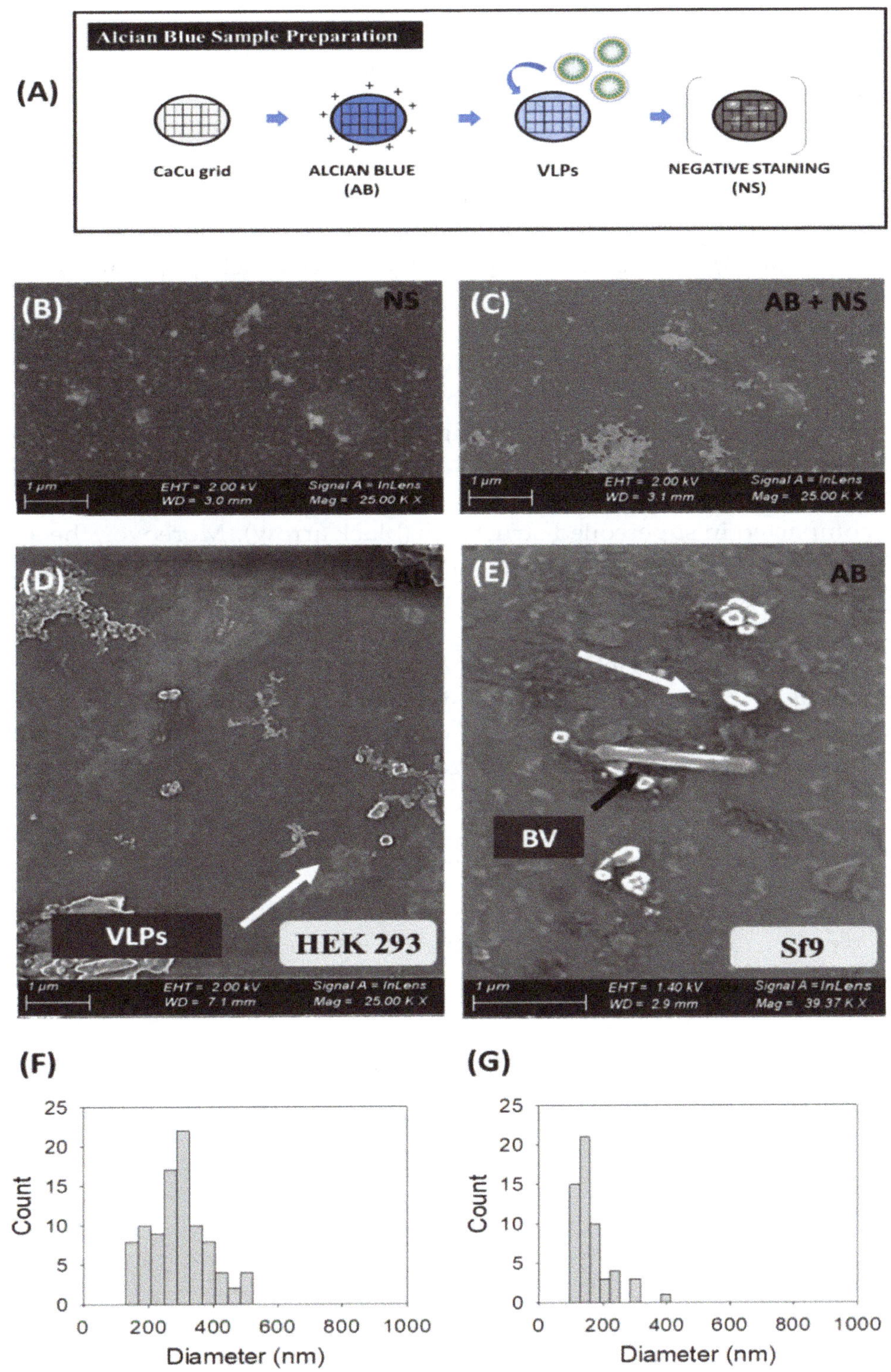

Figure 2. Scanning electron microscopy analysis of HIV-1 Gag-eGFP VLPs produced in HEK 293 and Sf9 cell lines harvested at 72 hpt and 72 hpi, respectively. (**A**) Sample preparation protocol; (**B–E**) Comparison of different sample preparation methods: (**B**) negative staining (NS) (**C**), combining Alcian Blue solution and negative staining (AB + NS) on HEK 293 supernatants; (**D**) Supernatant from transfected HEK 293 cells and (**E**) supernatant from BV infected Sf9 cells treated with Alcian Blue (AB) for 1 min in a Holey carbon 200 mesh grid. (**F–G**) PSD analysis of HEK 293 and Sf9 supernatants, respectively. White arrows indicate the presence of nanoparticles in HEK 293 and Sf9 supernatants and black arrows indicate the presence of BV. Negative controls were analyzed using the same conditions as in VLP samples (Supplementary materials S1).

3.3. *Cryogenic Transmission Electron Microscopy (cryo-TEM)*

Ultrastructural analysis of VLP, EV and BV populations was conducted in harvested supernatants by cryo-TEM (Figure 3B–F). Gag-eGFP VLPs were observed as electrodense nanoparticles surrounded by a lipid envelope with a granular-like heterogeneous internal structure (Figure 3B,C, white arrows). Gag-eGFP VLPs produced in both platforms displayed an average size of 202 ± 68 nm (n = 59) for HEK 293 and 146 ± 42 nm (n = 188) for Sf9 cells (Figure 3G,H, respectively). In parallel, different EV subpopulations could be detected, including exosomes (30–100 nm), microvesicles (50–2000 nm) and multivesicular bodies (MVB) (Figure 3D–F) [6]. Similar nanoparticle populations were detected in conditioned medium samples from both cell lines (Supplementary materials S1), indicating a basal expression of EVs in these cell lines. As for infected Sf9 supernatants, a large concentration of BVs was detected (black arrows), encompassing different BV phenotypes: the occlusion-derived BV (ODV), a relaxed form of the BV (rBV) (Figure 3E) and the typical infective BV (budded virus) (Figure 3F). ODVs presented several rod-shaped nucleocapsids arranged in parallel disposition inside vesicular bodies (light blue arrow), while a spiral-like nucleocapsid organization could be clearly distinguished in rBV (mid blue arrow) [7]. Budded BVs displayed ovoid-like structures containing one nucleocapsid, with the DNA highly compacted in supercoiled structures (black arrow). Moreover, the apical spikes and the BV lateral pocket, which is the space between the lipid bilayer and the nucleocapsid, were resolved using this technique (Figure 3G) [7]. Other BV forms could be identified in infected Sf9 samples and consisted of BV containing vesicles or protein structures besides the nucleocapsid (cBV, dark blue arrow, Figure 3E). Differences in Gag-eGFP VLPs (green) and Gag VLPs (brown) were also evaluated by cryo-TEM (Figure 3I,J). Gag VLPs evidenced a higher internal degree of ordered Gag arrangement in comparison to Gag-eGFP VLPs, similar to that of immature HIV-1 virions [38], while Gag-eGFP VLPs did not attain such level of structural organization.

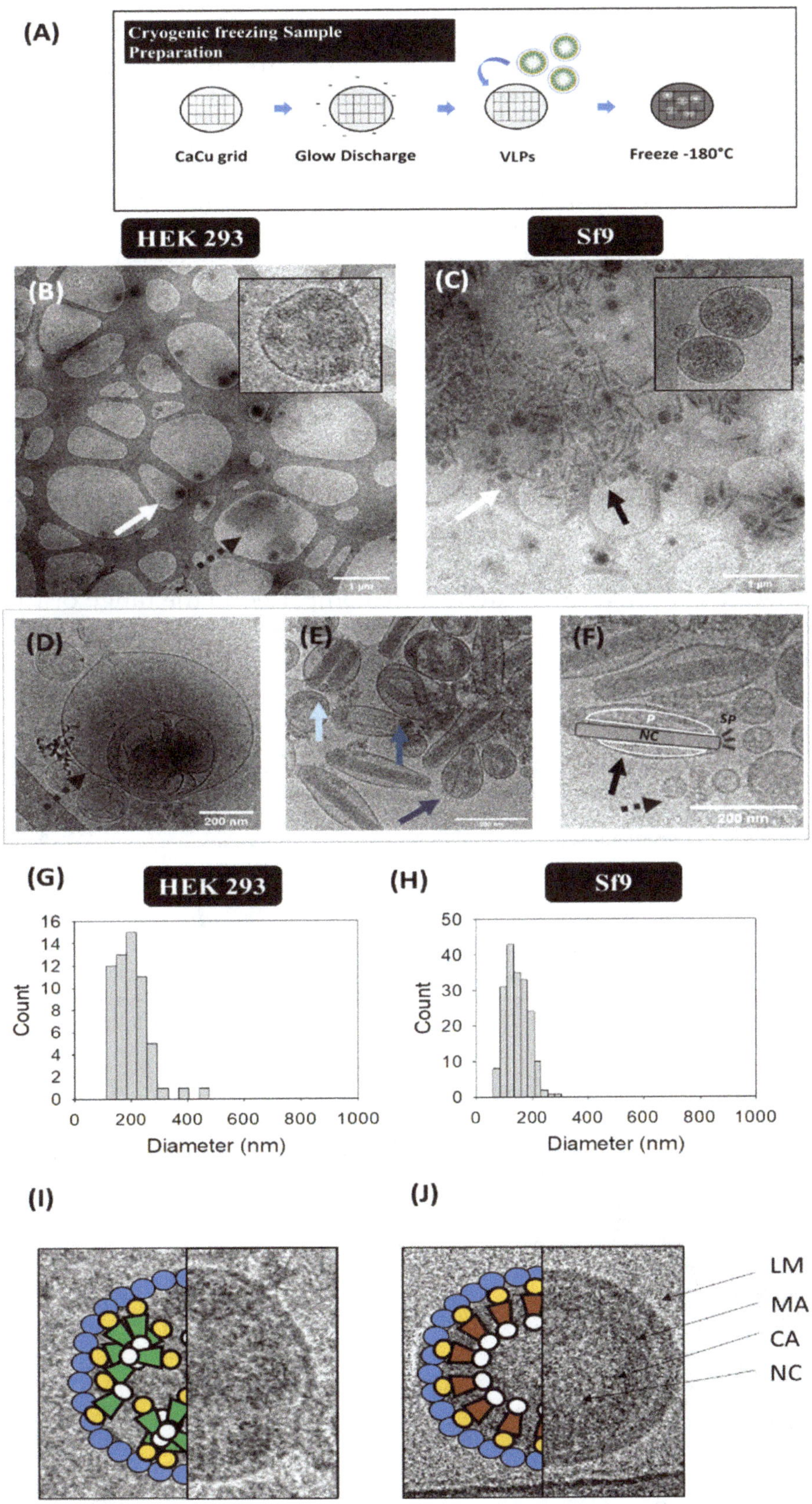

Figure 3. Cryo-TEM analysis of HIV-1 Gag-eGFP VLPs produced in HEK 293 and Sf9 cells harvested at 72 hpt and 72 hpi, respectively. (**A**) Sample preparation protocol. Supernatant from HEK 293 (**B**) and Sf9 cells (**C**). Both samples were prepared and visualized in Holey carbon grids. (**D–F**) Morphological

characterization of contaminant particles including multivesicular bodies (MVB) (**D**), occlusion-derived BV (ODV, light blue), a relaxed-form of the BV (rBV, mid blue) or BV-containing vesicles or protein structures (cBV, dark blue) (**E**), and analysis of the infective BV (budded virus) structure: nucleocapsid (NC), lateral pocket side (P) and apical spikes (SP) (**F**). (**G–H**) PSD analysis of HEK 293 and Sf9 supernatants, respectively. White arrows indicate the presence of VLPs, dashed grey arrows point EVs and infective BVs are shown in black arrows. (**I,J**) Ultrastructural organization of an HIV-1 Gag-eGFP VLP (**I**) and an HIV-1 Gag VLP (**J**) produced in Sf9 cells by BV infection. LM: lipid membrane, MA: matrix; CA: capsid, NC: nucleocapsid. Negative controls were assessed using the same conditions as in VLP samples (Supplementary materials S1).

3.4. Super-Resolution Fluorescence Microscopy (SRFM)

HyVolution2 SRFM nanoparticle analyses were conducted in HEK 293 and Sf9 supernatants by a simple preparation strategy similar to common cell visualization methods used in confocal microscopy. Images were acquired at 100 X magnification as depicted in Figure 4B, where VLPs correspond to green dots. VLPs presented an elongated structure in the Z plane while a smaller diameter was observed in the XY axis due to the convolution effect of light. A mean VLP diameter of 268 ± 77 nm (n = 371) was obtained in HEK 293 samples, whereas an average of 261 ± 104 nm (n = 794) was measured for Sf9 supernatants (Figure 4C,D). VLP concentrations were comprised in the range of 10^9–10^{10} VLPs/mL in both platforms, representing a 1.7-fold difference for Sf9 over HEK 293-derived VLPs (Table 2). The same acquisition strategy was performed in conditioned medium samples from both cell lines, and no detection of GFP signal was observed (Supplementary materials S1).

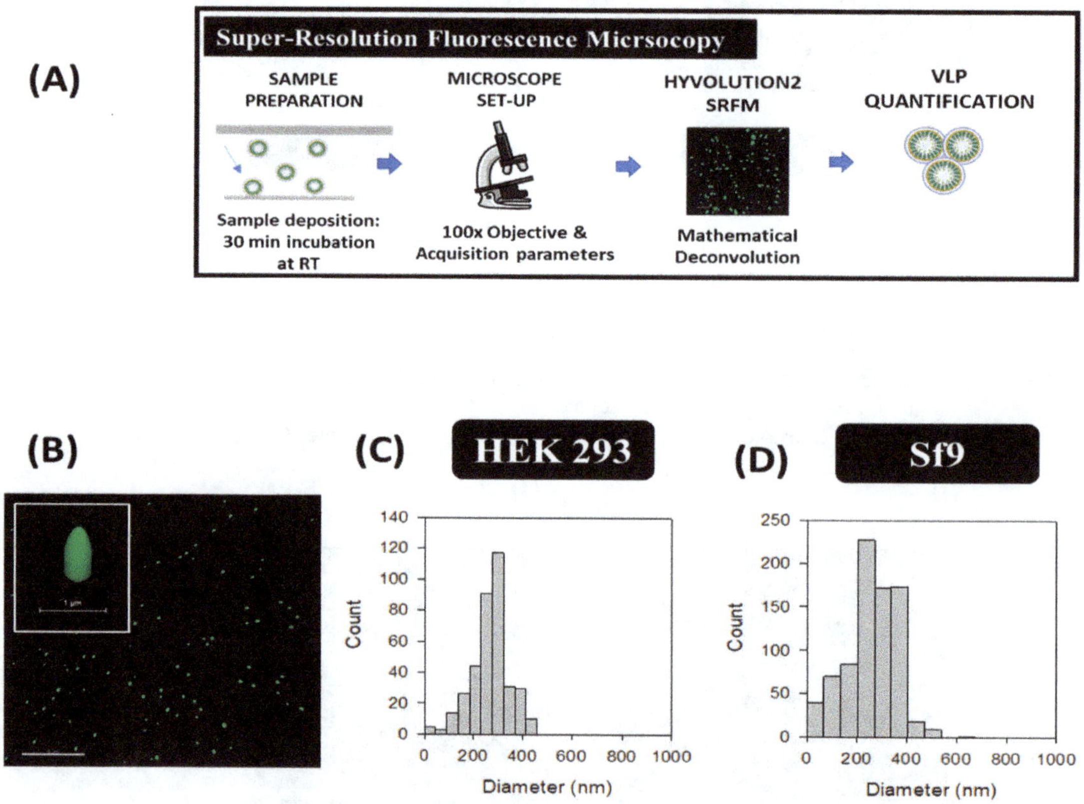

Figure 4. Super-resolution fluorescence microscopy analysis of HIV-1 Gag-eGFP VLPs produced in HEK 293 and Sf9 cells harvested at 72 hpt and 40 hpi, respectively. (**A**) Sample preparation and analysis workflow and (**B**) Gag-eGFP VLP imaging. (**C,D**) PSD analysis of HEK 293 and Sf9 supernatants directly quantified after their addition to the microscope slide, respectively. Negative controls were analyzed in the same conditions as in VLP samples (Supplementary materials S1).

Table 2. Quantification of VLP and EV concentrations in transfected HEK 293 and BV infected Sf9 supernatants using different analytical methods.

Technique	VLPs (10^9/mL)			EVs (10^9/mL)	
	FV	NTA	SRFM	FV	NTA
HEK 293	0.2 ± 0.0	5.0 ± 0.5 *	4.0–43.0 *	0.2 ± 0.0	16.6 ± 2.9 *
Sf9	0.2 ± 0.0	8.6 ± 2.1 *	6.6–74.5 *	0.3 ± 0.0	9.7 ± 1.6 *
Fold difference (Sf9:HEK 293)	1.5	1.7	1.7	1.2	0.6

* From González-Domínguez et al. [24].

3.5. *Nanoparticle Tracking Analysis (NTA)*

The total amount of nanoparticles produced in each platform was evaluated by NTA with the light scattering mode and VLPs were analyzed with the fluorescent filter module (Figure 5A). The PSD and concentration of the different nanoparticle populations was conducted by the combination of both modules. An average diameter of 143 ± 39 nm for VLPs and 161 ± 66 nm considering all nanoparticles as a single population was measured in HEK 293 samples. As for Sf9 supernatants, an average diameter of 213 ± 95 nm was measured for VLPs and 194 ± 75 nm for total nanoparticles. Comparison of VLP concentrations in both platforms resulted in a 1.7-fold increase in Sf9 compared to HEK 293 samples (Figure 5C,D). On the contrary, a higher EV content was found in HEK 293 samples (Table 2). Analysis of original FreeStyle and Sf900III cell culture media by light scattering NTA resulted in a concentration of $0.6 \pm 0.1 \times 10^9$ and $24.4 \pm 1.1 \times 10^9$ diffracting particles/mL, respectively, with a mean size diameter of 174 ± 39 nm and 92.7 ± 74.6 nm. Thus, a difference of two orders of magnitude in particle concentration was obtained in Sf900III over FreeStyle medium. Evaluation of conditioned FreeStyle and Sf900III media was also assessed by NTA and yielded a concentration of $17.6 \pm 0.9 \times 10^9$ and $27.3 \pm 1.5 \times 10^9$ diffracting particles/ml, respectively, with a mean diameter of 174 ± 65 nm and 101 ± 47 nm for HEK 293 and Sf9 samples, respectively.

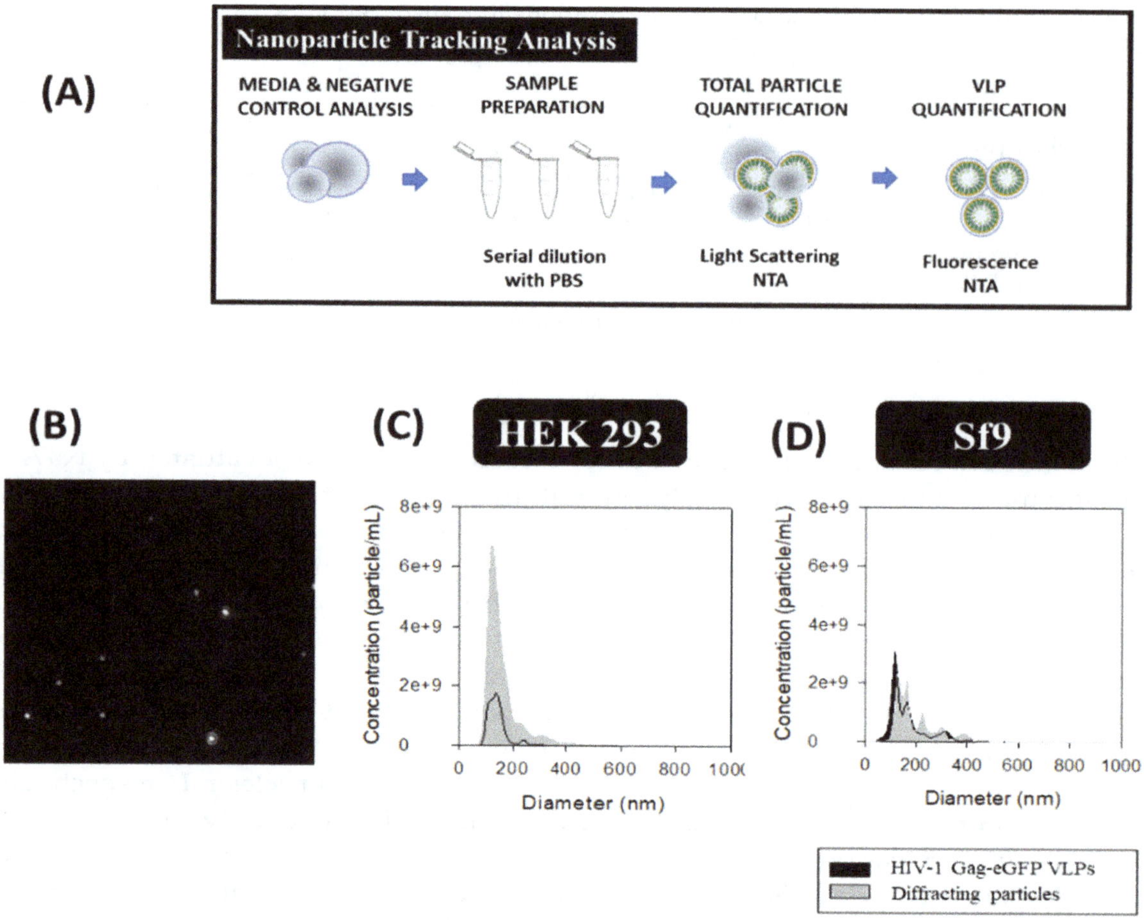

Figure 5. Nanoparticle tracking analysis of HIV-1 Gag-eGFP VLPs produced in HEK 293 and Sf9 cells harvested at 72 hpt and 40 hpi, respectively. (**A**) Sample preparation and analysis workflow. (**B**) Image of nanoparticles tracked by NTA. (**C**,**D**) PSD analysis of HEK 293 and Sf9 supernatants, respectively. HEK 293 and Sf9 supernatants were diluted with filtered DPBS to adjust their concentration prior to analysis. Negative controls were analyzed in the same conditions as in VLP samples (Supplementary materials S1).

3.6. Flow Virometry

The production of HIV-1 Gag-eGFP VLPs and other nanoparticle populations was simultaneously analyzed by flow virometry. Equipment calibration for VLP analysis was performed with commercial beads of known diameter (100, 160, 200, 240, 300, 500 and 900 nm) in order to calculate the mean nanoparticle diameter (Figure 6B, B.1 and B.2). Mie scatter modelling allowed to convert V-SSC intensities of VLPs and EVs to their corresponding size with FCM_{PASS} software developed by Welsh and co-authors (Figures 3 and 6 and Supplementary materials S2) [33]. By doing so, the detection of nanoparticles with diameters down to 100 nm could be achieved.

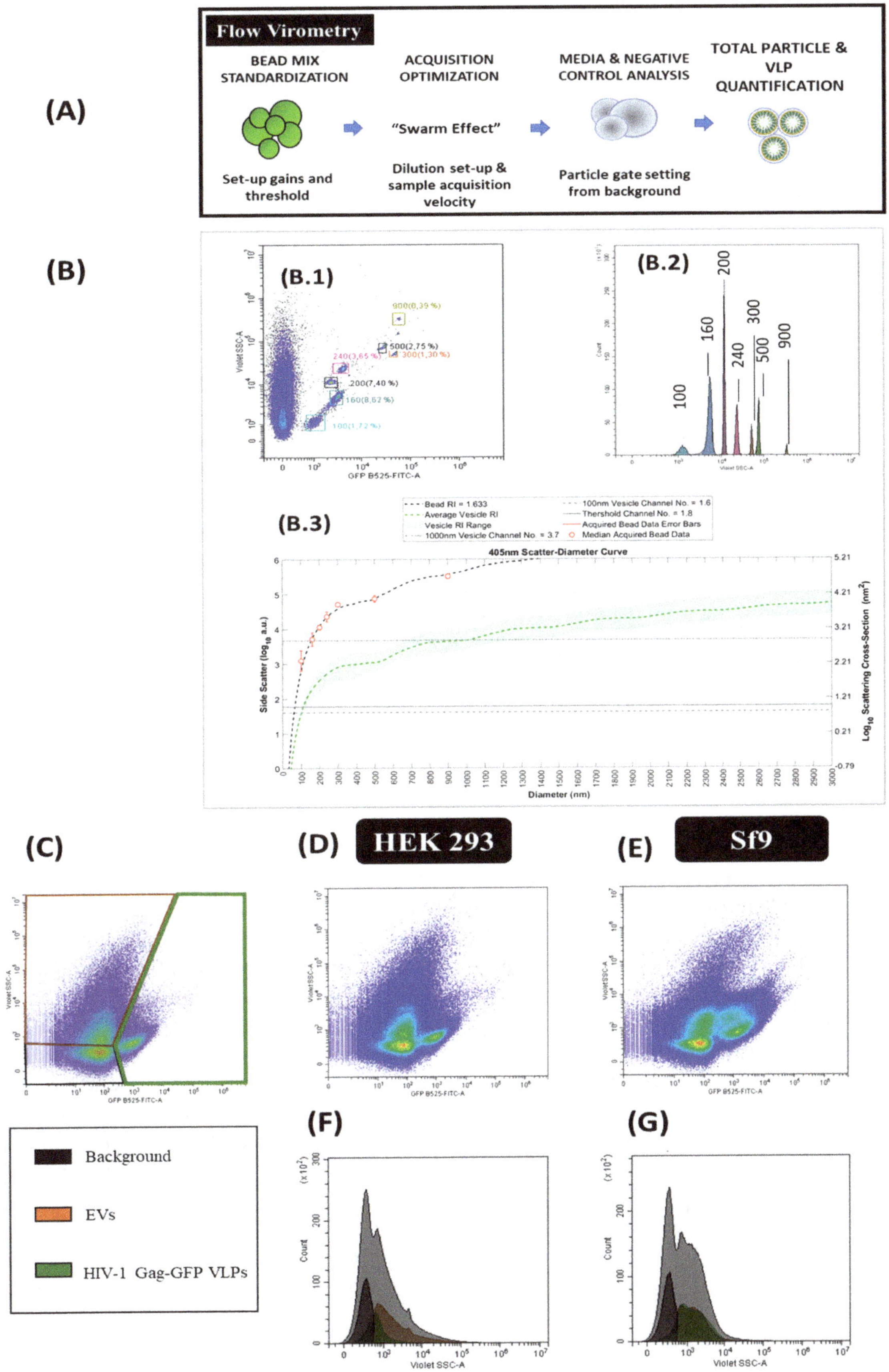

Figure 6. Flow virometry analysis of HIV-1 Gag-eGFP VLPs produced in HEK 293 and Sf9 cells harvested at 72 hpt and 40 hpi, respectively. (**A**) Sample preparation and analysis workflow and (**B**) equipment calibration using beads with a known diameter. Megamix-Plus fluorescent beads of 100,

160, 200, 240, 300, 500 and 900 nm were used. (B.1) GFP B525-FITC-A vs. V-SSC density plots of the beads, (B.2) GFP B525-FITC-A histogram of the beads and (B.3) Mie correlation of the beads with FCM_{PASS} software [33]. (**C**) Gating of the different nanoparticle populations in a density plot and defined as EVs, HIV-1 Gag-eGFP VLPs and background signal of the equipment. (**D–G**) Density plots and histograms of nanoparticles produced in HEK 293 (**D**,**F**) and Sf9 supernatants (**E**,**G**), respectively. HEK 293 and Sf9 supernatants were diluted with filtered DPBS prior to analysis. Negative controls were analyzed using the same conditions as in VLP samples (Supplementary materials S1).

After equipment set-up, different nanoparticle populations could be assessed in one single analysis. Three main populations were detected in transfected HEK 293 and BV infected Sf9 samples (Figure 6G). Two of these populations corresponded to EVs, classified as small and large EVs, and the third one was related to VLPs (fluorescent particles). EVs displayed a high level of heterogeneity in the V-SSC, with values ranging from 10^2 to 10^5 a.u. Interestingly, a second subpopulation of VLPs with a higher V-SSC intensity was detected in BV infected Sf9 samples, which could be probably associated to the aggregation of VLPs or the interaction of VLPs with other cellular compounds released to the medium. This second VLP subpopulation displayed a more pronounced right-skewed V-SSC distribution compared to the more homogeneous VLP population observed in HEK 293 samples (Figure 6F). In terms of quantification, VLP concentrations in the range of 10^8 particles/mL were measured with a 1.5-fold increase in VLP concentration in Sf9 over HEK 293 supernatants (Table 2). As regards EVs, higher levels of these nanoparticles were quantified in conditioned media from Sf9 over HEK 293 cells, respectively (Supplementary materials S1). Mean size analysis of VLPs and EVs by Mie correlation resulted in 114 ± 26 nm for VLPs and 115 ± 26 nm for EVs in HEK 293 supernatants, respectively, while a mean diameter of 117 ± 22 nm and 115 ± 24 nm was measured for VLPs and EVs in Sf9 supernatants (Figure 6D–G).

4. Discussion

4.1. Sample Preparation and Equipment Set-up

Among the different techniques used, the cost, technical requirements and the time needed for sample analysis are practical issues that have to be considered to select an adequate analytical technique for nanoparticle characterization (Table 3) [12]. Regarding sample preparation, purified VLPs were loaded and stained by the addition of uranyl acetate in TEM-Negative staining. Altogether, sample preparation time required less than 10 min per sample, without considering the previous ultracentrifugation step, which required one day of experimentation. Compared to the TEM-Negative staining protocol (Figure 1A), SEM-Alcian Blue grids were not treated by glow discharge before the addition of Alcian Blue solution. The VLP-containing supernatant was directly loaded, representing an overall process duration of 15 min. As for cryo-TEM, sample preparation required an approximate time of 10 min; however, the equipment set-up required a longer time of pre-conditioning compared to TEM and SEM due to the low temperature conditions employed. In SRFM, acquisition of 3D VLP images took around 10 min per field and data analysis with Imaris software required 15–20 min to process the different channels and construct the final image. As for NTA, the time needed to conduct a complete analysis lasted 1 h due to sample preparation and software analysis (Figure 5A), while in flow virometry the different nanoparticle populations could be analyzed in one single run (Table 3).

Table 3. Comparison of the different analytical technologies assessed in this work.

Parameter	TEM	SEM	Cryo-TEM	HyVolution2 SRFM	NTA	Flow Virometry
Expertise	+++	+++	+++++	+++	++	++
Time of measurement	++++	++++	+++++	+++	++	+
Resolution	Nanometric (<10 nm) [14]	Nanometric (<10 nm) [48]	Atomic [13]	Nanometric (140 nm) [26]	Nanometric (30 nm) [29]	Nanometric (100–200 nm) [5]
Pros	Widely used, ultrastructural analysis	Surface analysis of nanoparticle populations	Ultrastructural analysis in its native form	Direct visualization, compatible with fluorescence	Easy handling, compatible with fluorescence	Simultaneous analysis of light scattering and fluorescence labelling
Cons	Staining required, working under vacuum conditions	Working under vacuum conditions	Time consuming, working at cryogenic temperatures	Data analysis, convolution effect of light	Screening effect, variability due to acquisition settings	Sensitivity, inter-equipment variability

In most cases, sample preparation and equipment set-up are based on trial-and-error, which can introduce a certain degree of variability in the characterization of nanoparticles. In the case of TEM, the low electron density present in biological samples as well as the need to work under vacuum conditions require the addition of contrast agents for a better resolution of the specimens under evaluation. Uranium strongly reacts with phosphate and amino groups [44], thus conferring a higher level of electron density to biological samples and VLPs are observed as round structures surrounded by a bright corona. Despite the simplicity of negative staining, the presence of artifacts and background due to the composition of the contrast medium are detected (Figure 1B–D), as reported in the literature [3,15]. Depending on the sample origin, this can have a major impact, as observed in Sf9 cell micrographs in comparison to HEK 293 samples, where a higher level of background was identified and EVs could not be distinguished from VLPs (Figure 1C). This background is probably caused by the larger load of particles present in insect cell culture media [49]. In this sense, new commercially available chemically defined insect cell culture media could alleviate this problem [50]. Different approaches have been investigated to overcome the drawbacks of negative staining [1]. SEM-Alcian Blue has been studied in this work as a possible alternative. On the one hand, TEM has been traditionally used for viral intraparticle characterization, while SEM is generally applied for a broader screening of biological populations [48,51]. Novel preparation methods, such as ionic liquid infiltration [51] or virus quantification by Prep/g [52] have been reported as strategies to assess bacterial and viral preparations with SEM in the recent years. In the same line, the use of Alcian Blue as a solution for grid pre-treatment was shown to increase the adsorption of nanoparticles in this work, thus allowing to improve the detection of these particles avoiding negative staining (Figure 2). Nevertheless, the differentiation of VLPs from EVs was not possible due their similar morphology, but this new label-free method has a potential applicability in combination with X-ray spectroscopy [31], SRFM [53], or "wet" SEM [51] to deepen into nanoparticle characterization. Alternatively, the low contrast present in biological samples can also be overcome in EM by using cryo-TEM, which does not require sample staining (Figure 3). However, an adjustment of the cryogenic freezing protocol for each sample depending on its physicochemical properties is required [21]. Overall, all EM techniques demand a high expertise by the user and often entail long sample analysis times (Table 3). Therefore, the development of more automatic and high throughput complementary methods is required to process nanoparticle samples in a faster manner.

SRFM, NTA and flow virometry can be implemented to this purpose since they allow mass quantification of nanoparticles. Nonetheless, sample standardization and technical expertise is still critical for an adequate nanoparticle assessment (Table 3). A microscope equipped with advanced capture and image processing modules, and the optimization of acquisition conditions together with different imaging software are required in SRFM. Additional process automatization should be developed to widen its application since the time required for sample analysis is still high and operator-dependent. In NTA, relevant parameters to be considered during nanoparticle analysis are the camera level and the detection threshold [5]. These settings need to be manually adjusted in each sample for an adequate tracking of the nanoparticles recorded and their automatic quantification. NTA measurements depend on the refractive index (RI) of each particle and the nanoparticle containing solution. Thus, different specific settings were applied to measure HEK 293 and Sf9 supernatants (Table 1). Another important feature affecting the final output with NTA is size heterogeneity of nanoparticle populations in the sample, which hinder the quantification of the small subpopulations due to the screening effect of higher particles, as reported by van der Pol et al. [5]. Regarding flow virometry, differences in the measurements due to inter-equipment variability have been pointed as one of the major challenges of this technique. Nevertheless, the use of commercial beads as standard nanoparticles and the implementation of Mie correlations have contributed to solve this problem [33,52,54]. Similarly, tunable resistive pulse sensing (TRPS), Atomic Force Microscopy (AFM) and field-flow fractionation coupled to multiangle light scattering (FFF-MALS) are single particle analysis methods that can be implemented for nanoparticle characterization [12]. However, none of these techniques enable to differentiate VLPs from EVs without additional sample treatments.

4.2. Ultrastructural Analysis

Single particle evaluation conducted by SRFM, NTA and flow virometry is an interesting option for characterization analyses since specific labeling can be applied to study different nanoparticle populations [27,55]. The use of the fluorescently tagged Gag polyprotein enabled the differentiation of VLPs from the other co-produced nanoparticle populations in this work. These analytical methods have also been successfully used in combination with immunolabeling to quantitatively asses viral populations [27]. A step further has been recently achieved in SRFM with the possibility to detect nucleic acids and the lipid membrane in VLPs [25]. The commercially available ViroCyt®flow cytometer has been similarly used to quantify different viral isolates, including the Ebola virus [56]. Still, the detection of VLPs with ViroCyt® has not been reported [57]. Nevertheless, none of these techniques achieve the levels of nanoparticle resolution of EM methods (Table 3).

Among the different EM methods evaluated, cryo-TEM showed a higher benefit compared to TEM and SEM since the native conformation of the different nanoparticles could be assessed. The ultrastructural analysis of the different VLP, EV and BV subpopulations could be described in detail, with remarkable differences detected between Gag-eGFP and Gag VLPs. The Gag polyprotein is known to travel to the vicinity of the plasma membrane, aggregate with other Gag monomers, and bud to the extracellular space as an immature HIV-1 particle (Figure 3J) [38,58]. Interestingly, Gag-eGFP VLPs do not achieve the expected organized structure as Gag VLPs probably due to the eGFP fusion that alters the native budding process [59]. These differences could not be detected by TEM due to the interference of negative staining with the samples [11,36,60]. To our knowledge, this is the first time were Gag-eGFP VLP intraparticle organization is observed. Therefore, it is shown that fusion proteins can introduce morphological alterations in the structure of the nanoparticles produced and cryo-TEM is an interesting method to identify them.

4.3. Particle Size Distribution

The PSD of VLPs has been studied with the six methods evaluated in this work. Typically, the VLP mean diameter is comprised between 100 and 200 nm, as observed by TEM, cryo-TEM, NTA and flow virometry [61]. Non-symmetric right-skewed distributions were observed for VLPs measured with the different techniques. Similar PSDs of HIV-1 Gag VLPs produced in CAP-T and CHO cells were shown by Gutierrez-Granados et al. and Steppert et al., respectively [37,62]. The presence of larger population of VLPs, especially when measuring Sf9 samples by NTA and flow virometry, could be related to the aggregation of VLPs or their interaction with other cellular compounds released to the medium. SEM and SRFM presented higher PSD in comparison to the rest of analytical technologies. SEM analysis of HEK 293 samples resulted in a PSD of 296 ± 88 nm, which could indicate that several EVs were quantified instead of VLPs since microvesicles can reach up to 2000 nm [6]. HyVolution2 SRFM yielded the highest VLP PSD values in both cell platforms (>250 nm), which has also been observed by Xiao and co-workers when analyzing Cy5-labeled adeno-associated viruses [63], and could be attributed to the convolution effect of light. In this case, the individual fluorochrome intensity does not necessarily correlate with the real particle size and might result in particle size diameter overestimation [64]. The use of more powerful SRFM techniques, such as stimulated emission depletion (STED) or stochastic optical reconstruction microscopy (STORM) could reduce this effect [65]. However, STED and STORM require specific fluorophores that tolerate the high laser intensities applied and also a higher level of expertise and equipment infrastructure in comparison to HyVolution2 SRFM.

The PSD of EVs was assessed by NTA and flow virometry (Figures 5 and 6). In both cases, EVs presented an average diameter comprised between 100 and 200 nm, similar to that of VLPs. Nonetheless, a right-skewed distribution with vesicles diameters from 45 to 500 nm was observed, especially in Sf9 samples. These results correlate with the existence of several types of EVs, encompassing exosomes and microvesicles, and BVs as visualized in cryo-TEM micrographs (Figure 3). Of note, the PSD of rod-shaped baculoviruses could not be accurately characterized by any of these methods since they assume that all nanoparticles are spherical. Van der Pol and coworkers also observed the size heterogeneity of EVs, with diameters ranging between 70 and 800 nm. They report a minimum detection limit for EVs of 70–90 nm with NTA and 150–190 nm by flow virometry [5]. Lower EV detection limits of 45 nm with NTA and 100 nm by flow virometry were reported in this work. The sample composition and also the implementation of the V-SSC instead of the 488 nm SSC in flow virometry could contribute to explain these differences [34]. Still, a higher level of accuracy is possible by using National Institute of Standards and Technology (NIST)-traceable beads in the Mie correlation with flow virometry.

4.4. Particle Concentration

SRFM, NTA and flow virometry were compared for the quantification of nanoparticles in HEK 293 and Sf9 samples (Figures 4–6 and Table 2). Compared to SRFM and NTA, flow virometry yielded a lower concentration of nanoparticles being around 30-fold lower for VLPs and >60-fold lower for EVs (Table 2). Similar differences in quantification by flow virometry have also been reported by van der Pol and co-authors in the analysis of urinary vesicles [5]. Differences in nanoparticle quantification between techniques could be related to the swarm effect, which is based on the fact that more than one particle passes through the detector simultaneously. However, the analysis of the same sample dilutions by flow virometry and NTA resulted in a linear correlation between both methods (VLPs, $R^2 > 0.99$; total particles $R^2 > 0.91$), indicating that the swarm effect could not be the main reason behind these results (Supplementary materials S3). On the other hand, it is also possible that the detection of small particles fell in the range of the background signal of the cytometer, thus contributing to reduce the final titers. Even though the average particle size of EVs and VLPs was above the minimum detection particle diameter of flow virometry, additional refinement of the Mie correlation could still be required to adequately explain these data.

Analysis of the different nanoparticle populations in each platform revealed that at least 50% of the total particles produced did not correspond to VLPs (Table 2). The possibility to discriminate but also simultaneously quantify VLPs and the rest of specimens by NTA and flow virometry represents a remarkable advantage for nanoparticle-based bioprocesses. However, further refinement of light scattered-based methodologies is required since a remarkable background signal is detected in medium solutions devoid of particles (Supplementary materials S1).

5. Conclusions

The selection of an adequate analytical method is essential in VLP characterization processes. Among the six methodologies studied in this work, cryo-TEM was shown as the best method to resolve nanoparticle structures while maintaining its native conformation. This technique allowed for a detailed characterization of the different EV and BV subpopulations co-produced with VLPs in HEK293 and Sf9 productions. Alternatively, the high-throughput analysis of VLPs and their differentiation from other contaminant particles was achieved by flow virometry, SRFM and NTA. Among them, flow virometry showed to be the fastest method for PSD analysis while also allowing to simultaneously quantify different nanoparticle subpopulations. Nonetheless, further improvements of these methods are required since different quantification results are observed between techniques.

Author Contributions: Conceptualization, I.G.-D. and E.P.-M.; methodology, I.G.-D. and E.P.-M.; formal analysis, I.G.-D. and E.P.-M.; investigation, I.G.-D. and E.P.-M.; writing—original draft preparation, I.G.-D. and E.P.-M.; review, editing and supervision, L.C. and F.G. All authors have read and agreed to the published version of the manuscript.

Acknowledgments: The help of Manuela Costa (Servei de Cultius Cel·lulars, Producció d'Anticossos i Citometria, UAB) and Ángel Calvache and Jorge Fomaro (Beckman Coulter) for facilitating access to the Cytoflex LX equipment and the Megamix-Plus beads is very appreciated. The authors would like to acknowledge the help of Marti de Cabo and Emma Rossinyol (Servei de Microscòpia, UAB, Barcelona, Spain) for the assistance with EM methodologies, Mònica Roldan for the support with SRFM (Servei d'Anatomia Patològica, Hospital Sant Joan de Déu, Barcelona, Spain) and Joshua Welsh (NIH, Bethesda, MD, USA) for the help with FCM_{PASS} Software.

Abbreviations

AB	Alcian Blue
AFM	Atomic Force Microscopy
BV	Baculovirus
CQA	Critical Quality Attributes
Cryo-TEM	Cryogenic Transmission Electron Microscopy
DLS	Dynamic Light Scattering
EM	Electron Microscopy
EV	Extracellular Vesicle
cBV	filled baculovirus with vesicle-like or protein content
LM	Lipid Membrane
MVB	Multivesicular Body
NS	Negative Staining
NTA	Nanoparticle Tracking Analysis
ODV	Occlusion-Derived Baculovirus
PSD	Particle Size Distribution
RI	Refractive Index
rBV	relaxed-form of baculovirus
RT	Room Temperature
SEM	Scanning Electron Microscopy
SRFM	Super-Resolution Fluorescence Microscopy
TEM	Transmission Electron Microscopy
TRPS	Tunable Resistive Pulse Sensing
V-SSC	Violet Side Scatter
VLP	Virus-Like Particle

References

1. Charlton Hume, H.K.; Vidigal, J.; Carrondo, M.J.T.; Middelberg, A.P.J.; Roldão, A.; Lua, L.H.L. Synthetic biology for bioengineering virus-like particle vaccines. *Biotechnol. Bioeng.* **2019**, *116*, 919–935. [CrossRef]
2. Cervera, L.; Gòdia, F.; Tarrés-Freixas, F.; Aguilar-Gurrieri, C.; Carrillo, J.; Blanco, J.; Gutiérrez-Granados, S. Production of HIV-1-based virus-like particles for vaccination: Achievements and limits. *Appl. Microbiol. Biotechnol.* **2019**, *103*, 7367–7384. [CrossRef] [PubMed]

3. Lua, L.H.L.; Connors, N.K.; Sainsbury, F.; Chuan, Y.P.; Wibowo, N.; Middelberg, A.P.J. Bioengineering virus-like particles as vaccines. *Biotechnol. Bioeng.* **2014**, *111*, 425–440. [CrossRef] [PubMed]
4. Jain, N.K.; Sahni, N.; Kumru, O.S.; Joshi, S.B.; Volkin, D.B.; Russell Middaugh, C. Formulation and stabilization of recombinant protein based virus-like particle vaccines. *Adv. Drug Deliv. Rev.* **2015**, *93*, 42–55. [CrossRef] [PubMed]
5. Van der Pol, E.; Coumans, F.a.W.; Grootemaat, a.E.; Gardiner, C.; Sargent, I.L.; Harrison, P.; Sturk, A.; van Leeuwen, T.G.; Nieuwland, R. Particle size distribution of exosomes and microvesicles determined by transmission electron microscopy, flow cytometry, nanoparticle tracking analysis, and resistive pulse sensing. *J. Thromb. Haemost.* **2014**, *12*, 1182–1192. [CrossRef] [PubMed]
6. Akers, J.C.; Gonda, D.; Kim, R.; Carter, B.S.; Chen, C.C. Biogenesis of extracellular vesicles (EV): Exosomes, microvesicles, retrovirus-like vesicles, and apoptotic bodies. *J. Neurooncol.* **2013**, *113*, 1–11. [CrossRef] [PubMed]
7. Wang, Q.; Bosch, B.-J.; Vlak, J.M.; van Oers, M.M.; Rottier, P.J.; van Lent, J.W.M. Budded baculovirus particle structure revisited. *J. Invertebr. Pathol.* **2016**, *134*, 15–22. [CrossRef]
8. Transfiguracion, J.; Manceur, A.P.; Petiot, E.; Thompson, C.M.; Kamen, A.A. Particle quantification of influenza viruses by high performance liquid chromatography. *Vaccine* **2015**, *33*, 78–84. [CrossRef]
9. Steppert, P.; Burgstaller, D.; Klausberger, M.; Tover, A.; Berger, E.; Jungbauer, A. Quantification and characterization of virus-like particles by size-exclusion chromatography and nanoparticle tracking analysis. *J. Chromatogr. A* **2017**, *1487*, 89–99. [CrossRef]
10. Gutiérrez-Granados, S.; Cervera, L.; Gòdia, F.; Carrillo, J.; Segura, M.M. Development and validation of a quantitation assay for fluorescently tagged HIV-1 virus-like particles. *J. Virol. Methods* **2013**, *193*, 85–95. [CrossRef]
11. Venereo-Sanchez, A.; Gilbert, R.; Simoneau, M.; Caron, A.; Chahal, P.; Chen, W.; Ansorge, S.; Li, X.; Henry, O.; Kamen, A. Hemagglutinin and neuraminidase containing virus-like particles produced in HEK-293 suspension culture: An effective influenza vaccine candidate. *Vaccine* **2016**, *34*, 3371–3380. [CrossRef] [PubMed]
12. Heider, S.; Metzner, C. Quantitative real-time single particle analysis of virions. *Virology* **2014**, *462–463*, 199–206. [CrossRef] [PubMed]
13. Jiang, W.; Tang, L. Atomic cryo-EM structures of viruses. *Curr. Opin. Struct. Biol.* **2017**, *46*, 122–129. [CrossRef]
14. Popov, V.L.; Tesh, R.B.; Weaver, S.C.; Vasilakis, N.; Popov, V.L.; Tesh, R.B.; Weaver, S.C.; Vasilakis, N. Electron Microscopy in Discovery of Novel and Emerging Viruses from the Collection of the World Reference Center for Emerging Viruses and Arboviruses (WRCEVA). *Viruses* **2019**, *11*, 477. [CrossRef]
15. De Carlo, S.; Harris, J.R. Negative staining and cryo-negative staining of macromolecules and viruses for TEM. *Micron* **2011**, *42*, 117–131. [CrossRef]
16. Kalsoom, A.; Khan, S.A.; Khan, S.B.; Asiri, A.M. Chapter 4. Scanning Electron Microscopy: Principle and Applications in Nanomaterials Characterization. In *Handbook of Materials Characterization*; Sharma, S.K., Ed.; Springer International Publishing: Cham, Switzerland, 2018; pp. 113–146. ISBN 978-3-319-92954-5.
17. Gállego Ossul, I. *Estructura y propiedades de las placas de cromatina de los cromosomas metafásicos: Estudio mediante técnicas de microscopía TEM, AFM y Espectroscopia de Fuerza Atómica*; Universitat Autònoma de Barcelona: Bellaterra, Spain, 2010.
18. Michen, B.; Graule, T. Isoelectric points of viruses. *J. Appl. Microbiol.* **2010**, *109*, 388–397. [CrossRef]
19. Deregibus, M.C.; Figliolini, F.; D'antico, S.; Manzini, P.M.; Pasquino, C.; De Lena, M.; Tetta, C.; Brizzi, M.F.; Camussi, G. Charge-based precipitation of extracellular vesicles. *Int. J. Mol. Med.* **2016**, *38*, 1359–1366. [CrossRef]
20. Murata, K.; Wolf, M. Cryo-electron microscopy for structural analysis of dynamic biological macromolecules. *Biochim. Biophys. Acta Gen. Subj.* **2018**, *1862*, 324–334. [CrossRef]
21. Thompson, R.F.; Walker, M.; Siebert, C.A.; Muench, S.P.; Ranson, N.A. An introduction to sample preparation and imaging by cryo-electron microscopy for structural biology. *Methods* **2016**, *100*, 3–15. [CrossRef]
22. Hanne, J.; Zila, V.; Heilemann, M.; Müller, B.; Kräusslich, H.-G. Super-resolved insights into human immunodeficiency virus biology. *FEBS Lett.* **2016**, *590*, 1858–1876. [CrossRef] [PubMed]

23. Godin, A.G.; Lounis, B.; Cognet, L. Super-resolution Microscopy Approaches for Live Cell Imaging. *Biophysj* **2014**, *107*, 1777–1784. [CrossRef] [PubMed]
24. González-Domínguez, I.; Puente-Massaguer, E.; Cervera, L.; Gòdia, F. Quantification of the HIV-1 virus-like particle production process by super-resolution imaging: From VLP budding to nanoparticle analysis. **2020**. Under review.
25. Puente-Massaguer, E.; Lecina, M.; Gòdia, F. Application of advanced quantification techniques in nanoparticle-based vaccine development with the Sf9 cell baculovirus expression system. *Vaccine* **2020**, *38*, 1849–1859. [CrossRef] [PubMed]
26. Borlinghaus, R.T.; Kappel, C. HyVolution—The smart path to confocal super-resolution. *Nat. Methods* **2016**, *13*, i. [CrossRef]
27. Zamora, J.L.R.; Aguilar, H.C. Flow virometry as a tool to study viruses. *Methods* **2017**, *134–135*, 87–97. [CrossRef]
28. Maguire, C.M.; Rösslein, M.; Wick, P.; Prina-Mello, A. Characterisation of particles in solution—A perspective on light scattering and comparative technologies. *Sci. Technol. Adv. Mater.* **2018**, *19*, 732–745. [CrossRef]
29. Kramberger, P.; Ciringer, M.; Štrancar, A.; Peterka, M. Evaluation of nanoparticle tracking analysis for total virus particle determination. *Virol. J.* **2012**, *9*, 265. [CrossRef]
30. Aguilar, P.P.; González-Domínguez, I.; Schneider, T.A.; Gòdia, F.; Cervera, L.; Jungbauer, A. At-line multi-angle light scattering detector for faster process development in enveloped virus-like particle purification. *J. Sep. Sci.* **2019**, *42*, 2640–2648. [CrossRef]
31. González-Domínguez, I.; Grimaldi, N.; Cervera, L.; Ventosa, N.; Gòdia, F. Impact of physicochemical properties of DNA/PEI complexes on transient transfection of mammalian cells. *N. Biotechnol.* **2019**, *49*, 88–97. [CrossRef]
32. Nolan, J.P.; Duggan, E. Analysis of Individual Extracellular Vesicles by Flow Cytometry. In *Flow Cytometry Protocols, Methods in Molecular Biology*; Hawley, T.S., Hawley, R.G., Eds.; Springer Science+Business Media LLC: Berlin, Germany, 2018; Volume 1678, pp. 79–92. ISBN 978-1-4939-7346-0.
33. Welsh, J.A.; Horak, P.; Wilkinson, J.S.; Ford, V.J.; Jones, J.C.; Smith, D.; Holloway, J.A.; Englyst, N.A. FCM PASS Software Aids Extracellular Vesicle Light Scatter Standardization. *Cytom. Part A* **2019**. [CrossRef]
34. McVey, M.J.; Spring, C.M.; Kuebler, W.M. Improved resolution in extracellular vesicle populations using 405 instead of 488 nm side scatter. *J. Extracell. Vesicles* **2018**, *7*, 1–11. [CrossRef] [PubMed]
35. Charlton Hume, H.K.; Lua, L.H.L. Platform technologies for modern vaccine manufacturing. *Vaccine* **2017**, *35*, 4480–4485. [CrossRef]
36. Cervera, L.; Gutiérrez-Granados, S.; Martínez, M.; Blanco, J.; Gòdia, F.; Segura, M.M. Generation of HIV-1 Gag VLPs by transient transfection of HEK 293 suspension cell cultures using an optimized animal-derived component free medium. *J. Biotechnol.* **2013**, *166*, 152–165. [CrossRef] [PubMed]
37. Gutiérrez-Granados, S.; Cervera, L.; de L.M. Segura, M.; Wölfel, J.; Gòdia, F. Optimized production of HIV-1 virus-like particles by transient transfection in CAP-T cells. *Appl. Microbiol. Biotechnol.* **2016**, *100*, 3935–3947. [CrossRef] [PubMed]
38. Göttlinger, H.G. HIV-1 Gag: A Molecular Machine Driving Viral Particle Assembly and Release. In *HIV Sequence Compendium 2011*; Kuiken, C., Foley, B., Leitner, T., Apetrei, C., Hahn, B., Mizrachi, I., Mullins, J., Rambaut, A., Wolinsky, S., Korber, B., Eds.; Los Alamos National Laboratory, Theoretical Biology and Biophysics: Los Alamos, NM, USA, 2011; pp. 2–28, LA-UR-11-11440.
39. Thompson, C.M.; Petiot, E.; Mullick, A.; Aucoin, M.G.; Henry, O.; Kamen, A.A. Critical assessment of influenza VLP production in Sf9 and HEK293 expression systems. *BMC Biotechnol.* **2015**, *15*, 1–12. [CrossRef] [PubMed]
40. Genzel, Y. Designing cell lines for viral vaccine production: Where do we stand? *Biotechnol. J.* **2015**, *10*, 728–740. [CrossRef]
41. Puente-Massaguer, E.; Lecina, M.; Gòdia, F. Integrating nanoparticle quantification and statistical design of experiments for efficient HIV-1 virus-like particle production in High Five cells. *Appl. Microbiol. Biotechnol.* **2020**, *104*, 1569–1582. [CrossRef]
42. De Rond, L.; Coumans, F.A.W.; Nieuwland, R.; van Leeuwen, T.G.; van der Pol, E. Deriving Extracellular Vesicle Size From Scatter Intensities Measured by Flow Cytometry. *Curr. Protoc. Cytom.* **2018**, *86*, 1–14. [CrossRef]

43. Malvern Instruments Limited. Determining Fluorescence Limit of Detection with Nanoparticle Tracking Analysis (NTA). 2015. Available online: https://www.malvernpanalytical.com/en/learn/knowledge-center/application-notes/AN150507FluorescenceLOD (accessed on 17 February 2020).
44. Ellis, E.A. Staining Sectioned Biological Specimens for Transmission Electron Microscopy: Conventional and En Bloc Stains. In *Electron Microscopy: Methods and Protocols, Methods in Molecular Biology*; Kuo, J., Ed.; Humana Press: Totowa, NJ, USA, 2014; pp. 57–72. ISBN 978-1-62703-776-1.
45. Cervera, L.; Fuenmayor, J.; González-Domínguez, I.; Gutiérrez-Granados, S.; Segura, M.M.; Gòdia, F. Selection and optimization of transfection enhancer additives for increased virus-like particle production in HEK293 suspension cell cultures. *Appl. Microbiol. Biotechnol.* **2015**, *99*, 9935–9949. [CrossRef]
46. González-Domínguez, I.; Gutiérrez-Granados, S.; Cervera, L.; Gòdia, F.; Domingo, N. Identification of HIV-1–Based Virus-like Particles by Multifrequency Atomic Force Microscopy. *Biophys. J.* **2016**, *111*, 1173–1179. [CrossRef]
47. Puente-Massaguer, E.; González-Domínguez, I.; Universitat Autònoma de Barcelona, Barcelona, Spain. Preliminary experiments on HIV-1 Gag-eGFP VLP characterization by Scanning Electron Microscopy. Personal communication, 2020.
48. Gencer, D.; Bayramoglu, Z.; Nalcacioglu, R.; Kleespies, R.G.; Demirbag, Z.; Demir, I. Characterisation of three Alphabaculovirus isolates from the gypsy moth, Lymantria dispar dispar (Lepidoptera: Erebidae), in Turkey. *Biocontrol Sci. Technol.* **2018**, *28*, 107–121. [CrossRef]
49. Palomares, L.A.; Realpe, M.; Ramírez, O.T. An Overview of Cell Culture Engineering for the Insect Cell-Baculovirus Expression Vector System (BEVS). In *Methods in Molecular Biology*; Humana Press: Totowa, NJ, USA, 2015; Volume 5, pp. 501–519. ISBN 978-3-319-10319-8.
50. Thermo Fisher Scientific. ExpiSfTM Expression System. 2020. Available online: https://assets.thermofisher.com/TFSAssets/LSG/manuals/MAN0017532_ExpiSfExpressionSystem_UG.pdf (accessed on 17 February 2020).
51. Golding, C.G.; Lamboo, L.L.; Beniac, D.R.; Booth, T.F. The scanning electron microscope in microbiology and diagnosis of infectious disease. *Sci. Rep.* **2016**, *6*, 26516. [CrossRef] [PubMed]
52. Van Der Pol, E.; Hoekstra, A.G.; Sturk, A.; Otto, C.; Van Leeuwen, T.G.; Nieuwland, R. Optical and non-optical methods for detection and characterization of microparticles and exosomes. *J. Thromb. Haemost.* **2010**, *8*, 2596–2607. [CrossRef] [PubMed]
53. Pedersen, M.; Jamali, S.; Saha, I.; Daum, R.; Bendjennat, M.; Saffarian, S. Correlative iPALM and SEM resolves virus cavity and Gag lattice defects in HIV virions. *Eur. Biophys. J.* **2019**, *48*, 15–23. [CrossRef] [PubMed]
54. Welsh, J.A.; Holloway, J.A.; Wilkinson, J.S.; Englyst, N.A. Extracellular Vesicle Flow Cytometry Analysis and Standardization. *Front. Cell Dev. Biol.* **2017**, *5*, 1–7. [CrossRef]
55. Yang, Z.; Sharma, A.; Qi, J.; Peng, X.; Lee, D.Y.; Hu, R.; Lin, D.; Qu, J.; Kim, J.S. Super-resolution fluorescent materials: An insight into design and bioimaging applications. *Chem. Soc. Rev.* **2016**, *45*, 4651–4667. [CrossRef]
56. Rossi, C.; Kearney, B.; Olschner, S.; Williams, P.; Robinson, C.; Heinrich, M.; Zovanyi, A.; Ingram, M.; Norwood, D.; Schoepp, R. Evaluation of ViroCyt® Virus Counter for Rapid Filovirus Quantitation. *Viruses* **2015**, *7*, 857–872. [CrossRef]
57. Blancett, C.D.; Fetterer, D.P.; Koistinen, K.A.; Morazzani, E.M.; Monninger, M.K.; Piper, A.E.; Kuehl, K.A.; Kearney, B.J.; Norris, S.L.; Rossi, C.A.; et al. Accurate virus quantitation using a Scanning Transmission Electron Microscopy (STEM) detector in a scanning electron microscope. *J. Virol. Methods* **2017**, *248*, 136–144. [CrossRef]
58. Strauss, J.D.; Hammonds, J.E.; Yi, H.; Ding, L.; Spearman, P.; Wright, E.R. Three-Dimensional Structural Characterization of HIV-1 Tethered to Human Cells. *J. Virol.* **2016**, *90*, 1507–1521. [CrossRef]
59. Pornillos, O.; Higginson, D.S.; Stray, K.M.; Fisher, R.D.; Garrus, J.E.; Payne, M.; He, G.P.; Wang, H.E.; Morham, S.G.; Sundquist, W.I. HIV Gag mimics the Tsg101-recruiting activity of the human Hrs protein. *J. Cell Biol.* **2003**, *162*, 425–434. [CrossRef]
60. Chen, Y.; Wu, B.; Musier-Forsyth, K.; Mansky, L.M.; Mueller, J.D. Fluorescence fluctuation spectroscopy on viral-like particles reveals variable Gag stoichiometry. *Biophys. J.* **2009**, *96*, 1961–1969. [CrossRef] [PubMed]

61. Inamdar, K.; Floderer, C.; Favard, C.; Muriaux, D. Monitoring HIV-1 Assembly in Living Cells: Insights from Dynamic and Single Molecule Microscopy. *Viruses* **2019**, *11*, 72. [CrossRef] [PubMed]
62. Steppert, P.; Burgstaller, D.; Klausberger, M.; Berger, E.; Aguilar, P.P.; Schneider, T.A.; Kramberger, P.; Tover, A.; Nöbauer, K.; Razzazi-Fazeli, E.; et al. Purification of HIV-1 gag virus-like particles and separation of other extracellular particles. *J. Chromatogr. A* **2016**, *1455*, 93–101. [CrossRef] [PubMed]
63. Xiao, P.J.; Li, C.; Neumann, A.; Samulski, R.J. Quantitative 3D tracing of gene-delivery viral vectors in human cells and animal tissues. *Mol. Ther.* **2012**, *20*, 317–328. [CrossRef]
64. Sarder, P.; Nehorai, A. Deconvolution methods for 3-D fluorescence microscopy images. *IEEE Signal Process. Mag.* **2006**, *23*, 32–45. [CrossRef]
65. Schermelleh, L.; Ferrand, A.; Huser, T.; Eggeling, C.; Sauer, M.; Biehlmaier, O.; Drummen, G.P.C. Super-resolution microscopy demystified. *Nat. Cell Biol.* **2019**, *21*, 72–84. [CrossRef]

12

A Single Dose of Dendrimer B2T Peptide Vaccine Partially Protects Pigs against Foot-and-Mouth Disease Virus Infection

Rodrigo Cañas-Arranz [1], Mar Forner [2], Sira Defaus [2], Patricia de León [1], María J. Bustos [1], Elisa Torres [1], Francisco Sobrino [1,*], David Andreu [2,*] and Esther Blanco [3,*]

1 Centro de Biología Molecular "Severo Ochoa" (CSIC-UAM), 28049 Madrid, Spain; rcannas@cbm.csic.es (R.C.-A.); pdeleon@cbm.csic.es (P.d.L.); mjbustos@cbm.csic.es (M.J.B.); elisa.torres@cbm.csic.es (E.T.)

2 Departament de Ciències Experimentals i de la Salut, Universitat Pompeu Fabra, 08003 Barcelona, Spain; mar.forner@upf.edu (M.F.); sira.defaus@upf.edu (S.D.)

3 Centro de Investigación en Sanidad Animal (CISA-INIA), Valdeolmos, 28130 Madrid, Spain

* Correspondence: fsobrino@cbm.csic.es (F.S.); david.andreu@upf.edu (D.A.); blanco@inia.es (E.B.)

Abstract: Foot-and-mouth disease virus (FMDV) causes a highly contagious disease of cloven-hoofed animals whose control relies on efficient vaccination. We have reported that dendrimer peptide B_2T, with two copies of FMDV B-cell epitope VP1 (136–154) linked through maleimide units to T-cell epitope 3A (21–35)], elicits potent B- and T-cell specific responses and confers solid protection in pigs to type-O FMDV challenge after two doses of peptide. Herein we now show that B_2T evokes specific protective immune responses after administration of a single dose of either 2 or 0.5 mg of peptide. High titers of ELISA and neutralizing antibodies against FMDV were detectable at day 15 post-immunization. Likewise, activated T cells and induced IFN-γ response to in vitro recall with FMDV peptides were also detected by the same day. Further, in 70% of B_2T-vaccinated pigs, full protection—no clinical signs of disease—was observed upon virus challenge at day 25 post-immunization. These results strengthen the potential of B_2T as a safe, cost-effective candidate vaccine conferring adequate protection against FMDV with a single dose. The finding is particularly relevant to emergency scenarios permitting only a single shot immunization.

Keywords: FMDV; peptide vaccine; single dose; amount; pig

1. Introduction

Vaccination remains the most effective approach to prevent human and animal diseases [1]. In animal health, development of safe, cost-effective and marker vaccines, capable of telling infected from vaccinated animals (DIVA), remains a challenge for many diseases, particularly viral ones [2,3]. Conventional vaccines based on inactivated or attenuated viruses entail risks such as accidental escape or incomplete inactivation of infectious viruses, as well as possible reversion of attenuated into virulent forms. Subunit or epitopic vaccines represent an alternative that solves most such problems by excluding the infectious agent and allowing targeting to well characterized viral epitopes relevant for protection [4–6].

Foot-and-mouth disease virus (FMDV) is the prototype member of the *Aphthovirus* genus within the *Picornaviridae* family [7] and the etiological agent of FMD, a highly transmissible infection of pigs and other cloven-hoofed animals, with huge economic impact worldwide [8,9]. FMD underscores paradigmatically the challenge of finding alternative strategies to the classic vaccines still used to prevent this highly contagious disease [10]. The massive amplification and shedding of FMDV in infected pigs turns this species to a key epidemiological factor for the spread of the virus over the course of outbreaks in many regions of the world [11]. In addition, the growing numbers of domestic pigs worldwide, particularly in Asian countries, make the development of pig-suited FMD vaccines a strategic task.

Conventional FMDV vaccines based on chemically inactivated virus have allowed FMD control and eradication in some countries, although their manufacturing process—not upgraded over recent decades—poses significant biosafety concerns that have been related to occasional escape episodes of diverse consequence [12–14]. This risk plus other limitations, such as the need for a strict cold chain to preserve stability, and the use of updated vaccine strains, because of the high potential antigenic diversity of the virus, underlie the adoption of non-vaccination policies in FMDV-free countries, a controversial and by no means risk-free practice, as borne out by not infrequent outbreaks in those locations. In crisis scenarios of this kind [15], vaccines incorporating outbreak-relevant epitopes, eliciting protective responses and generated as a quick response to the epidemic, can become an invaluable emergency resource for FMD containment [16]. Among such emergency vaccines, those based on synthetic peptides [6] are particularly appealing because of their (i) total lack of biological hazard; (ii) possibility of displaying various epitopes on a single platform; (iii) DIVA compliance; (iv) efficient synthetic production and characterization as pharmaceuticals, and (v) no cold-chain required; easy transport and storage [17].

The main B-cell antigenic site in FMDV, located at the GH loop of capsid protein VP1 (residues ca. 140–160), is structurally continuous [18,19]. Linear peptides reproducing this loop, either alone or in combination with T-cell FMDV epitopes, have been shown to confer limited protection in natural hosts [20–23].

A substantial enhancement in immunogenicity can be achieved by multiple display of B- and/or T-cell epitopes on a single molecular scaffold [17] inspired on the multiple antigenic peptide (MAP) platform of Tam [24]. In an initial realization in this regard, a peptide spanning residues 21–35 of FMDV protein 3A [thereafter T3A], which delimit an immunodominant T-cell epitope in domestic pigs [25], was N-terminally elongated into a Lys tree to which four copies of a B-cell epitope (residues 140–158 of VP1; containing the RGD motif that mediates binding to integrins, the cell receptors) were covalently linked in a dendrimeric (branched) fashion. The sequence of the B-cell epitope corresponded to that of the epidemiologically relevant O/UKG/11/01 isolate, belonging to serotype O the most prevalent worldwide [26]. This multivalent construct (named B_4T) elicited high titers of FMDV-neutralizing antibodies, activated specific T cells, and fully protected pigs against FMDV challenge [27]. Interestingly, a simpler version (i.e., two B-cell epitope branches) of the peptide vaccine candidate, termed B_2T, also elicited potent specific responses and conferred solid protection in pigs to challenge [28] (Table 1). In both B_4T and B_2T trials, animals were immunized with two 2-mg doses of peptide (3 weeks apart from each other) before challenge.

Table 1. Synthetic peptides used in this study.

Peptide	FMDV Protein (Residues)	Sequence
B	VP1 (136–154)	PVTNVRGDLQVLAQKAART-amide
T	3A (21–35)	AAIEFFEGMVHDSIK-amide
B_2T	VP1 (136–154), 3A (21–35)	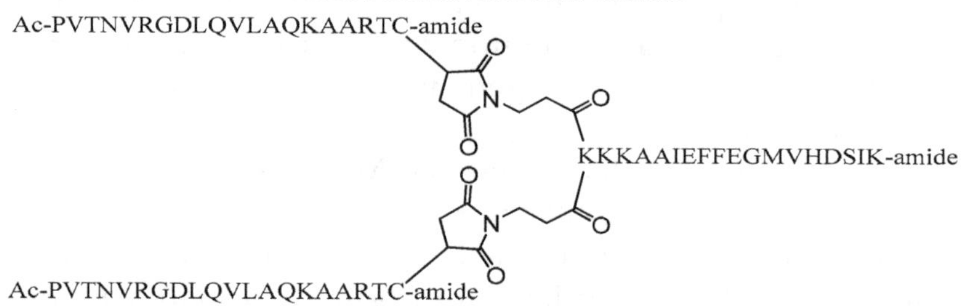

As mentioned above, emergency FMD vaccines, eliciting protective responses upon a single shot, are particularly valuable in containing uncontrolled FMDV outbreaks [14]. The modular nature of B_2T affords considerable versatility in the sequences that can be integrated into the constructions, either as part of a single molecule or as mixtures of different molecules. Thus, incorporation of VP1 GH-loop sequences from different FMDV isolates can modulate/enhance the protective spectrum of the candidates. This is particularly relevant because of the high FMDV antigenic diversity reflected in seven serotypes and many variants within each of them, which makes matching of vaccine strains with circulating virus a critical issue for vaccine efficacy [11,15]. On the other hand, the T3A sequence mentioned above is highly conserved among FMDV serotypes and therefore can evoke heterologous responses, again contributing to broaden the protective response conferred by B_2T. In addition to versatile, readily adaptable responses to new virus threats, emergency vaccines require fast and cost-effective manufacturing programs, which are ideally met by the expediency and flexibility inherent to chemical synthesis production.

Herein we have explored the possibility of: (i) Eliciting protective responses in pigs upon administration of a single B_2T dose, and (ii) reducing the amount of antigen required to elicit protective responses. Thus, we report results with both the 2 mg dose of previous experiments [28] and with a reduced 0.5 mg inoculum. Remarkably, the latter dose elicits a rapid immune response involving high titers of FMDV neutralizing antibodies and specific IFN-γ secreting T cells at 15 days post-immunization (dpi). In addition, solid protection is observed in 80% of pigs vaccinated with 0.5 mg B_2T, with no clinical signs upon viral challenge at day 25 dpi. Taken together, our results highlight the value of B_2T as candidate FMD vaccine for pigs in emergency scenarios.

2. Results

2.1. A Single B_2T Dose Elicits Rapid Humoral Specific Responses Including FMDV Neutralizing Antibodies

Domestic pigs, in two different groups of five animals each, were immunized once with 2 or 0.5 mg of B_2T (pigs 1 to 5 and 6 to 10, respectively), and two additional non-immunized animals were kept as controls (pigs 11 and 12 inoculated with PBS). Total FMDV-specific IgG antibodies were determined by ELISA at 0, 15, and 21 dpi. Both 2 and 0.5 mg doses elicited consistent and comparable IgG titers ($\log_{10}$) at 15 (4.3 ± 0.4 vs. 3.7 ± 0.3) and 21 (4.2 ± 0.2 vs. 4.3 ± 0.3) dpi (Figure 1A). Upon FMDV challenge (day 25) these titers were not boosted up, remaining similar in both B_2T-immunized groups (4.3 ± 0.1 vs. 4.6 ± 0.5). Non-immunized control pig 11 that survived 10 days post-challenge (dpc) showed anti-FMDV titers >2$\log_{10}$ units lower than those of the immunized and challenged groups (Figure 1A).

Regarding induction of FMDV neutralizing antibodies, as observed with the ELISA results, no major differences were noticed between virus neutralization titers (VNT) in the groups immunized with either 2 or 0.5 mg B_2T at day 15 (1.5 ± 0.2 vs. 1.4 ± 0.4) or day 21 pi (1.9 ± 0.4 vs. 2 ± 0.5) (Figure 1B). On the other hand, and in contrast to ELISA antibody titers, post-challenge VNT increased at 10 dpc (35 dpi) in both groups (3.1 ± 0.3 vs. 3.2 ± 0.4). As expected, no neutralizing antibodies were detected in the two control animals before challenge. The non-vaccinated animal that survived the challenge (pig 11), showed VNT (3.1) similar to those in immunized groups (Figure 1B), showing that neutralizing antibody levels in B_2T-immunized/challenged pigs—including those found to be protected—were as high as those in infected and recovered animals.

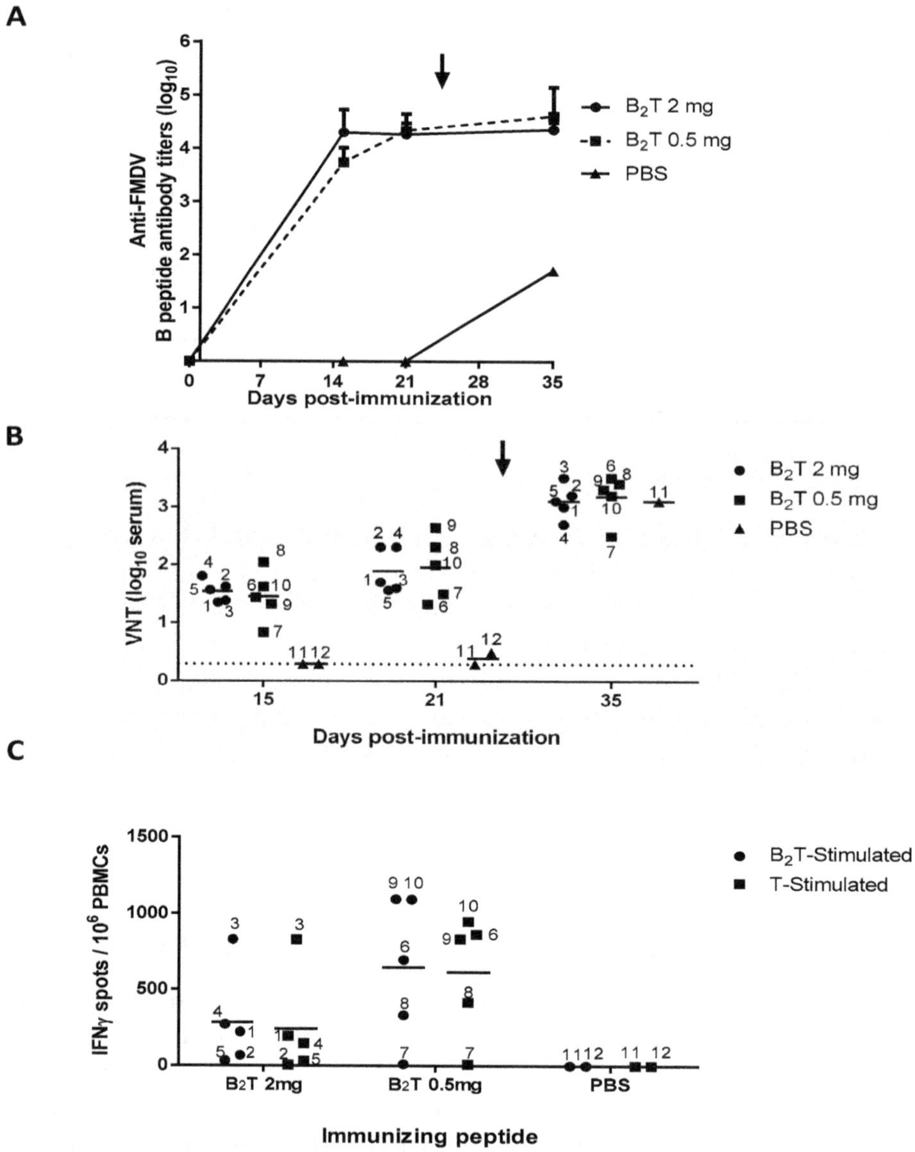

Figure 1. B- and T-cell responses in pigs immunized with a single dose and different amounts of B_2T. Time course of the specific antibody responses in sera collected on the indicated days pi. (**A**) Total anti peptide B IgG titers analyzed by ELISA. Each point depicts mean antibody titers (calculated as described in Methods) ± SD for each group of pigs (n = 5). (**B**) Virus neutralization titers, VNT, expressed as the reciprocal log10 of the last serum dilution that neutralized 100 TCID50 of FMDV isolate O/UKG 11/01. Each symbol represents the value for an individual pig (numbering is included). Horizontal lines indicate the geometric mean for each animal group. In no case individual spontaneous reactivity was observed in the titers determined at day 0. Dotted lines denotes the assay detection limit. In (**A**,**B**) arrows point FMDV challenge (day 25 pi). (**C**) Specific T-cell responses measured by an ex vivo IFN-γ ELISPOT at days 15 pi. The frequency of FMDV-specific IFN-γ secreting cells was determined as detailed in Methods. Horizontal bars represent the mean frequencies of IFN-γ release spots of triplicates of peripheral blood mononuclear cells (PBMCs) from pigs stimulated in vitro with B_2T (circles) or T (T3A) (squares) peptides (pig numbering is included).

2.2. B_2T Elicits Early FMDV-Specific IFN-γ Responses

Specific T cell responses elicited by B_2T at 15 dpi were determined by ELISPOT analysis of IFNγ-expressing PBMCs. High frequencies of spot-forming cells were found at day 15 in pigs immunized with either dose of B_2T in response to in vitro recall with homologous peptide (284.8 ± 321.1 vs. 645.6 ± 467.9). On average, pigs in the 0.5 mg group showed higher frequencies of IFNγ-expressing

PBMCs than those in the 2 mg group (Figure 1C). All responses were specific, as no peptide-driven IFN-γ-producing cells were detected in the two non-immunized pigs. PBMC stimulation with T3A peptide paralleled those observed with B_2T (241.3 ± 365.8 vs. 614.4 ± 403.1) (Figure 1C), supporting the recognition of T3A as a T-cell epitope.

2.3. A Single Dose of B_2T Peptide Confers Clinical Protection against FMDV Challenge

At 25 dpi, pigs in all three groups were challenged with FMDV. Animals were examined daily for clinical signs (see Methods) and considered protected when lesions were not observed or appeared only at the inoculation site [29]. As expected, PBS-inoculated control pigs 11 and 12 showed full FMD signs upon challenge, developing vesicular lesions on all four feet at 4 dpc and on the snout at 7 and 5 dpc, respectively (Table 2). The acute FMDV infection caused myocarditis, leading to heart failure and sudden death, of pig 12 at 5 dpc. In contrast, only 3 out of 10 peptide-immunized animals developed lesions outside the inoculation site: two pigs (3 and 5) in the 2 mg group and one (pig 10) in the 0.5 mg group. The remaining immunized animals did not develop any clinical signs, the cumulative lesion score of immunized groups being significantly lower than that of the non-immunized one (Table 2). In general, a correlation between lower body temperature and protection was observed, being the protected animals immunized with 0.5 mg B_2T those that did not develop fever.

Table 2. Evidences for protection in immunized pigs.

Inoculum	Pig	VNT/IFNγ [a]	Fever [b]	Lesion Score [c]	Protected [d]	RNA [e]
B_2T (2 mg)	1	1.7/221	39.8 (6)	0	++	ND
	2	2.3/68	39.7 (6)	0	++	ND
	3	1.6/830	41.7 (7)	3 (7)	−	1.8×10^4 (5)
	4	2.3/270	39.6 (7)	0	++	ND
	5	1.6/33	39.9 (10)	2 (10)	+	ND
B_2T (0.5 mg)	6	1.3/696	No fever	0	++	ND
	7	1.5/10	No fever	0	++	ND
	8	2.3/332	No fever	0	++	ND
	9	2.6/1096	No fever	0	++	ND
	10	2/1093	39.6 (8)	5 (7)	−	10^8 (3); 2×10^6 (5)
Non-immunized	11		40.7 (5)	7 (5)	−	1.4×10^8 (3); 4.5×10^6 (5)
	12		No fever	7 (5)	− [f]	1.1×10^8 (3)

[a] VNT and IFNγ spots/10^6 PBMCs determined at day 21 and 15 post-immunization, respectively. [b] Temperature (°C) and (in parenthesis) day pi when maximum temperature registered. No fever: ≤39.0–39.5 °C. [c] Animals were monitored up to 10 days pc for lesions. Lesion score (maximum value of 7): 1 point/vesicle in foot (up to 4 points); 1 point/mouth, tongue or snout lesion; 1 point/>2 lesions of diameter ≥10 mm. In parenthesis, day pc when lesion(s) was first observed. [d] Animals were considered fully protected (++) if lesion score ≤ 1; partially protected (mild/delayed disease) (+) if lesion score ≤ 2, or non-protected (−) if lesion score > 2. [e] Detection of FMDV RNA in serum samples. ND: RNA not detected. The amount of RNA in positive animals are expressed as viral RNA copies (VRC)/mL serum. Detection limit: 5×10^3 VRC/mL serum. The values from RNA positive animals are presented as VRC/mL serum. The day(s) post-challenge when RNA was detected is shown in brackets. [f] Animal died on day 5 pc.

Detection of FMDV RNA in serum samples from challenged pigs by RT-qPCR showed the presence of viral RNA in non-immunized control pigs 11 (days 3 and 5 pc) and 12 (day 3 pc), as well as in the two immunized but non-protected pigs 10 (days 3 and 5 pc) and 3 (only at day 5 pc), which showed the higher lesion score at day 7 pc (Table 2). Hence, virus detection in sera associated with the severity of the lesions of challenged pigs. Further work is necessary to assess the potential contribution of viruses circulating in non-protected animals, and to a lesser extent in protected animals, to the spread of the disease under field conditions.

In conclusion, immunization with a single 2 mg dose and, remarkably, even more with a 0.5 mg dose of B_2T dendrimer afforded substantial protection against conventional FMDV challenge.

3. Discussion

Protection after a single inoculation is a must for effective FMD vaccines, as it reduces both the cost of the vaccine as well as the logistics and labor expenses associated with the double immunization schedules. The application of a single dose vaccination program to the pig population can favor disease eradication, considering that pigs serve as amplifiers of FMDV and therefore a rapid control of the infection in swine is essential for disease control [11]. This is particularly relevant in settings such as diseases outbreaks occurring in areas where FMD is not enzootic and livestock remains unvaccinated [30]. To our knowledge, with the exception of adenovirus-vectored vaccines expressing FMDV empty capsids [31], few studies exist on the capability of FMD subunit vaccines alternative to classical ones to confer protection in relevant hosts after a single administration [32]. In this context, our optimization of the minimal amount of B_2T dendrimer still conferring protection is pertinent, both for understanding the response mechanisms to B_2T and for scaling down production costs, a relevant issue for FMD vaccine development.

We had previously shown that two 2 mg doses of B_2T conferred solid protection to FMDV challenge in swine, and that protection correlated with the induction of strong B- and T-cell specific responses [28]. Here, we explore the feasibility of B_2T as a protective, single dose subunit vaccine alternative to conventional FMD formulations. To this end, the original 2 mg dose and a four-fold lower one (0.5 mg) have been compared.

The challenge protocol followed in our experiment was as recommended by the OIE manual, for evaluation of protection against podal generalization (PPG) test, except that virus was inoculated 3 days earlier than indicated [33]. Under such conditions, full protection, considered as the absence of lesions at points other than the inoculation site, was observed in 70% of pigs vaccinated with B_2T; 3 out of 5 in the 2 mg dose group, and 4 out of 5 in the 0.5 mg group. This level of protection correlated with an average increase in virus neutralizing (VN) antibodies that was not observed for B-specific IgG antibodies detected by ELISA (Figure 1), suggesting the recall upon viral infection of a subset of FMDV-specific memory B cells, as well as of memory T cells capable to promote B-cell maturation. This increment of VN antibodies in protected animals, matching that of a non-immunized pig, might reflect virus multiplication to a limited extent not resulting in detectable viremia (Table 2). Similar levels of VN antibodies boost upon virus challenge have been reported in pigs and cattle immunized with live-vectored vaccines or FMDV-like particles [34,35].

Non-protected (pigs 3 and 10) and partially protected (pig 5) animals showed lower levels of VN antibodies at the day of challenge, albeit animals with lower VNT yet protected were also observed (Figure 1B); the lack of correlation in a fraction of protected animals immunized with different FMDV vaccines has been described [21,36]. Experiments aimed at assessing the amount of antibodies that may target the FMDV receptor [37] as well as at examining cross-neutralization among other type O FMDVs will be foreseen to further characterize the antibody response evoked by the dendrimer peptide vaccines.

In addition, and supporting T3A recognition as a T-cell epitope, specific IFN-γ releasing activated T cells were detected rather early, at 15 dpi, in 7 of the 10 immunized pigs. The average frequencies of IFN-γ releasing cells in PBMCs from pigs in the 0.5 mg dose group were higher than those in the 2 mg group (Figure 1C and Table 2), possibly reflecting differences in the in vitro dose-effect of peptide stimulation and/or on the MHC allele composition of the animals analyzed. High doses of antigen might also facilitate its capture by APC/DC subsets with suboptimal costimulatory capacity that favor the development of regulatory T cells, which could limit the activation of B cells and subsequent antibody production as well as the development of IFN-γ producing cells [38]. In any case, additional studies of the effector mechanisms triggered by the dendrimers will be necessary to understand the effect on the protective responses of different peptide vaccine doses. One animal that was low responder at 15 dpi (pig 7), turned out to be protected upon challenge and pig 5, also low responder, was partially protected. Among responder animals, no clear correlation between IFN-γ releasing cell frequency at 15 dpi and protection to FMDV challenge was observed, i.e., non-protected pigs 3 and 10 showed high responses. Thus, as previously observed [21], VNT and T-cell stimulation do not fully correlate with the protection conferred by FMD peptide vaccines.

A potential problem of epitopic vaccines such us the dendrimeric peptides used in this study is the selection in non-protected animals of escape viruses capable to avoid antibody neutralization [21] and/or T cell recognition. In our experiment, we could not rule out that possibility since the limited number and size of the vesicles developed by non-protected animals did not allow virus recovery for sequencing analyses.

Our evidence of the level of full protection conferred by a single B_2T dose upon challenge at 25 dpi is particularly remarkable with regard to the 0.5 mg dose group (80% of the pigs), as it opens the way to significant savings in manufacturing costs. Incidentally, on a related note, we have found that long-lasting (up to 19/20 weeks post-boost) reduced susceptibility to FMDV infection can be attained with two B_2T doses and, remarkably, a similarly lasting protective response with a single dose of B_2T (Cañas-Arranz et al., submitted).

Attempts to use B_2T and B_4T dendrimer peptides as vaccines in cattle showed a trend toward a reduced capacity to confer protection relative to swine, including the need for a third immunization to elicit protective levels on neutralizing antibodies [39,40]. Failure in conferring protection in cattle has been described for linear FMDV peptide vaccines containing a heterologous T cell epitope [41]. Further work on the requirements of the interactions between neutralizing epitopes and B cells, as well as the identification of new, effective T helper epitopes frequently recognized by individuals will contribute to the improvement of the effectiveness of this kind of vaccines for cattle and, eventually, other host species.

In summary, our findings portray the B_2T peptide as a safe, potentially cost-effective candidate to be included in FMD vaccine formulations conferring single-shot protection in pigs. Formulation of dendrimers with alternative adjuvants as well as the incorporation of peptides corresponding to other T cell epitopes previously identified in pigs [42,43] can contribute to improve their immunogenicity in swine.

4. Methods

4.1. Peptides

Peptides identified as B- and T-cell epitopes of FMDV O/UKG/11/01 (Table 1) were assembled by Fmoc-solid phase synthesis, purified by reverse-phase liquid chromatography, and characterized by mass spectrometry. Dendrimeric B_2T construct was conjugated in solution using two previously synthesized precursors: (i) B epitope (VP1, residues 136–154) plus a C-terminal Cys residue (free thiol form) and (ii) T epitope (3A, residues 21–35) elongated at the N-terminal with two Lys residues followed by an additional Lys branching derivatized as two maleimide groups. The B_2T peptide was efficiently obtained after the thiol-maleimide ligation at pH = 6, RP-HPLC purification and MS characterization [27,28,44].

4.2. Virus

A virus stock derived from FMDV isolate O/UKG/11/01 [45] by two amplifications in swine kidney cells (IB-RS-2 cells) was used. The resulting virus maintained the consensus sequences at the capsid region [46].

4.3. Animals and Experimental Design

The immune response to B_2T dendrimer peptide was assessed in ten 9-weeks-old white cross-bred Landrace female pigs (Agropardal SA breed), free of antibodies to FMDV. The study was approved (CBS2014/015 and CEEA2014/018) by the INIA Committees on Ethics of Animal Experiments and Biosafety, and by the National Committee on Ethics and Animal Welfare (PROEX 218/14). Pigs were randomly assigned to two groups of five animals each and immunized once (days 0) by intramuscular injection with 2 mL of Montanide ISA 50V2 emulsion (Seppic, Paris, France) containing 2 or 0.5 mg of B_2T peptide. Two additional non-vaccinated pigs were kept as infection controls (#11 and 12). Animals were housed in separate units of the high-containment facility and challenged at day 25 with 1.6×10^4 plaque forming units (pfu) of FMDV O/UKG/11/01, by inoculation at two sites of both main claws of the left-hindfoot pad (0.1 mL/site). Animals were monitored for clinical signs of disease during the 10 days (Table 2), and then euthanized at day 35.

4.4. *Viral RNA Detection after Challenge*

Serum samples were examined for the presence of viral RNA by real time RT-qPCR. Briefly, the cDNA obtained in a RT reaction using primer A (5′-CACACGGCGTTCACCCA(A/T)CGC-3′) [47] was amplified by qPCR using the "Light Cycler RNA Master SYBR Green I" kit (Roche, Basel, Switzerland) and LightCycler equipment following the instructions of the manufacturer. The amplicon synthesized spanned a conserved region of 290 pb length in the 3D protein coding sequence, and was amplified using primers A (5′-CACACGGCGTTCACCCA(A/T)CGC-3′) and B (5′-GACAAAGGTTTTGTTCTTGGTC-3′). The values for the quantification of the samples were obtained from a standard curve from a RNA transcript derived from the infectious clone pMT-28 codifying the genomic RNA from FMDV C-S8c1 [48].

4.5. *Virus Neutralization Test (VNT)*

Serial two-fold dilutions of sera were incubated with 100 infection units—50% tissue culture infective doses (TCID50) of FMDV O/UKG 11/01, for 1 h at 37 °C. End-point titers were calculated as the reciprocal of the serum dilution that neutralized FMDV infection in 50% of the wells [28].

4.6. *Detection of Specific Anti-FMDV Antibodies by ELISA*

Total anti-FMDV antibodies were determined by ELISA. Briefly, 96-well plates (Nunc, Rochester, NY, USA) were coated with peptide B (1 μg) overnight at 4 °C. Duplicate three-fold dilution series of each serum sample were prepared in 50 μL, starting at 1/100. Pre-immune sera from peptide-immunized pigs and sera from non-immunized animals were used as negative controls. Specific antibodies were detected with HRP-conjugated protein A (Thermo Fisher, Rochester, NY, USA), diluted 1/4000. Color development was obtained after addition of 100 μL/well of TMB (Sigma Aldrich, St. Louis, MO, USA) and stopped by an equal volume of 1M H_2SO_4. Plates were read at 450 nm, titers expressed as the reciprocal of the last dilution giving the absorbance recorded in the control wells (serum at day 0) plus 2 SD.

4.7. *PBMC Isolation and IFN-γ Detection by ELISPOT*

Porcine peripheral blood mononuclear cells (PBMCs) were isolated by density gradient centrifugation using Histopaque-1077 (Sigma, St. Louis, MO, USA) and cryopreserved prior to assay. Vials were defrosted and resuspended in complete RPMI 1640 and incubated overnight at 37 °C, 5% CO_2. Cell counting and viability were tested by Trypan blue staining. For the IFN-γ ELISPOT assay 2.5×10^5 PBMCs were shed in triplicate wells of Immobilon-P plates (Merck Millipore, Burlington, MA, USA) coated with 5 μg/mL of anti-pig IFN-γ antibody (clone P2G10, Becton Dickinson, Franklin Lakes, NJ, USA). For in vitro antigen recall, PBMCs were stimulated with 25 μg/mL of the peptide used for pig immunization [49]. As positive control, PBMCs were incubated with 5 μg/mL of phytohaemagglutinin (Sigma) using cells incubated without antigen as negative control. After 48 h at 37 °C, 5% CO_2, plates were washed and incubated with 2 μg/mL of biotinylated anti-mouse IFN-γ antibody (clone P2C11, BD) and HRP-streptavidin (BD). Antibody was visualized with 3-amino-9-ethyl carbazole (BD). The frequency of peptide-specific T cells in was expressed as the mean number of spot-forming cells/10^6 PBMCs, with background values (number of spots in negative control wells) subtracted from the respective counts of stimulated cells.

4.8. Statistical Analyses

Differences among the peptide-immunized groups in FMDV-antibody titers and number of IFN-γ producing cells were analyzed by two-way ANOVA, followed by Tukey's post-hoc comparisons tests. Values are cited in the text as means ± SD. All p values are two sided, and p values < 0.05 were considered significant. Statistical analyses were conducted using GraphPad Prism Software 5.0 (Graphpad Software, San Diego, CA, USA).

Author Contributions: Conception, design and funding of the work (D.A., E.B. and F.S.). Data Acquisition and analysis (R.C.-A., M.F., S.D., P.d.L., M.J.B. and E.T.). Interpretation of data for the work (R.C.-A., M.F., S.D., P.d.L., D.A., F.S. and E.B.). Drafting the work (R.C.-A., M.F., S.D., P.d.L., F.S. and E.B.). Revising the data critically for important intellectual content (D.A., E.B. and F.S.). All authors have read and agreed to the published version of the manuscript.

Acknowledgments: We thank P. Pallarés for her advice and support.

References

1. Sallusto, F.; Lanzavecchia, A.; Araki, K.; Ahmed, R. From vaccines to memory and back. *Immunity* **2010**, *33*, 451–463. [CrossRef] [PubMed]
2. van Oirschot, J.T. Present and future of veterinary viral vaccinology: A review. *Vet. Q.* **2001**, *23*, 100–108. [CrossRef] [PubMed]
3. Brun, A.; Barcena, J.; Blanco, E.; Borrego, B.; Dory, D.; Escribano, J.M.; Le Gall-Recule, G.; Ortego, J.; Dixon, L.K. Current strategies for subunit and genetic viral veterinary vaccine development. *Virus Res.* **2011**, *157*, 1–12. [CrossRef] [PubMed]
4. Correia, B.E.; Bates, J.T.; Loomis, R.J.; Baneyx, G.; Carrico, C.; Jardine, J.G.; Rupert, P.; Correnti, C.; Kalyuzhniy, O.; Vittal, V.; et al. Proof of principle for epitope-focused vaccine design. *Nature* **2014**, *507*, 201–206. [CrossRef] [PubMed]
5. Sette, A.; Fikes, J. Epitope-based vaccines: An update on epitope identification, vaccine design and delivery. *Curr. Opin. Immunol.* **2003**, *15*, 461–470. [CrossRef]
6. Purcell, A.W.; McCluskey, J.; Rossjohn, J. More than one reason to rethink the use of peptides in vaccine design. *Nat. Rev. Drug Discov.* **2007**, *6*, 404–414. [CrossRef]
7. Saiz, M.; Nunez, J.I.; Jimenez-Clavero, M.A.; Baranowski, E.; Sobrino, F. Foot-and-mouth disease virus: Biology and prospects for disease control. *Microbes Infect.* **2002**, *4*, 1183–1192. [CrossRef]
8. Rweyemamu, M.; Roeder, P.; MacKay, D.; Sumption, K.; Brownlie, J.; Leforban, Y. Planning for the progressive control of foot-and-mouth disease worldwide. *Transbound. Emerg. Dis.* **2008**, *55*, 73–87. [CrossRef]
9. Knight-Jones, T.J.; Rushton, J. The economic impacts of foot and mouth disease—What are they, how big are they and where do they occur? *Prev. Vet. Med.* **2013**, *112*, 161–173. [CrossRef]
10. Grubman, M.J.; Baxt, B. Foot-and-mouth disease. *Clin. Microbiol. Rev.* **2004**, *17*, 465–493. [CrossRef]
11. Perez, A.M.; Willeberg, P.W. Editorial: Foot-and-Mouth Disease in Swine. *Front. Vet. Sci.* **2017**, *4*, 133. [CrossRef] [PubMed]
12. Rodriguez, L.L.; Gay, C.G. Development of vaccines toward the global control and eradication of foot-and-mouth disease. *Expert Rev. Vaccines* **2011**, *10*, 377–387. [CrossRef] [PubMed]
13. Doel, T.R. Natural and vaccine induced immunity to FMD. *Curr. Top. Microbiol. Immunol.* **2005**, *288*, 103–131. [PubMed]
14. Robinson, L.; Knight-Jones, T.J.; Charleston, B.; Rodriguez, L.L.; Gay, C.G.; Sumption, K.J.; Vosloo, W. Global Foot-and-Mouth Disease Research Update and Gap Analysis: 3—Vaccines. *Transbound. Emerg. Dis.* **2016**, *63* (Suppl. 1), 30–41. [CrossRef]
15. Kitching, R.P. Diagnosis and Control of Foot-and-Mouth Disease. In *Foot and Mouth Disease: Current Perspectives*; Sobrino, F., Domingo, E., Eds.; Horizon Press: Norfolk, UK, 2004.
16. Lyons, N.A.; Lyoo, Y.S.; King, D.P.; Paton, D.J. Challenges of Generating and Maintaining Protective Vaccine-Induced Immune Responses for Foot-and-Mouth Disease Virus in Pigs. *Front. Vet. Sci.* **2016**, *3*, 102. [CrossRef]
17. Blanco, E.; Andreu, D.; Sobrino, F. Peptide vaccines against foot-and-mouth disease. In *Foot-and-Mouth Disease Virus. Current Research and Emerging Trends*; Sobrino, F., Domingo, E., Eds.; Caister Academis Press: Norfolk, UK, 2017; pp. 231–317.

18. Acharya, R.; Fry, E.; Stuart, D.; Fox, G.; Rowlands, D.; Brown, F. The three-dimensional structure of foot-and-mouth disease virus at 2.9 A resolution. *Nature* **1989**, *337*, 709–716. [CrossRef] [PubMed]
19. Mateu, M.G.; Verdaguer, N.; Sobrino, F.; Domingo, E. Functional and structural aspects of the interaction of foo-and-outh disease virus with antibodies. In *Foot-and-Mouth Disease: Current Perspectives*; Mateu, M.G., Verdaguer, N., Eds.; Horizon Bioscience: Norfolk, UK, 2004; p. 37.
20. Bittle, J.L.; Houghten, R.A.; Alexander, H.; Shinnick, T.M.; Sutcliffe, J.G.; Lerner, R.A.; Rowlands, D.J.; Brown, F. Protection against foot-and-mouth disease by immunization with a chemically synthesized peptide predicted from the viral nucleotide sequence. *Nature* **1982**, *298*, 30–33. [CrossRef] [PubMed]
21. Taboga, O.; Tami, C.; Carrillo, E.; Nunez, J.I.; Rodriguez, A.; Saiz, J.C.; Blanco, E.; Valero, M.L.; Roig, X.; Camarero, J.A.; et al. A large-scale evaluation of peptide vaccines against foot-and-mouth disease: Lack of solid protection in cattle and isolation of escape mutants. *J. Virol.* **1997**, *71*, 2606–2614. [CrossRef]
22. Cubillos, C.; de la Torre, B.G.; Barcena, J.; Andreu, D.; Sobrino, F.; Blanco, E. Inclusion of a specific T cell epitope increases the protection conferred against foot-and-mouth disease virus in pigs by a linear peptide containing an immunodominant B cell site. *Virol. J.* **2012**, *9*, 66. [CrossRef]
23. Collen, T.; Dimarchi, R.; Doel, T.R. A T cell epitope in VP1 of foot-and-mouth disease virus is immunodominant for vaccinated cattle. *J. Immunol.* **1991**, *146*, 749–755.
24. Tam, J.P. Synthetic peptide vaccine design: Synthesis and properties of a high-density multiple antigenic peptide system. *Proc. Natl. Acad. Sci. USA* **1988**, *85*, 5409–5413. [CrossRef] [PubMed]
25. Blanco, E.; Garcia-Briones, M.; Sanz-Parra, A.; Gomes, P.; De Oliveira, E.; Valero, M.L.; Andreu, D.; Ley, V.; Sobrino, F. Identification of T-cell epitopes in nonstructural proteins of foot-and-mouth disease virus. *J. Virol.* **2001**, *75*, 3164–3174. [CrossRef]
26. Mahapatra, M.; Parida, S. Foot and mouth disease vaccine strain selection: Current approaches and future perspectives. *Expert Rev. Vaccines* **2018**, *17*, 577–591. [CrossRef] [PubMed]
27. Cubillos, C.; de la Torre, B.G.; Jakab, A.; Clementi, G.; Borras, E.; Barcena, J.; Andreu, D.; Sobrino, F.; Blanco, E. Enhanced mucosal immunoglobulin A response and solid protection against foot-and-mouth disease virus challenge induced by a novel dendrimeric peptide. *J. Virol.* **2008**, *82*, 7223–7230. [CrossRef] [PubMed]
28. Blanco, E.; Guerra, B.; de la Torre, B.G.; Defaus, S.; Dekker, A.; Andreu, D.; Sobrino, F. Full protection of swine against foot-and-mouth disease by a bivalent B-cell epitope dendrimer peptide. *Antivir. Res.* **2016**, *129*, 74–80. [CrossRef] [PubMed]
29. Francis, M.J.; Black, L. Response of young pigs to foot-and-mouth disease oil emulsion vaccination in the presence and absence of maternally derived neutralising antibodies. *Res. Vet. Sci.* **1986**, *41*, 33–39. [CrossRef]
30. Smitsaart, E.; Bergmann, I. Quality and attributes of current inactivated foot-and-mouth disease vaccines and their effects on the success of vaccination programmes. In *Foot-and-Mouth Disease Virus. Current Research and Emerging Trends*; Sobrino, F., Domingo, E., Eds.; Caister Academic Press: Norfolk, UK, 2017; pp. 287–316.
31. Pacheco, J.M.; Brum, M.C.; Moraes, M.P.; Golde, W.T.; Grubman, M.J. Rapid protection of cattle from direct challenge with foot-and-mouth disease virus (FMDV) by a single inoculation with an adenovirus-vectored FMDV subunit vaccine. *Virology* **2005**, *337*, 205–209. [CrossRef]
32. Lyons, N.A.; Knight-Jones, T.J.D.; Bartels, C.; Paton, D.J.; Ferrari, G.; Vermillion, M.S.; Brooks, A.W.; Motroni, R.; Parker, E.; Hefferin Berquist, M.L.; et al. Considerations for design and implementation of vaccine field trials for novel foot-and-mouth disease vaccines. *Vaccine* **2019**, *37*, 1007–1015. [CrossRef]
33. OIE. *Manual of Diagnositic Tests and Vaccines for Terrestrial Animals (Terrestrial Manual)*; OIE: Paris, France, 2017.
34. Sitt, T.; Kenney, M.; Barrera, J.; Pandya, M.; Eckstrom, K.; Warner, M.; Pacheco, J.M.; LaRocco, M.; Palarea-Albaladejo, J.; Brake, D.; et al. Duration of protection and humoral immunity induced by an adenovirus-vectored subunit vaccine for foot-and-mouth disease (FMD) in Holstein steers. *Vaccine* **2019**, *37*, 6221–6231. [CrossRef]
35. Guo, H.C.; Sun, S.Q.; Jin, Y.; Yang, S.L.; Wei, Y.Q.; Sun, D.H.; Yin, S.H.; Ma, J.W.; Liu, Z.X.; Guo, J.H.; et al. Foot-and-mouth disease virus-like particles produced by a SUMO fusion protein system in Escherichia coli induce potent protective immune responses in guinea pigs, swine and cattle. *Vet. Res.* **2013**, *44*, 48. [CrossRef]
36. McCullough, K.C.; Bruckner, L.; Schaffner, R.; Fraefel, W.; Muller, H.K.; Kihm, U. Relationship between the anti-FMD virus antibody reaction as measured by different assays, and protection in vivo against challenge infection. *Vet. Microbiol.* **1992**, *30*, 99–112. [CrossRef]

37. Polacek, C.; Gullberg, M.; Li, J.; Belsham, G.J. Low levels of foot-and-mouth disease virus 3C protease expression are required to achieve optimal capsid protein expression and processing in mammalian cells. *J. Gen. Virol.* **2013**, *94*, 1249–1258. [CrossRef]
38. Bilate, A.M.; Lafaille, J.J. Induced CD4+Foxp3+ regulatory T cells in immune tolerance. *Annu. Rev. Immunol.* **2012**, *30*, 733–758. [CrossRef]
39. Soria, I.; Quattrocchi, V.; Langellotti, C.; Gammella, M.; Digiacomo, S.; Garcia de la Torre, B.; Andreu, D.; Montoya, M.; Sobrino, F.; Blanco, E.; et al. Dendrimeric peptides can confer protection against foot-and-mouth disease virus in cattle. *PLoS ONE* **2017**, *12*, e0185184. [CrossRef] [PubMed]
40. Soria, I.; Quattrocchi, V.; Langellotti, C.; Perez-Filgueira, M.; Pega, J.; Gnazzo, V.; Romera, S.; Schammas, J.; Bucafusco, D.; Di Giacomo, S.; et al. Immune Response and Partial Protection against Heterologous Foot-and-Mouth Disease Virus Induced by Dendrimer Peptides in Cattle. *J. Immunol. Res.* **2018**, *2018*, 3497401. [CrossRef] [PubMed]
41. Rodriguez, L.L.; Barrera, J.; Kramer, E.; Lubroth, J.; Brown, F.; Golde, W.T. A synthetic peptide containing the consensus sequence of the G-H loop region of foot-and-mouth disease virus type-O VP1 and a promiscuous T-helper epitope induces peptide-specific antibodies but fails to protect cattle against viral challenge. *Vaccine* **2003**, *21*, 3751–3756. [CrossRef]
42. Blanco, E.; McCullough, K.; Summerfield, A.; Fiorini, J.; Andreu, D.; Chiva, C.; Borras, E.; Barnett, P.; Sobrino, F. Interspecies major histocompatibility complex-restricted Th cell epitope on foot-and-mouth disease virus capsid protein VP4. *J. Virol.* **2000**, *74*, 4902–4907. [CrossRef]
43. Garcia-Briones, M.M.; Blanco, E.; Chiva, C.; Andreu, D.; Ley, V.; Sobrino, F. Immunogenicity and T cell recognition in swine of foot-and-mouth disease virus polymerase 3D. *Virology* **2004**, *322*, 264–275. [CrossRef]
44. Monso, M.; de la Torre, B.G.; Blanco, E.; Moreno, N.; Andreu, D. Influence of conjugation chemistry and B epitope orientation on the immune response of branched peptide antigens. *Bioconjug. Chem.* **2013**, *24*, 578–585. [CrossRef]
45. Sumption, K.; Rweyemamu, M.; Wint, W. Incidence and distribution of foot-and-mouth disease in Asia, Africa and South America; combining expert opinion, official disease information and livestock populations to assist risk assessment. *Transbound. Emerg. Dis.* **2008**, *55*, 5–13. [CrossRef]
46. Nunez, J.I.; Molina, N.; Baranowski, E.; Domingo, E.; Clark, S.; Burman, A.; Berryman, S.; Jackson, T.; Sobrino, F. Guinea pig-adapted foot-and-mouth disease virus with altered receptor recognition can productively infect a natural host. *J. Virol.* **2007**, *81*, 8497–8506. [CrossRef] [PubMed]
47. Saiz, M.; De La Morena, D.B.; Blanco, E.; Nunez, J.I.; Fernandez, R.; Sanchez-Vizcaino, J.M. Detection of foot-and-mouth disease virus from culture and clinical samples by reverse transcription-PCR coupled to restriction enzyme and sequence analysis. *Vet. Res.* **2003**, *34*, 105–117. [CrossRef] [PubMed]
48. García-Arriaza, J.; Manrubia, S.C.; Toja, M.; Domingo, E.; Escarmís, C. Evolutionary transition toward defective RNAs that are infectious by complementation. *J. Virol.* **2004**, *78*, 11678–11685. [CrossRef] [PubMed]
49. Saiz, J.C.; Rodriguez, A.; Gonzalez, M.; Alonso, F.; Sobrino, F. Heterotypic lymphoproliferative response in pigs vaccinated with foot-and-mouth disease virus. Involvement of isolated capsid proteins. *J. Gen. Virol.* **1992**, *73*, 2601–2607. [CrossRef] [PubMed]

13

Medical Outcomes in Women Who Became Pregnant after Vaccination with a Virus-Like Particle Experimental Vaccine against Influenza A (H1N1) 2009 Virus Tested during 2009 Pandemic Outbreak

Arturo Cérbulo-Vázquez [1], Lourdes Arriaga-Pizano [2], Gabriela Cruz-Cureño [3], Ilka Boscó-Gárate [2], Eduardo Ferat-Osorio [4], Rodolfo Pastelin-Palacios [5], Ricardo Figueroa-Damian [6], Denisse Castro-Eguiluz [7], Javier Mancilla-Ramirez [8], Armando Isibasi [2] and Constantino López-Macías [2,9,10,*]

[1] Facultad de Medicina, Plan de Estudios Combinados en Medicina (MD, PhD Program), Universidad Nacional Autónoma de México, Mexico City CP 04510, Mexico; cerbulo@unam.mx
[2] Unidad de Investigación Médica en Inmunoquímica, Hospital de Especialidades del Centro Médico Nacional Siglo XXI, Instituto Mexicano del Seguro Social (IMSS), Mexico City CP 06720, Mexico; landapi@hotmail.com (L.A.-P.); ibosco45@hotmail.com (I.B.-G.); isibasi@prodigy.net.mx (A.I.)
[3] Escuela Nacional de Ciencias Biológicas, Programa de Inmunología, Instituto Politécnico Nacional, Mexico City CP 11340, Mexico; gabrielacruz30@gmail.com
[4] Servicio de Cirugía Gastrointestinal, Unidad Médica de Alta Especialidad, Hospital de Especialidades Dr Bernardo Sepúlveda Gutiérrez, Centro Médico Nacional Siglo XXI, Instituto Mexicano del Seguro Social (IMSS), Mexico City CP 06720, Mexico; eduardoferat@prodigy.net.mx
[5] Departamento de Biología, Facultad de Química, Universidad Nacional Autónoma de México, Mexico City CP 04510, Mexico; rodolfop@unam.mx
[6] Departamento de Infectología, Instituto Nacional de Perinatología, Mexico City CP 11000, Mexico; rfd6102@yahoo.com.mx
[7] Consejo Nacional de Ciencia y Tecnología (CONACYT)- Departamento de Investigación Clínica, Instituto Nacional de Cancerología, Mexico City CP 14080, Mexico; angeldenisse@gmail.com
[8] Escuela Superior de Medicina, Instituto Politécnico Nacional; Hospital de la Mujer, Secretaria de Sauld, Mexico City CP 11340, Mexico; javiermancilla@hotmail.com
[9] Visiting Professor of Immunology, Nuffield Department of Medicine, University of Oxford, Oxford OX3 7LF, UK
[10] Mexican Translational Immunology Research Group, Federation of Clinical Immunology Societies Centers of Excellence, National Autonomous University of Mexico, Mexico City 04510, Mexico
* Correspondence: constantino@sminmunologia.mx or constantino.lopez@imss.gob.mx

Abstract: The clinical effects and immunological response to the influenza vaccine in women who later become pregnant remain to be thoroughly studied. Here, we report the medical outcomes of 40 women volunteers who became pregnant after vaccination with an experimental virus-like particle (VLP) vaccine against pandemic influenza A(H1N1)2009 (influenza A(H1N1)pdm09) and their infants. When included in the VLP vaccine trial, none of the women were pregnant and were randomly assigned to one of the following groups: (1) placebo, (2) 15 μg dose of VLP vaccine, or (3) 45 μg dose of VLP vaccine. These 40 women reported becoming pregnant during the follow-up phase after receiving the placebo or VLP vaccine. Women were monitored throughout pregnancy and their infants were monitored until one year after birth. Antibody titers against VLP were measured in the mothers and infants at delivery and at six months and one year after birth. The incidence of preeclampsia, fetal death, preterm delivery, and premature rupture of membranes was similar among groups. All vaccinated women and their infants elicited antibody titers (≥1:40). Women vaccinated prior to pregnancy had no adverse events that were different from the nonvaccinated population. Even though this study is limited by the sample size, the results suggest that the anti-influenza A(H1N1)pdm09 VLP experimental vaccine applied before pregnancy is safe for both mothers and their infants.

Keywords: virus-like particle; influenza A(H1N1)pdm09; vaccination; pregnant women; antibody titers

---

1. Introduction

Vaccination against pandemic influenza A is crucial for limiting the incidence and severity of infection in the general population [1,2]. Influenza A infection in pregnant women has been associated with higher admission rates to intensive care units and severe disease compared with nonpregnant women [3]. Studies in animal models show that the seasonal influenza virus infection in pregnant mice initiates a powerful pro-abortive mechanism and adverse outcomes in fetal health [4], highlighting the importance of vaccination in protecting both pregnant women and their infants to whom immunity may also be passively transferred [5,6].

In 2009, our group conducted a phase 2 clinical trial following Good Clinical Practices according to the International Conference of Harmonization (ICH-GCP) to evaluate the safety and immunogenicity of a virus-like particle (VLP) vaccine against influenza A(H1N1)pdm09. That study was a randomized, placebo-controlled, double-blind clinical trial that included 4555 male and female volunteers. Healthy nonpregnant women (confirmed by a negative pregnancy test) were included in the study [7,8], and by written informed consent, women were requested to avoid pregnancy for the duration of the trial. The use of a contraceptive method was instructed and provided to female participants upon request; however, some of the volunteers became pregnant in the postvaccination follow-up period. As indicated by our institutional Ethics Committee recommendations and local regulations, the pregnant women and their infants remained under the intention to treat protocol, so they were closely monitored. The medical outcomes and antibody response to the vaccine in both the women and their infants were registered. Here, we report, in a nested cohort study, the results of the surveillance of the 40 pregnant women who agreed to take part and provided their informed consent.

2. Materials and Methods

While conducting an ICH-GCP phase 2 clinical trial using a VLP vaccine against pandemic influenza A at the Mexican Institute of Social Security (IMSS, Mexico City, Mexico), 4555 male and nonpregnant female (confirmed by a negative pregnancy test) volunteers were included. Despite the use of contraceptive methods—as stated by the participants—40 women reported pregnancy in the postvaccination period (Table 1). We reported these events to the IMSS Ethics Committee and Comisión Federal para la Prevención de Riesgos Sanitarios (COFEPRIS) (the Mexican equivalent of the US Food and Drug Administration), and they both recommended that the pregnant women and their infants should remain under medical surveillance and be closely monitored according to local regulations.

The design of this study was a nested cohort study that included the 40 women who became pregnant after the influenza A(H1N1)pdm09 virus vaccination and their infants (Figure 1).

Table 1. Characteristics of the study population (women).

	Placebo (n = 16)	VLP 15 µg (n = 23)	p	VLP 45 µg (n = 1)
Age (mean ± SD)	24.25 ± 2.43	27.44 ± 5.79	0.14 *	19
	Personal history of diseases			
Denied, n (%)	16 (100%)	23 (100%)	1 **	1 (100%)

Table 1. *Cont.*

	Placebo (n = 16)	VLP 15 µg (n = 23)	p	VLP 45 µg (n = 1)
Family history				
Type 2 diabetes mellitus, n (%)	1 (6.25%)	4 (17.4%)		1 (100%)
Hypertension, n (%)				1 (100%)
Cancer, n (%)		1 (4.34%)		
Cardiovascular disease, n (%)				1 (100%)
Renal insufficiency, n (%)				1 (100%)
Hypothyroidism, n (%)				1 (100%)
Epilepsy, n (%)		1 (4.34%)		
Time elapsed from vaccination to pregnancy				
1 month, n (%)		6 (26%)		1 (100%)
2 months, n (%)		3 (13%)		
3 months, n (%)		3 (13%)		
4 months, n (%)		2 (8.6%)		
5 months, n (%)		2 (8.6%)		
6 months, n (%)		3 (13%)		
7–9 months, n (%)		2 (8.6%)		
>9 months, n (%)		2 (8.6%)		
Breastfed the child				
Yes, n (%)	4 (25%)	14 (60.8%)	0.049 **	1 (100%)
No, n (%)	12 (75%)	9 (39.2%)		

* Student's t test comparing placebo vs. VLP 15 µg; ** Fisher's exact test comparing placebo vs. VLP 15 µg. VLP—virus-like particle.

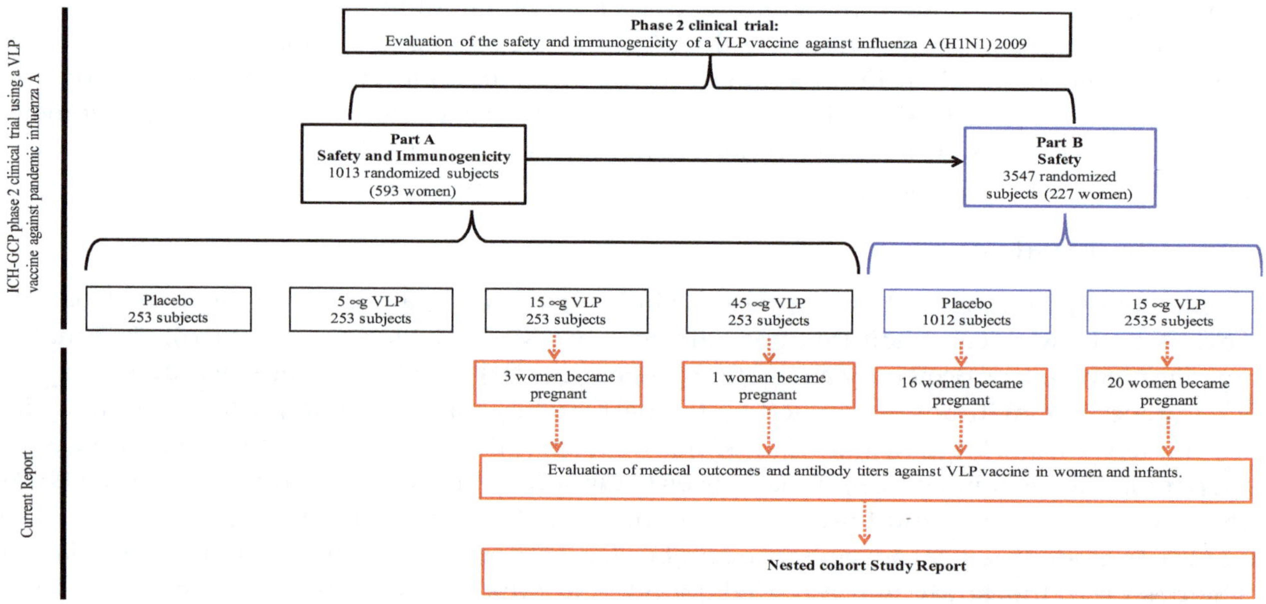

Figure 1. Flow and details of the subjects in the trial. A total of 820 women volunteers participated in the phase 2 clinical trial to evaluate the safety and immunogenicity (part A) and safety (part B) of the VLP vaccine against influenza A(H1N1)pdm09 [6]. After vaccination, 40 women became pregnant—16 from the placebo group, 23 from the 15 µg VLP vaccine dose, and 1 from the 45 µg VLP vaccine dose. All these volunteers were provided with medical surveillance and close monitoring; clinical outcomes and VLP vaccine specific antibody titers in both mothers and their infants were evaluated. Both the Mexican Institute of Social Security and the National Institute of Perinatology Ethic Committees approved the study (IMSS:R-2011-785-040, INPer:212250-06181).

2.1. Participant Characteristics

The 40 women who became pregnant after vaccination were recruited from the VLP vaccine clinical trial groups—16 (40%) pregnant women from the placebo group, 23 (57.5%) from the 15 μg dose of VLP vaccine group, and 1 (2.5%) woman from the 45 μg dose of VLP vaccine group (Figure 1). None of the women had documented an infection with pandemic influenza A (H1N1) 2009 or a vaccination against seasonal or pandemic influenza A (other than the experimental vaccine), and none of them reported a medical history of chronic diseases.

The pregnant women were monitored medically until delivery, following the standard protocol for medical care in Mexico [9]. Both mothers and infants remained under medical surveillance and safety follow-up at 3, 6, and 12 months after delivery. Any adverse medical or perinatal event experienced by the mothers or infants was recorded in detail. The newborn surveillance included anthropometry, gestational age at birth, nutritional status, and congenital disease.

The IMSS and the National Institute of Perinatology Ethic Committees approved the study (IMSS:R-2011-785-040, INPer:212250-06181). All participants signed a written informed consent for the study.

2.2. Sample Collection

Whole blood samples (5 mL) from the pregnant women or umbilical cord blood (10 mL) were collected at birth. At 3, 6, and 12 months of age, 5 mL of peripheral blood was collected from the mothers and 1 mL from the infants. Serum was obtained from the blood samples by centrifugation, and the aliquots were stored at −20 °C until analysis.

2.3. Hemagglutination Inhibition (HAI) Test

The serum samples were tested in triplicate. Assays were conducted as previously described [10,11]. The aliquots of each serum sample were treated using the receptor-destroying enzyme. The samples were diluted (1:2) into V-bottom 96-well microtiter plates. Eight units of 50 μL of hemagglutinin (HA) were added to each well, plated, and incubated for 30 min at room temperature, followed by the addition of in-house, freshly prepared turkey erythrocytes (1% in phosphate-buffered saline). The plates were mixed by agitation, covered, and allowed to set for 30 min at 25 °C. The HAI titer was determined by the reciprocal of the last dilution of nonagglutinated red blood cells. Samples with HAI titers of ≥1:40 were considered to have a positive antibody response to the influenza A(H1N1)pdm09 virus.

2.4. Statistical Analysis

Descriptive statistics were used for the characterization of the patients studied. We compared the placebo and VLP 15 μg dose. The statistical analysis was performed using StataCorp software (2011 Stata Statistical Software—Release 12, College Station, TX: StataCorp LP). Descriptive statistics were used to characterize the categorical variables, expressed as a percentage. A bivariate analysis was performed for comparison among groups, using Fisher's exact test or chi-square test; $p < 0.05$ was considered statistically significant.

3. Results

3.1. Medical Outcomes in Women Who Became Pregnant after Vaccination with VLP Vaccine against Influenza A(H1N1)pdm09 Virus and Their Infants

Table 1 describes the characteristics of the women studied. All volunteers included in the study were residents of the metropolitan area of Mexico City and were rightful claimants of full cover medical attention provided by the public health system; all were homemakers, literate, and none reported a medical history of chronic diseases (Table 1). The mean age was 26.1 ± 5.4 years (see Table 1 for the differences in characteristics among the placebo and 15 μg VLP groups). The mean time to become pregnant after vaccination was 130 ± 115 days; the details on the elapsed time from vaccination to pregnancy are described in Table 1.

The gestational age of the newborns and the frequency of the delivery type were similar between the placebo and 15 μg VLP vaccine groups (Table 2). A similar average birth weight of newborns was observed between the placebo group (2878 ± 554 g) and the 15 μg VLP vaccine group (3081 ± 398 g; $p > 0.05$). The woman from the 45 μg VLP vaccine group delivered via cesarean section at 38 weeks of gestational age, the newborn had a birth weight of 3000 g and an Apgar score typical for a healthy newborn (8/9, 1 min and 5 min).

Table 2. Gestational age and delivery type in the placebo and 15 mg VLP vaccine groups.

Condition	Placebo, *n* (%)	VLP 15 μg, *n* (%)	*p* *
	16 (40)	23 (57.5)	
Gestational age			
Preterm	1 (5.5)	2 (8.7)	0.2
Term	15 (83.3)	20 (86.9)	0.8
Post-term	0	1 (4.3)	0.4
Delivery type			
Vaginal	8 (50)	11 (47.8)	0.9
Cesarean	8 (50)	12 (52.2)	0.9

* Fisher's test.

None of the pregnant women from the placebo group were diagnosed with preeclampsia, fetal death, premature rupture of membranes, oligohydramnios, or gestational hypertension (Table 3). Two of the women from the VLP 15 μg group received a second immunization (28 days after the first dose); no obstetric complications or adverse events developed in these two women. Six (26%) of the women in the 15 μg VLP group experienced adverse events. These events were preeclampsia ($n = 2$), fetal death ($n = 1$), premature rupture of membranes ($n = 1$), oligohydramnios ($n = 1$), and gestational hypertension ($n = 1$). Table 3 describes the obstetric complications for both the placebo and 15 μg VLP groups; the epidemiological reference of obstetric adverse events reported for the Mexican population is also provided [12]. In all cases, the frequency of the above-mentioned events was not significantly different among the placebo and 15 μg VLP groups (Table 3). The patient who received the 45 μg VLP vaccine did not have any pathology during her pregnancy. In the placebo group, one patient had a preterm birth delivered by cesarean section at 36 weeks, whereas 2 out of 23 (8.7%) women in the 15 μg VLP vaccine group had a cesarean preterm birth at 35 and 36 weeks of gestational age. The woman in the 45 μg VLP vaccine group delivered at term gestational age.

Table 3. Obstetric complications in placebo and vaccinated women compared with the Mexican population.

Obstetric Complication	Placebo, *n* (%)	15 μg VLP, *n* (%)	*p* **	Reference Value *
	16 (40)	23 (57.5)		%
Preeclampsia	0	2 (8.6)	0.6	8
Fetal death	0	1 (4.3)	0.7	1.5
Premature rupture of membranes	0	1 (4.3)	0.7	5
Oligohydramnios	0	1 (4.3)	0.7	1.5
Gestational hypertension	0	1 (4.3)	0.7	10

* COMEGO: Clinic Gynecology and Obstetrics Guides in Mexico 2015, Mexico, Nieto Eds.; ** Fisher's test comparing the placebo and the 15 μg VLP groups.

We evaluated 32 infants during the first year of life. Seven abandoned the study during follow-up, and in one case, consent was withdrawn. One infant (6.2%) from the placebo group was diagnosed with pneumonia during the surveillance period. In the 15 μg VLP group, one infant (4.3%) was diagnosed with a hydrocele, one infant (4.3%) was diagnosed with an umbilical hernia, and one infant (4.3%) was diagnosed with gastroesophageal reflux and bacterial pneumonia during medical surveillance (Table 4). Low birth weight and fetal distress were not statistically different between the placebo and 15 μg VLP vaccine groups (Table 4). The infant exposed to the 45 μg VLP dose did not present any pathology.

Table 4. Neonatal and one-year surveillance adverse events in infants of women in the vaccinated and placebo groups.

Condition	**Placebo, *n* (%)**	**15 μg VLP, *n* (%)**	***p* ***
	16 (40)	**23 (57.5)**	
	Neonatal diagnosis		
Low birth weight (<2500 g)	0	3 (13.0)	0.51
Fetal distress	0	2 (8.7)	0.6
	One-year surveillance period		
Pneumonia	1 (6.25)	1 (4.3)	0.7
Hydrocele	0	1 (4.3)	0.1
Umbilical hernia	0	1 (4.3)	0.1
Gastroesophageal reflux	0	1 (4.3)	0.1

* Fisher's test.

3.2. *Vaccination Elicited Humoral Response in Pregnant Women and Infants*

Figure 2 shows the titer of antibodies against pandemic influenza in the peripheral blood of women who were vaccinated before becoming pregnant. Women in the placebo group showed low levels of antibodies against pandemic influenza at the beginning of the trial; however, these levels increased from delivery up to one year after delivery, and the titer reached high levels (>1:40) at 12 months after delivery. The titer was less than 1:40 in the placebo infants, reaching the highest levels at six months after birth. In the 15 μg VLP vaccine group, the antibody titer in women increased as early as 20 days after vaccination and reached high levels at 36 days after the vaccination, whereas at delivery, the titer was higher than 1:80 and then decreased to 1:40 at 12 months after delivery. The titer in the infants from the 15 μg VLP group was 1:40 at the moment of birth and remained elevated at six months of age; however, the titer fell below 1:40 at 12 months after birth (Figure 2). In the woman from the 45 μg VLP vaccine group, the initial titer was 1:160 and remained protective from the moment of vaccination until one year after delivery; the infant from this group showed a similar titer as the mother at birth, but it diminished at six months of age and remained below 1:40 at 12 months after birth (Figure 2).

To understand the elevated antibody titers observed in women and infants from the placebo group, we determined the antibody titers against pandemic influenza in 249 pregnant women who did not participate in the vaccination trial (Figure 3). About 30% of Mexican women who became pregnant in the period from July 2009 to August 2010 expressed natural immunity and antibody titers of 1:40 against pandemic influenza, which is similar to the antibody titers described for the placebo group.

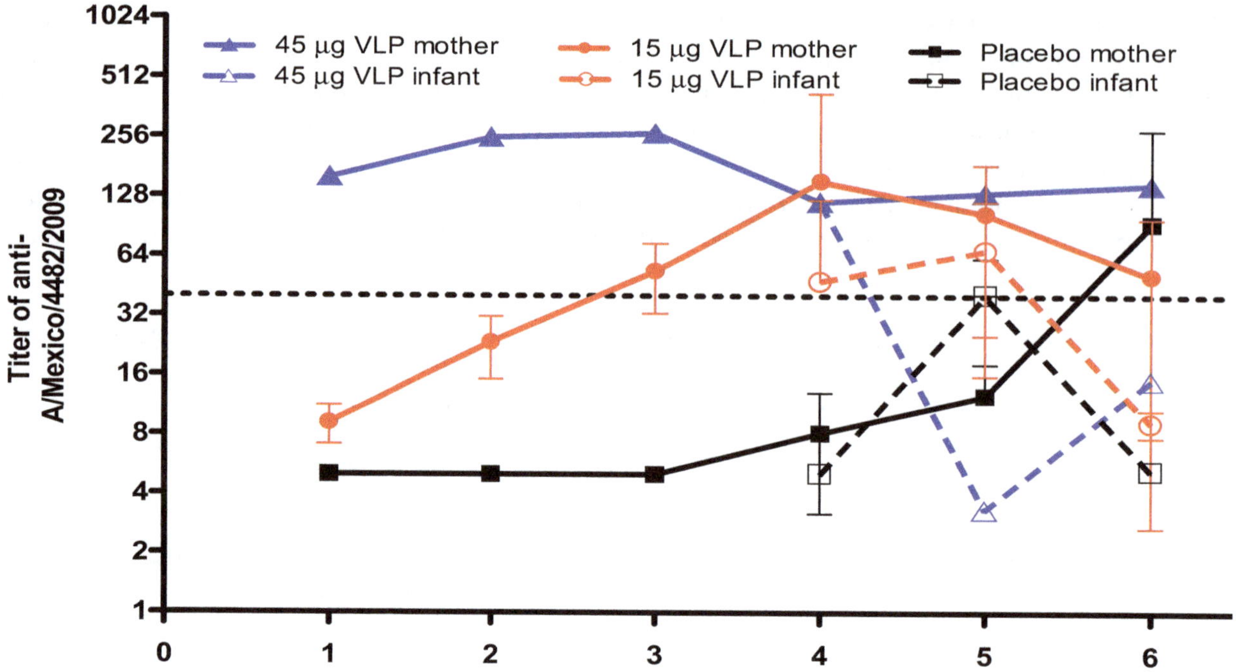

Figure 2. VLP vaccination induces humoral response against the anti-A/Mexico/4482/2009 virus in mothers and infants. Antibody titers in women volunteers vaccinated with 15 µg VLP (n = 23), 45 µg VLP (n = 1), or placebo (n = 16). D0—day of vaccination (first dose); D22—day 22 after vaccination (also, two women in the 15 µg group received a second dose); D36—day 36 after vaccination; birth—day of delivery of the newborns; 6 months—6 months after birth; and 12 months—12 months after birth. Closed symbols and continuous lines show antibody titers in women. Open symbols and dashed lines show antibody titers in infants. Mean ± SD.

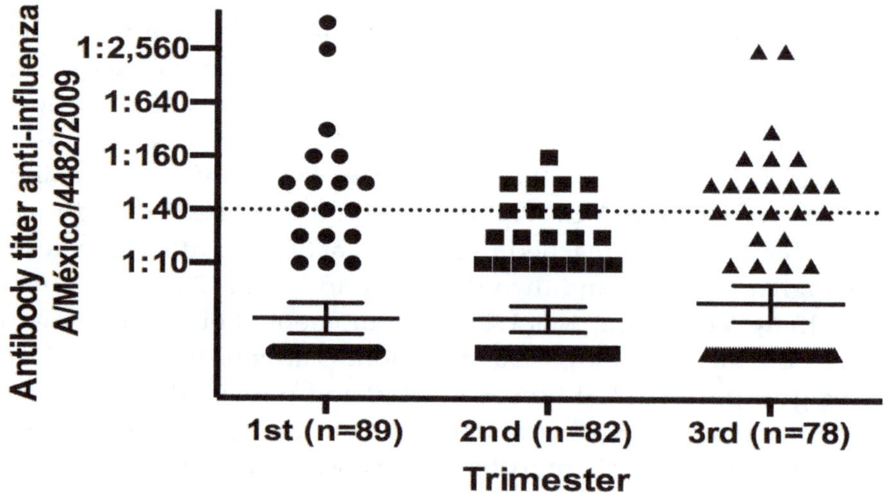

Figure 3. Protective antibody titer against pandemic influenza in healthy Mexican pregnant women. We collected 249 peripheral blood samples from healthy pregnant women who did not participate in the vaccination clinical trial—12 out of 89 women (13%) in the first trimester, 9 out of 82 (12%) in the second trimester, and 18 out of 78 (30%) in the third trimester had an antibody titer ≥1:40. Mean ± SD.

4. Discussion

Here we have reported the results of a nested cohort study that evaluated the potential effect of the anti-influenza A(H1N1)pdm09 VLP experimental vaccine in women who later became pregnant on medical outcomes as well as on the antibody response of the women and their infants [7]. Tavares et al. [13] reported similar results in their study of the effect of a pandemic vaccine against influenza A (H1N1) in pregnant women using an AS03-adjuvanted split virion H1N1 (2009) pandemic influenza vaccine. They did not observe an increase in the frequency of obstetric complications, infection, or teratogenicity. Tamma and Muñoz [14,15] reported no adverse effects in the infants of mothers vaccinated using an inactivated virus.

We monitored 40 women from early gestation to delivery and 32 infants during the first year of life. Although this study may lack statistical power due to the small sample size, our results showed that most women in this cohort reached term gestational age (37–42 weeks); this could suggest that the VLP vaccination does not result in a higher risk of preterm birth than occurs in the nonvaccinated population, as the average gestational age was similar to the Mexican national epidemiological data of term newborns [16].

We did not observe an increase in the rates of maternal obstetric complications or infection. The incidences of preeclampsia, fetal death, and premature rupture of membranes were not significantly higher in the VLP-vaccinated women compared to nonvaccinated women, suggesting that the VLP vaccine is safe in the pregnant population even under conditions of influenza outbreak. A prospective and larger study should be conducted to ascertain the safety of the VLP vaccine in the pregnant population.

The rates of congenital disease, fetal death, preterm delivery, and low birth weight in the neonates of VLP-vaccinated women were similar to that of the nonvaccinated population, suggesting that the VLP vaccine does not result in a higher risk to the fetus. In the VLP vaccine group, there were three cases of low birth weight and two cases of fetal distress, even though no statistical significance was reached, this finding may be clinically relevant and considered for further studies. Pediatric monitoring showed no negative effects on the exposed infants; cases of hydroceles, umbilical hernias, and gastroesophageal reflux are common in Mexican newborn infants, and it was not possible to establish a causal factor between the application of the influenza vaccine prior to pregnancy and the occurrence of these complications. However, the effect of the VLP vaccine applied in pregnant women must be studied to provide confidence in the safety of this type of vaccination.

Vaccination with an inactivated or attenuated virus for influenza A has some disadvantages, such as the risk of anaphylactic reactions and requirements for annual boosters or high doses to reach protection [17–20]. We observed specific antibody titers to A/Mexico/4482/2009 in pregnant women in the placebo group; these antibodies may be passively transferred to the fetus. As we observed, these antibody titers are maintained up to 12 months after birth. About 30% of Mexican women who became pregnant during the period of the pandemic showed elevated antibody titers; accordingly, our data suggest that some women in the placebo group may have been naturally infected by the influenza virus and developed an antibody response that could be transferred to the fetus. One dose of 15 μg VLP vaccine was shown to elicit a transitory but protective titer in the perinatal period, which was maintained 12 months after delivery. A similar titer was detected in infants during the newborn period up to six months after birth, suggesting that one dose of 15 μg VLP is sufficient to elicit an antibody response. Considering 60% of these infants were breastfed throughout the first year of life, it is possible that antibodies may have been passively transferred during this period; thus, the 15 μg VLP dose may be considered sufficient to support passive immunity in the fetus and infant. Finally, the high titer that we found in the woman who was exposed to one dose of 45 μg VLP vaccine suggests an asymptomatic infection with the pandemic influenza virus, and this condition may have interfered with the response to the 45 μg VLP vaccine. However, the titer remained elevated and the antibodies were passively transferred to the neonate at the moment of delivery but were not sustained at six months. Taken together, our data suggest that 15 μg may be an adequate dose of VLP vaccine to elicit an adequate antibody titer in both mother and infant. Another clinical trial is necessary to demonstrate if the 15 μg dose of the VLP vaccine could be considered protective against pandemic influenza in women who become pregnant.

Although vaccination was performed prior to pregnancy, our data indicate that this VLP vaccine does not induce negative side effects in either women or their infants during pregnancy. The vaccine induced a specific antibody response that was observed 21 months after immunization (the last time point observed) and was transferred to the newborns, showing that the VLP vaccine induced a long-lasting antibody response. Although more studies must be conducted to determine if VLP vaccination is safe during pregnancy, these data could be useful as a precedent to support safety and immunogenicity studies of this vaccine platform during pregnancy.

There were limitations in this study. Firstly, the sample size was limited in the placebo and intervention arms, so the statistical power was insufficient to measure the differences in pregnancy complications and birth outcomes. A second limitation was the collection of pregnancy-specific information, since this was not part of the initial clinical trial. Therefore, the information was heterogeneous and the results inconclusive. The most important confounding factor was the exposure to the natural influenza A(H1N1)pdm09 virus infection. Volunteers did not present clinical symptoms suggesting an influenza infection; however, since they were residents of the Mexico City metropolitan area during the pandemic outbreak, they were likely to have been exposed to the virus. This study was importantly limited by the lack of design—the clinical trial was not designed to include pregnant women. Avoiding pregnancy during the study was requested in the written informed consent. Here, we have reported the observations that we could perform on the volunteers who gained the added risk of becoming pregnant as well as observations on their infants. Nonetheless, this study represents a unique opportunity to understand the effect of an experimental anti-influenza VLP vaccine administered prior to pregnancy. Notably, the trial was performed during the particular conditions of a pandemic outbreak at the epicenter of the emergency. Although this study was limited by its sample size, these results could suggest that it is safe to be vaccinated with the anti-influenza A(H1N1)pdm09 VLP experimental vaccine before pregnancy.

Author Contributions: Conceptualization, C.L.-M.; data curation, G.C.-C., I.B.-G., and R.F.-D.; formal analysis, A.C.-V., L.A.A.-P., E.F.-O., R.P.-P., R.F.-D., and D.C.-E.; funding acquisition, C.L.-M. and A.C.-V.; methodology, L.A.A.-P., G.C.-C., and I.B.-G.; project administration, A.I. and C.L.-M.; resources, R.P.-P., J.M.-R., C.L.-M., and A.I.; supervision, A.C.-V., E.F.-O., and J.M.-R.; validation, L.A.A.-P. and A.I.; writing—original draft, A.C.-V. and D.C.-E.; writing—review and editing, C.L.-M.

Acknowledgments: The authors thank the neonatologists and pediatricians in the labor room of the INPer who helped us to obtain cord blood samples. We also appreciate the technical assistance provided by R. Montecillo-Sandoval.

References

1. Milne, G.J.; Halder, N.; Kelso, J.K. The cost effectiveness of pandemic influenza interventions: A pandemic severity based analysis. *PLoS ONE* **2013**, *8*, e61504. [CrossRef] [PubMed]
2. Kelso, J.K.; Halder, N.; Milne, G.J. Vaccination strategies for future influenza pandemics: A severity-based cost effectiveness analysis. *BMC Infect Dis.* **2013**, *13*, 81. [CrossRef] [PubMed]
3. Creanga, A.A.; Johnson, T.F.; Graitcer, S.B.; Hartman, L.K.; Al-Samarrai, T.; Schwarz, A.G.; Chu, S.Y.; Sackoff, J.E.; Jamieson, D.J.; Fine, A.D.; et al. Severity of 2009 pandemic influenza A (H1N1) virus infection in pregnant women. *Obstet. Gynecol.* **2010**, *115*, 717–726. [CrossRef] [PubMed]
4. Littauer, E.Q.; Esser, E.S.; Antao, O.Q.; Vassilieva, E.V.; Compans, R.W.; Skountzou, I. H1N1 influenza virus infection results in adverse pregnancy outcomes by disrupting tissue-specific hormonal regulation. *PLoS Pathog.* **2017**, *13*, e1006757. [CrossRef] [PubMed]
5. Linder, N.; Ohel, G. In utero vaccination. *Clin. Perinatol.* **1994**, *21*, 663–674. [CrossRef]
6. Zuccotti, G.; Pogliani, L.; Pariani, E.; Amendola, A.; Zanetti, A. Transplacental antibody transfer following maternal immunization with a pandemic 2009 influenza A(H1N1) MF59-adjuvanted vaccine. *JAMA* **2010**, *304*, 2360–2361. [CrossRef] [PubMed]
7. Lopez-Macias, C.; Ferat-Osorio, E.; Tenorio-Calvo, A.; Isibasi, A.; Talavera, J.; Arteaga-Ruiz, O.; Arriaga-Pizano, L.; Hickman, S.P.; Allende, M.; Lenhard, K.; et al. Safety and immunogenicity of a virus-like particle pandemic influenza A (H1N1) 2009 vaccine in a blinded, randomized, placebo-controlled trial of adults in Mexico. *Vaccine* **2011**, *29*, 7826–7834. [CrossRef] [PubMed]
8. Lopez-Macias, C. Virus-like particle (VLP)-based vaccines for pandemic influenza: performance of a VLP vaccine during the 2009 influenza pandemic. *Hum. Vaccin Immunother.* **2012**, *8*, 411–414. [CrossRef] [PubMed]
9. Mexicanos, S.d.S.E.U. Atención de la mujer durante el embarazo, parto y puerperio y del recién nacido. Criterios y procedimientos para la prestación del servicio. In *NOM-007-SSA2-1993*; Salud, S.d., Ed.; Comité Consultivo Nacional de Normalización de Servicios de Salud. Available online: http://www.salud.gob.mx/unidades/cdi/nom/007ssa23.html (accessed on 6 January 1995).

10. Pushko, P.; Tumpey, T.M.; Bu, F.; Knell, J.; Robinson, R.; Smith, G. Influenza virus-like particles comprised of the HA, NA, and M1 proteins of H9N2 influenza virus induce protective immune responses in BALB/c mice. *Vaccine* **2005**, *23*, 5751–5759. [CrossRef] [PubMed]
11. Yan, D.; Wei, Y.Q.; Guo, H.C.; Sun, S.Q. The application of virus-like particles as vaccines and biological vehicles. *Appl. Microbiol. Biotechnol.* **2015**, *99*, 10415–10432. [CrossRef] [PubMed]
12. COMEGO. Clinic Gynecology and Obstetrics Guides in Mexico 2015. Available online: http://tv.comego.org.mx/session.php?pag=session05.php&BUSCAR001=3 (accessed on 15 September 2019).
13. Tavares, F.; Nazareth, I.; Monegal, J.S.; Kolte, I.; Verstraeten, T.; Bauchau, V. Pregnancy and safety outcomes in women vaccinated with an AS03-adjuvanted split virion H1N1 (2009) pandemic influenza vaccine during pregnancy: a prospective cohort study. *Vaccine* **2011**, *29*, 6358–6365. [CrossRef] [PubMed]
14. Tamma, P.D.; Steinhoff, M.C.; Omer, S.B. Influenza infection and vaccination in pregnant women. *Expert Rev. Respir. Med.* **2010**, *4*, 321–328. [CrossRef] [PubMed]
15. Munoz, F.M.; Greisinger, A.J.; Wehmanen, O.A.; Mouzoon, M.E.; Hoyle, J.C.; Smith, F.A.; Glezen, W.P. Safety of influenza vaccination during pregnancy. *Am. J. Obstet. Gynecol.* **2005**, *192*, 1098–1106. [CrossRef] [PubMed]
16. Flores-Huerta S, M.-S.H. Birth weight of male and female infants born in hospitals affiliated with the Instituto Mexicano del Seguro Social. *Bol. Med. Hosp. Infect. Mex.* **2012**, *69*, 30–39.
17. McNeil, M.M.; Weintraub, E.S.; Duffy, J.; Sukumaran, L.; Jacobsen, S.J.; Klein, N.P.; Hambidge, S.J.; Lee, G.M.; Jackson, L.A.; Irving, S.A.; et al. Risk of anaphylaxis after vaccination in children and adults. *J. Allergy. Clin. Immunol.* **2016**, *137*, 868–878. [CrossRef] [PubMed]
18. McNeil, M.M.; DeStefano, F. Vaccine-associated hypersensitivity. *J. Allergy Clin. Immunol.* **2018**, *141*, 463–472. [CrossRef]
19. Houser, K.; Subbarao, K. Influenza vaccines: challenges and solutions. *Cell Host Microbe* **2015**, *17*, 295–300. [CrossRef]
20. Shinjoh, M.; Sugaya, N.; Yamaguchi, Y.; Iibuchi, N.; Kamimaki, I.; Goto, A.; Kobayashi, H.; Kobayashi, Y.; Shibata, M.; Tamaoka, S.; et al. Inactivated influenza vaccine effectiveness and an analysis of repeated vaccination for children during the 2016/17 season. *Vaccine* **2018**, *36*, 5510–5518. [CrossRef]

Hepatitis C Virus Vaccine: Challenges and Prospects

Joshua D. Duncan [1,2,3,*], Richard A. Urbanowicz [1,2,3], Alexander W. Tarr [1,2,3] and Jonathan K. Ball [1,2,3]

1 School of Life Sciences, The University of Nottingham, Nottingham NG7 2UH, UK; richard.urbanowicz@nottingham.ac.uk (R.A.U.); alex.tarr@nottingham.ac.uk (A.W.T.); jonathan.ball@nottingham.ac.uk (J.K.B.)

2 NIHR Nottingham BRC, Nottingham University Hospitals NHS Trust and the University of Nottingham, Nottingham NG7 2UH, UK

3 Nottingham Digestive Diseases Centre, School of Medicine, University of Nottingham, Nottingham NG7 2UH, UK

* Correspondence: joshua.duncan@nottingham.ac.uk

Abstract: The hepatitis C virus (HCV) causes both acute and chronic infection and continues to be a global problem despite advances in antiviral therapeutics. Current treatments fail to prevent reinfection and remain expensive, limiting their use to developed countries, and the asymptomatic nature of acute infection can result in individuals not receiving treatment and unknowingly spreading HCV. A prophylactic vaccine is therefore needed to control this virus. Thirty years since the discovery of HCV, there have been major gains in understanding the molecular biology and elucidating the immunological mechanisms that underpin spontaneous viral clearance, aiding rational vaccine design. This review discusses the challenges facing HCV vaccine design and the most recent and promising candidates being investigated.

Keywords: hepatitis C virus; vaccines; neutralising antibodies; animal models; immune responses

---

1. Introduction

First discovered in 1989 [1], the hepatitis C virus (HCV) is a major global health burden. Current estimates of HCV prevalence state that approximately 1% of the world's population are infected [2]. Chronic infection with HCV leads to cirrhosis of the liver and is associated with the development of hepatocellular carcinoma (HCC). Annually, 400,000 deaths are attributed to HCV and in the US, deaths from HCV have now overtaken those attributed to the human immunodeficiency virus (HIV) [3]. The extensive damage resulting from chronic infection makes this virus the leading cause for liver transplantation, a procedure that ultimately results in reinfection of the transplanted organ [4,5]. In recent years, the growing problem of HCV prompted the World Health Organisation to set a target to eliminate HCV as a public health burden by 2030. However, in the absence of a vaccine against HCV, this will prove challenging.

Therapeutic treatment of HCV has been vastly improved over the past decade due to the development of direct acting antivirals (DAAs). These compounds act as inhibitors of either the NS3/4a serine protease, NS5a or the NS5b RNA-dependent polymerase [6] and can achieve a 95% cure rate [7]. However, there are limitations to this strategy. Firstly, in order to treat an infection, a diagnosis must be made which may not occur in asymptomatic cases. It has recently been reported that the diagnosis rate in 2014 in the United Kingdom was estimated at capturing less than half of infected individuals [8]. Secondly, the cost of these therapeutics limits their use in developed countries, and all but excludes their use in low and middle-income countries with high HCV burdens. Thirdly, the ability of HCV to rapidly respond to selective pressures means that the emergence of DAA-resistant strains is a major risk [9,10]. Indeed, resistance-associated substitutions (RAS) have been detected in circulating HCV strains in treatment naive patients [11,12]. One such example of a RAS that has been reported in treatment-naïve patients is the C316 mutation which has been associated with resistance to non-nucleotide NS5B inhibitors such as Nesbuvir [13]. Another example is the S282T RAS which is associated with sofosbuvir resistance in vitro [14] although at the time of writing this polymorphism is not prevalent in clinical cohorts. The risk of DAA-resistance is mitigated by using combinational therapies of DAAs that target different HCV proteins.

The ability to effectively treat HCV infection has been a major achievement. However, there is growing evidence that HCV can leave lasting impacts upon its host post infection. For example, during infection extensive liver fibrosis can occur, which can persist for several years after viral clearance. Furthermore, persistent hyperfunctional CD8+ T cell phenotype has been reported following successful treatment with DAAs, suggesting continued immunological impairment [15]. There are also conflicting reports about the risk of hepatocellular carcinoma after virus clearance [16,17]. Understanding the long-term effects following virus clearance will take years more research as more data become available from successful cases. However, it is now apparent that therapeutics alone are unlikely to achieve the 2030 elimination target and thus a vaccine is urgently needed.

Modelling based on viral kinetics in reinfected individuals with pre-existing immunity has shown that transmission risk can be greatly reduced when an immune response occurs, despite detectable virus RNA titres [18]. This is of particular importance when considering vaccination of people who inject drugs, a high-risk group for HCV infection and reinfection. This suggests that a successful vaccine could be used to reduce viral titres rather than inducing sterilising immunity. This is a key point as it provides a realistic goal for HCV vaccine research.

2. Host Immune Responses to Hepatitis C Virus

Virus-host interactions determine the outcome of acute HCV infection. This interplay is complex and includes components of both the adaptive and innate host immune system. The most common scenario is progression to chronic infection. However, 25%–40% of individuals undergo spontaneous viral clearance (SVC) [19,20] within 12 months of infection [21,22]. Approximately 80% of these individuals will achieve SVC a second time following reinfection [23] with a marked decrease in viral RNA titres and reduced infection times compared to the first infection [23,24]. This indicates that initial infection can lead to the establishment of an immunological memory which can control subsequent HCV infection. This protective response consists of both humoral and cellular adaptive immune responses that do not result in sterilising immunity but prevent chronic infection. This phenomenon provides a benchmark for HCV vaccine research and thus is vital to elucidate.

2.1. Innate Immune Reponses

Innate immunity provides a first line of defence against viral infection. The liver presents a unique microenvironment that is enriched with cells that participate in this response, namely Kupffer cells, natural killer (NK) cells, hepatic stellate cells (HSCs) and macrophages. Initial innate responses are triggered by HCV-derived pathogen-associated molecular patterns (PAMPs) that are recognised by pattern recognition receptors (PRRs). Virion-associated PAMPs are the E1 and E2 glycoproteins [25,26], while intracellular detection of viral PAMPs, including viral proteins and RNA, is mediated by toll-like receptors (TLRs), nucleotide-binding oligomerisation domain (NOD)-like receptors (NLRs) and retinoic acid-inducible gene-I-like receptors (RLRs) [27,28]. Activation of signalling cascades downstream of these receptors results in the production of proinflammatory cytokines including interleukin-1β (IL-1β), IL-18 and type I and type III interferons (IFNs). These IFNs mediate upregulation of interferon stimulated genes (ISGs) in an autocrine and paracrine manner leading to an antiviral response in the liver [29,30]. However, the HCV viral proteins core, E2, NS3/4a and NS5a all impair the expression of ISGs through disruption of signalling cascades, allowing the virus to overcome the host innate response [31,32]. This results in an innate immune response that is incapable of clearing HCV.

Successful SVC is influenced by the outcome of innate immune responses. A major example is the association of single nucleotide polymorphisms (SNP) rs12979860 present in the type III IFN gene *IFNλ4* with SVC. In this case approximately 50% of individuals with a C/C genotype achieve SVC [33,34]. Additionally, NK inhibitory receptor, killer immunoglobulin receptor 2DL3 (KIR2DL3) and human leukocyte antigen C group 1 (HLA-C1) are associated with SVC [35] due to a reduced inhibition of cytotoxic NK activity [36,37].

2.2. Ceullar Immune Responses

Cellular immunity has long been associated with spontaneous HCV clearance [38] and is mediated through two main T cell subsets, the cytolytic CD8+ T cells and CD4+ helper T cells. CD8+ T cells destroy infected cells in a manner restricted by MHCI presented epitopes [39]. In contrast, recognition by CD4+ helper T cells is MHCII restricted and their role is to aid the function of CD8+ T cells and the establishment of T cell memory through the secretion of cytokines such as IFN-γ [40,41]. CD4+ T cells also aid B cell activation and a CD4+ T cell subset, follicular helper T cells (T_{FH}) are required to establish a long-term antibody response [42,43]. HCV-specific T cells are detectable within the first 12 weeks of infection and target a broad range of HCV epitopes present on both structural and non-structural viral proteins [44]. During the progression to chronicity, the HCV-specific CD4+ T cells display an exhausted phenotype and the population collapses [45,46]. The decrease in CD4+ T cell function leads to a dysregulated CD8+ T cell response in which these cells become exhausted and dysfunctional with reports of continued IFN-γ secretion but an absence of cytolytic activity [47]. The reasons for this reduction in effective cellular responses are incompletely understood. The loss of functional HCV-specific T cells could be the result of host regulation of the immune system since persistent antigen stimulation could lead to the prolonged production of proinflammatory cytokines which in turn contributes to hepatic tissue damage.

The importance of T cells to SVC was first demonstrated in experimentally infected chimpanzee in which HCV persistence was observed in the absence of either a CD4+ or CD8+ T cell response [48,49]. Interestingly, when CD4+ T cells were depleted HCV persisted alongside functional CD8+ T cell responses. HCV-specific CD4+ T cells and CD8+ T cells are detectable during acute infection [45]. This provides strong evidence that the T cell responses have a major role in the outcome of HCV infection. HCV-specific CD4+ T cells are broadly targeting with the most common epitopes being found in the core, E2, NS3, NS4a, NS4b, NS5a and NS5b HCV proteins [44].

2.3. Humoral Immune Responses

Neutralising antibodies (nAbs) in the context of HCV infection were first described by Farci et al. [50], although their role in spontaneous clearance was disputed for many years due to reports of cell mediated clearance in seronegative individuals [51–53], suggesting that nAbs are not essential to achieve SVC. However, analysis of sera from individuals who cleared HCV has shown the presence of nAbs and these are detectable at earlier time points compared to acute infections that proceed to chronicity and are subsequently lost following viral clearance [54] suggesting that a rapid, short-lived humoral response is required for clearance [55–58]. It has recently been shown that nAbs generated within the first 100 days of infection often have a narrow neutralising capacity directed towards the founder virus [58]. The selective pressure exerted by nAbs upon the circulating strains can also drive the evolution of HCV towards escape mutations that compromise viral fitness further aiding clearance of the infection [59,60]. The delayed appearance of cross-reactive nAb responses are apparent in chronically infected individuals as isolated sera can neutralise circulating strains from previous infection time points with greater potency than the current dominant virus [56] and cross-reactive nAbs have been isolated from chronically infected individuals [61–64]. Although these nAbs cannot clear the infection, they have been associated with reduced liver fibrosis [65] and patients that experience hypogammaglobulinemia have a more severe disease progression [66].

Further insight into the humoral response has been obtained through characterising nAbs derived from patients. Bailey et al. [67] sequenced cross-reactive nAbs isolated from two individuals that cleared HCV and showed these nAbs shared >90% similarity with germline heavy chain variable (VH) genes and >92% similarity with germline light chain gene sequences revealing that generation of cross-reactive nAbs required limited somatic hypermutation. A common feature of these nAbs was the *VH1-69* gene which is found in potent cross-reactive nAbs that target antigenic region 3 (AR3) and is also present in nAbs targeting HIV and Influenza [68–71]. Structural investigation has also shown that cross-neutralising activity is a result of long complementarity-determining region H3 (CDRH3), typically 18–22 residues, that forms a β-hairpin structure that is stabilized by a disulphide bond allowing for interaction with conserved E2 epitopes [72,73]. This level of insight into how potent nAbs work can inform rational design of B-cell immunogens to favour the production of these types of antibodies in the host.

3. Hepatitis C Virus Envelope Proteins as Vaccine Targets

The HCV envelope glycoproteins, E1 and E2, are located at residues 192–746 of the polyprotein and are the targets of the humoral immune response, making them an attractive vaccine target [74] (Figure 1A). Both E1 and E2 are type I transmembrane proteins that form an intracellular non-covalent heterodimer that form higher order covalent structures on the mature virion [75,76]. The E2 ectodomain contains an immunoglobulin-like β-sandwich that is flanked by α-helices which form a front and back layer [77,78]. There are also regions that exhibit high levels of variability which are referred to as hypervariable regions (HVRs) 1 and 2, and a third intergenotypic variable region (IgVR; Figure 1A). The E1 protein is smaller, more conserved than E2 and less well characterized with partial crystal structures resolved for fragments encompassing residues 192-271 [79] and 314–324 [80].

The E1E2 heterodimer mediates entry into the hepatocytes through interactions with four essential host receptors, CD81 [81,82], scavenger receptor B1 (SRB1) [83], claudin [84] and occludin [85,86]. The first step in viral entry is the interaction between SRB1 and the HVR1 (Figure 1A) located at the N-terminus of E2 which induces a conformational change that exposes the conserved E2 core region and the CD81 binding loop (residues 519–535) [77]. The interaction between E2 and CD81 results in recruitment of claudin to CD81 which leads to clathrin-mediated endocytosis [87]. Membrane fusion occurs in low pH endosomes, which is thought to induce a conformational change in the E1E2 heterodimer [88]. This leads to membrane fusion, possibly mediated by E1 via the action of a putative fusion peptide located at residues 272–285 (Figure 1A) [89].

Antibody-mediated neutralisation of HCV is achieved through targeting the E1E2 heterodimer on the surface of the virus. To date, most characterized nAbs target the E2 protein. The are several linear and discontinuous regions of E2 that are targeted by Abs and these have varying nomenclature, being referred to as ARs1-5 [69], Epitopes I-III (Figure 1) [90], or domains A-E [91]. Importantly, AR4 and 5 are reliant on the presence of the E1E2 heterodimer for binding [69]. The epitope I, II and AR3 regions form the neutralising face of E2 which is targeted by some of the most potent cross-reactive nAbs described to date [92] arguing for their inclusion in a nAb-eliciting vaccine.

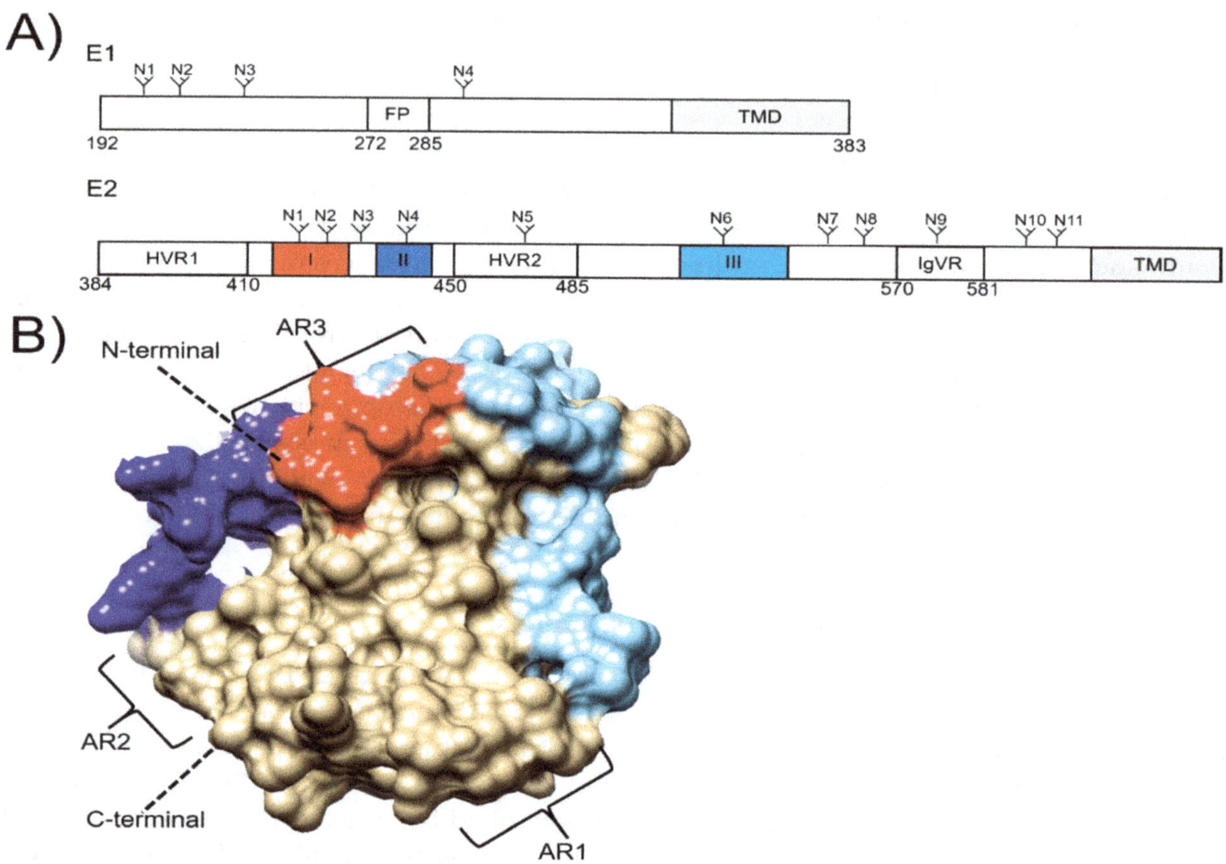

Figure 1. (**A**) Schematic diagrams of the hepatitis C virus envelope glycoproteins E1 and E2, showing N-linked glycosylation sites (N), transmembrane domains (TMDs), and the E1 fusion peptide (FP). E2 hypervariable regions (HVRs) 1 and 2, and the intergentypic variable region (IgVR) are also depicted. Linear epitopes I, II and III are highlighted in red, dark blue and light blue, respectively. (**B**) E2 structure (PDB: 6MEH). Linear epitopes I, II and III are highlighted in the corresponding schematic. Antigenic regions (ARs) are also shown.

4. Challenges to Hepatitis C Virus Vaccine Design

4.1. Genetic Diversity

As a species, HCV exhibits extensive genetic diversity is driven by a mutation rate in the order of 10^{-4} substitutions per site of the genome [93,94]. Mutations are acquired through the activity of the error prone NS5b RNA-dependent RNA polymerase and this coupled with high levels of virus production and selective pressures exerted by the host immune response has driven the diversification of HCV. There are currently eight genotypes (Gt1-8) reported which are defined by 30% difference in nucleotide sequence [95]. Gt1 HCV isolates have the highest prevalence, accounting for 49% of diagnosed cases globally followed by Gt3 accounting for 17.9% of cases [96], and are more prevalent in developed countries [96]. In contrast, Gt4 and Gt5 isolates are more prevalent in lower income countries in Africa and the Middle Eastern regions [96]. Genotypes are further classified into subtypes of which there are currently 90 confirmed groups. These exhibit a 15% variation in nucleotide sequence [95]. Gt1-7 contain multiple subtypes. However, the recently reported Gt8 group currently contains a single subtype isolated from four individuals [97]. Rapid evolution of HCV during the course of an infection leads to the establishment of a heterogeneous population [98]. The diversification of this population is driven by host immune selective pressure and the degree to which variation occurs in acute infection correlates with a progression to chronicity [99].

The extent of genetic diversity gives rise to genotype-specific immune responses. The E1E2 sequence shows the greatest level of variation as a result of the selective pressure exerted by the host immune response [100], leading to humoral responses that can have reduced heterologous neutralising activity [101]. However, cross-reactive nAbs that are capable of targeting isolates from different genotypes have been described in several studies [102], thus highlighting that this challenge can be overcome. Epitope variability also leads to genotype-specific cellular responses for example Luxenburger et al. [103] have recently shown CD8+ T cells from individuals chronically infected with a Gt4 HCV isolate failed to recognize Gt1 derived epitopes. Limited intergenotypic cross-reactivity of Gt3 HCV-specific T cells has also been reported in patients that successfully cleared Gt3 infections [104]. Limited cross-reactive immune responses to distantly related HCV isolates will be a key challenge to produce an effective vaccine

4.2. *Evading the Host Adaptive Immune Response*

The ability of HCV to establish a chronic infection highlights the efficiency in which this virus can subvert the host immune response. This is achieved through multiple strategies. Firstly, immunodominant epitopes such as the HVR1 of E2 elicit a response of non-neutralising antibodies. Currently it is thought that HVR1 acts as a shield of the more conserved epitopes in the E2 core that contain CD81 binding residues, since removal of HVR1 increases virus susceptibility to neutralisation [105,106]. Evidence also shows that HVR1 induces greater homologous nAbs and deletion induces broader heterologous nAbs [107].

Epitope masking is also achieved through the glycosylation of envelope proteins to form a glycan shield [108]. This mechanism diminishes the binding of nAbs and is used by other viruses such as HIV and Influenza although by comparison, HCV exhibits a reduced variability in the position of each glycan group. The E1 and E2 proteins contain 4 and 11 N-linked glycosylation sites which are highly conserved across different genotypes (Figure 1A) [109]. Deletion of E2 glycosylation sites increases HCV susceptibility to nAbs showing that glycosylation acts via steric hinderance to nAbs [109,110]. Interestingly, removal of E2 glycan sites or expression of this protein in systems that use smaller, less complex glycan groups enhance the immunogenicity compared to mammalian expressed E2 [111–113]. Another mechanism in which nAb resistance can be mediated through glycosylation is glycan shift. This arises through non-synonymous mutations that result in the deletion of a glycosylation site and the appearance of a new glycosylation site in a different position in the protein. Pantua et al. [114] reported this phenomenon after incubating cell cultured HCV (HCVcc) with the murine nAb, AP33 which targets residues within the E2 epitope I region [115]. After 5 days of incubation with AP33, escape mutants could be detected which contained either N417S or N417T residue variations coupled with a new glycosylation site at position 415 [114].

The evasion of nAbs can also be attributed to the presence of host derived factors. One such factor is high-density lipoproteins which are present in human serum and has been shown to increase HCV infectivity via SR-BI interactions which in turn decreases the time available for nAbs to bind to their target [116,117]. Additionally, the presence of host derived apolipoprotein E on the mature HCV virion has been shown to have a role in epitope masking the E2 protein abrogating nAb activity [118]. Another evasion method is through the use of decoys. Recently it has been reported that in a HCVcc system, infected cells produce lipid droplets coated with the E2 protein [119]. This may also be a strategy to subvert the immune system by using these E2-coated droplets to interact with nAbs, thereby reducing the availability of nAbs to target E2 present on the surface of the virus particle. Finally, evasion from nAbs has recently been shown to be associated with resistance to antiviral interferon-induced transmembrane (IFITM) proteins [120] showing that the innate immune response can also be a driving force for nAb evasion.

4.3. Models for Hepatitis C Virus Infection

4.3.1. In Vitro Models

Since the discovery of HCV, research was hampered by the lack of infection models both in vivo and in vitro. The use of models in vaccine research is essential for the assessment of sera and monoclonal antibodies arising from natural infection, experimental immunizations or vaccine trials. In the case of in vitro models, the key challenge was generating a cell culture-based system that could produce infectious HCV at titres suitable for further experimentation. This problem was solved with the discovery of two Gt2a isolates, JFH1 and J6 which produce high titres of infectious HCV from cultured Huh 7.5 cells [121]. Following this, it was found that intergenotypic recombinant viruses consisting of core-NS2 of an isolate of interest fused to NS3-NS5b of JFH-1 could produce viable chimeric viruses [121]. The developments in HCVcc techniques have allowed panels with representatives of the seven major genotypes to be set up [122–124]. Our group has recently described a method in which E1E2 patient derived sequences could be incorporated into chimeric HCVcc expression vectors [125,126], further aiding the ability to characterize isolates that have different neutralisation phenotypes.

Viral pseudotyping has also been used to study the entry mechanism of HCV. This approach utilizes the ability of retroviral gag/pol proteins to self-assemble into enveloped virus particles. Simultaneous expression of foreign viral envelope proteins in the same cells leads to the incorporation on to the surface of the retroviral particle whose entry properties are dictated by the envelope glycoprotein. Infectivity can be measured by the incorporation of a reporter gene, usually luciferase, which is introduced into target cells and expressed. Methods to generate HCV pseudoparticles (HCVpps) commonly use murine leukemia virus or HIV derived vectors [127,128]. Our group and others have utilized these systems to characterize extensive panels of patient-derived E1E2 sequences allowing important characterisation of these unique isolates [57,129–131]. These studies have shown that neutralisation sensitivity of patient derived isolates to both sera and monoclonal nAbs is markedly varied and not associated with genotype but is isolate dependent. Furthermore, it has been shown that the HCV reference isolate H77, a Gt1a isolate that was first adopted due to its ability to infect and cause disease in chimpanzees [132–134], is more susceptible to antibody-mediated neutralisation than many patient-derived isolates [102]. This finding is of significance since H77 neutralisation has been used to validate multiple vaccine candidates and therefore these data provide limited insight into how effective a candidate may be towards clinically relevant isolates. H77 has also been used in the design of immunogens with moderate success, although it could be argued that immunogen design based on more nAb-resistant isolates may elicit more potent nAbs.

The ability to generate both HCVcc and HCVpp provide essential tools for the in vitro study of HCV and assessing the neutralising breadth of sera and monoclonal nAbs. The importance of isolate panels for the validation of vaccine candidates is exemplified in the field of HIV vaccine research, in which candidates have been tested against an extensive panel of 109 isolates developed by Seaman et al. [135], which are grouped based on neutralisation susceptibility. In this way humoral responses following vaccination can be assessed in a standardized manner allowing for relevant comparisons between candidates and vaccines that induce responses capable of neutralising the most resistant isolates can be identified for further development. At the time of writing a consensus panel of isolates is yet to be widely adopted but doing so will greatly enhance our understanding of which candidates are promising and those that are not.

4.3.2. In Vivo Models

Humans are the natural host of HCV, and therefore it is imperative that suitable in vivo models are used in order to test the efficacy and safety of preclinical vaccine candidates. Arguably, the most successful model has been the chimpanzee, which is permissive to HCV infection under experimental conditions. However, ethical concerns over the use of this species has led to a ban on its use in experimental research. An alternative has been the use of chimeric humanized or transgenic mouse models which have humanized livers such as Alb-uPA/SCID mice [136,137] or those engineered to express human CD81 and occludin [138,139]. There are limitations to using chimeric mouse models, most notably that they do not exhibit cirrhosis or HCC, and are technically difficult to produce [140].

In light of the limited options available for the in vivo modelling of HCV, there has been increasing interest in other members of the *Hepacivirus* genus for use as analogues. At the time of writing there are two species of particular interest, the Rodent Hepacivirus (RHV) and the Equine Hepacivirus (EqHV). RHV was initially discovered in the species *Rattus norvegicus* in 2014 [141]. Experimental infection of different lab rat breeds leads to the establishment of permanent infection with features observed during HCV infection in humans such as hepatic fibrosis, steatosis and evidence of SVC in the Holtzman rat strain [142]. There are key contrasts between RHV and HCV infections, notably the lack of IFN-γ+ CD8+ T cell responses during RHV infection [143].

EqHV was initially discovered in canines and subsequent serology testing identified equines as the natural host [144,145]. This virus is the closest relative of HCV and there are shared features of both species such as similar levels of glycosylation of the E1E2 proteins and a conserved seed site in the 5′-UTR for the liver-specific microRNA-122 (miR-122) which contributes to stability, translation, and replication of the viral RNA [146]. Seroprevalence of EqHV is in the region of 30% of surveyed horses, with approximately 3% testing positive for viral RNA [147]. This discrepancy between serology and viral RNA may be indicative of a high viral clearance rate. Despite this potential high clearance rate, EqHV acute infection may proceed to chronicity after 6 months [148], further validating the relevancy of this virus as a model for HCV.

The use of analogous Hepacivirus species will allow for the testing of vaccine strategies and the experimental challenge in the natural host of that species, a feat that cannot currently be achieved for HCV. Whilst these approaches are likely to prove highly valuable to the field of HCV vaccine research it is important to acknowledge the differences in mammalian immune systems and how this will impact on our interpretation of experimental data. For example, the *IgVH 1-69* gene with an extended CDRH3 region has previously been described as a feature of anti-HCV specific nAbs that are elicited in SVC and therefore it is logical that a vaccine candidate could be assessed based on its ability to elicit these types of nAbs. With this in mind it is worth considering how comparable the antibodies of animal model species are to those of humans. One such difference is the length of the CDRH3 regions which are typically 16 residues long [149], however these are reduced to an average of 12 to 14 residues in rodent [149] and equine species [150], respectively. The CDRH3 region can be critical for the formation of the antigen-antibody complex and extended CDRH3 loops are effective at penetrating the glycan shield of viral envelope proteins, a favorable characteristic of anti-HCV nAbs. This raises an important question about the relevance and suitability of current animal models as predictors of the human antibody response. Similarly, the paradigm of vaccine research has been to test novel candidates in small animals followed by larger animal species before clinical testing in humans. This approach enables evaluation of immunogenicity and safety prior to exposure of an immunogen in humans. However, questions should be asked as to whether this approach has hindered the progress of at least some HCV vaccine candidates because of differences between the model and human antibody repertoires.

4.4. Rational Design of Immunogens to Elicit Cross-Reactive Neutralising Antibodies

The informed, rational design of immunogens will be vital in order to produce a successful HCV vaccine. As advances in the analysis of antibody repertoires are allowing deeper insight into the types of nAbs that are associated with SVC, there is potential to use this information to develop immunogens that favour the production of these types of antibodies. An example of this can be seen with the E2 epitope I region or antigenic site 412 (AS412). This linear epitope is structurally flexible and when in complex with nAbs and adopts three distinct conformations. Firstly epitope I forms an extended conformation in complex with the rat nAb 3/11, a β-hairpin conformation is observed when bound to AP33 or the human nAb HCV-1, and an intermediate conformation occurs when in complex with the human nAb HC33.1 [151]. As previously discussed, HCV may escape epitope I targeting nAbs by the mechanism of glycan shift. However, this mechanism does not abrogate and instead enhances the potency of HC33.1 [152]. With this in mind, rational design of an immunogen could strive to present the epitope I region in an intermediate conformation to bias the humoral response to elicit HC33.1-like nAbs. To date this has not been investigated however, efforts have been undertaken to present epitope I in the β-hairpin conformation using cyclic peptides based on θ-defensin which adopts a similar conformation [153]. This approach induced nAb responses when tested in mice however these were lower compared to mice immunized with E2 [153]. The rational design of HCV epitopes in this way is technically challenging and is limited to targeting linear epitopes. Additionally, delivery of cyclic peptides will require further development in order to enhance the immunogenicity and stimulate greater titers of nAbs.

5. Vaccine Prospects

Despite the challenges faced in HCV vaccine design, there have been a variety of different vaccine approaches investigated with a small number of these candidates reaching human trials (summarized in Table 1). Currently, DNA and peptide-based vaccine candidates are actively being investigated in murine models [154–158]. One recently reported peptide candidate consisted of overlapping peptides derived from the p7 protein which induced antigen-specific CD4+ T cells and cytotoxic CD8+ T cells capable of targeting p7 expressing hepatocytes in vivo [154]. This study has been the first to show the immunogenicity of p7 when used as the sole target in a vaccine. Additionally, a DNA-based vaccine has been shown to induce CD4+ T cell and CD8+ T cell responses and elicit T cell memory in mice; however, a non-neutralising Ab response was also observed [156]. These vaccine candidates are in an early stage of development and therefore the following sections will discuss candidates that have been more extensively studied.

5.1. Recombinant Subunit Vaccines

Recombinant subunit vaccines are an attractive technology as they have previously been utilized for a variety of pathogens [159] and are economical to produce on a commercial scale. In the field of HCV vaccine research, attempts to generate a subunit vaccine have focused exclusively on targeting the HCV E proteins. The most successful candidate has been the recombinant E1E2 protein (rE1E2) derived from a Gt1a isolate. Initially, HCV-1 derived rE1E2 was used to vaccinate seven chimpanzees which resulted in a humoral response [160]. Following homologous HCV challenge, five out of seven vaccinated chimpanzees exhibited sterilising immunity with the remaining two developing acute infections that were subsequently cleared [160,161]. This was further validated in small animal models and that immunisation rE1E2 derived from a single isolate could induce cross-reactive nAbs [161]. Following this work, a phase I human trial was performed in which rE1E2 derived from the Gt1a HCV-1 isolate was administered at different doses (4 μg, 20 μg and 100 μg of rE1E2) with the MF59 adjuvant to healthy volunteers [162]. Importantly this study showed that rE1E2 can be safely tolerated in humans, a finding of significance given that a successful HCV vaccine candidate will likely require these proteins or derivatives of them. Polyfunctional CD4+ T cell responses were detected and the magnitude of this response was inversely related to dosage. Humoral responses and nAbs were initially reported [162,163] and further testing using a diverse HCVcc panel with isolates from Gt1-7 showed that 3/16 volunteers had elicited cross reactive nAbs [164]. Additionally, post vaccination sera from 5 volunteers competed with nAbs AP33, AR3B, AR4A, AR5A and IGH526, showing that the humoral response targeted both E1, E2 and the E1E2 heterodimer [165]. The ability for rE1E2 from a single isolate to induce nAbs in humans is significant and encouraging although work should be undertaken to enhance the efficacy at which nAbs are generated. A key issue with rE1E2 was purification which relied on lectin-based affinity methods that were low affinity and non-specific [166]. Furthermore, efforts to improve rE1E2 production were made by removing the transmembrane domains of the E protein. However, this truncated E1E2 was found to be a weak immunogen that elicited low levels of nAbs [167]. In light of these issues, both flag-tagged and Fc-tagged rE1E2 have been investigated and elicit nAbs in mice at comparable levels to wild type rE1E2 [166,168].

Another subunit vaccine approach has been the use of truncated soluble E2 (sE2) which results in a secreted form of the E2 ectodomain. A candidate of particular note is the H77 derived sE2384-661 construct with deleted HVR1, HVR2 and IgVR ($sE2_{\Delta123}$) which can be expressed in a correct conformation which interacts with CD81 and conformation sensitive antibodies [169–171]. Vietheer et al. [170] reported that the expression of $sE2_{\Delta123}$ in mammalian cells results in biochemically and immunogenically distinct isoforms of this protein that exist as monomeric, dimeric, pentameric and a high molecular weight aggregate (HMW1; estimated at 51 protomers). Immunisation of guinea pigs with different isoforms showed that HMW1 elicited greater titres of cross-reactive nAbs that could neutralise isolates from Gt2a, 4a, 5a, 6a and 7a expressed in a HVCcc system [170]. Additionally, HMW1 had exhibited a reduced activity with non-neutralising antibodies, suggesting that this aggregate focuses the humoral immune response away from these epitopes, allowing for greater focusing to nAb epitopes [170]. Whilst this initial report is promising, it was noted that $sE2_{\Delta123}$ reduced homologous neutralisation activity, a likely result of the removal of HVR1 which was also observed by Law and colleagues [172].

5.2. Virus-Like Particles

Virus-like particles (VLPs) are a promising area of vaccine research and have been investigated extensively to design a HCV vaccine [173]. To date, there are two widely used commercial vaccines that utilize VLP technology, the hepatitis B virus (HBV) and human papilloma virus vaccines. VLPs are formed when the structural proteins of a virus assemble in a genome-independent manner to produce a particle that resembles the native virus whilst lacking the ability to replicate and are more immunogenic than soluble protein due to their repetitive structure and ability to drain into tissue lymph nodes [107,174].

HCV-LPs were first described by Baumert et al. [175] in which VLPs were expressed in the insect cell line Sf9 following transduction with a recombinant baculovirus containing the core E1 and E2 HCV structural proteins. These HCV-LPs elicited HCV-specific IgG production, IFN-γ secreting CD8+ T cell and CD4+ T cell mediated cellular responses in mice and baboons [176–178]. Immunisation of four chimpanzees with four doses of HCV-LPs resulted in CD4+ and CD8+ T cell responses in all animals [179]. Subsequent challenge with homologous HCV resulted in a reduced viremia in vaccinated animals compared to controls with two animals testing negative for HCV two years post challenge [179]. Interestingly, humoral responses in chimpanzees were not detectable in three of these animals and appear to have been absent during the reduction of viremia. Further work on this candidate has not been progressed since this first study in chimpanzees. However, it is an important example for future HCV vaccine work, as it showed that viral clearance can be achieved using an experimental VLP vaccine candidate. Despite work on this candidate ceasing, HCV-LPs continued to be investigated. Recently, a HCV-LP system has been established through the transduction of the human hepatoma cell line Huh 7 with recombinant adenovirus encoding the structural genes of HCV [180]. Initially designed using the H77 isolate, further development has expanded by generating HCV-LPs using the structural sequences of different isolates representing Gt1b, 2a and 3a subtypes to produce HCV-LPs with a conformation close to that the wild type virus [180–183]. Trials of this candidate in mice showed the induction of nAbs and activation of both CD4+ and CD8+ T cell responses and this has recently been reported in a vaccinated Landrace pigs [184]. To date, assessment of the humoral response has demonstrated that this vaccine elicits nAbs with activity towards homologous strains. Heterologous neutralisation data have not been reported for this candidate. Testing the sera from animals immunized with this quadrivalent vaccine against a diverse panel of HCV isolates would be of particular interest not only for this candidate but to inform future vaccine design.

5.3. Viral Vector Vaccines

Viral vectors have the capacity to induce high level cellular immune responses [185], making them an attractive approach for HCV candidates. Viral vectors of particular interest are human adenovirus 6 (HuAd6), chimpanzees Ad 3 (ChAd3) and modified vaccinia ankara (MVA) [186]. The only HCV vaccine candidates to be tested in phase I and phase I/II human trials has been ChAd3 and MVA which each encoded HCV NS3, NS4a, NS4b, NS5a and inactivated NS5b (NSmut) derived from the Gt1b BK isolate [187,188]. These candidates were tested together in a heterologous primer/boost strategy in which healthy human volunteers were primed with ChAd3-NSmut and boosted with MVA-NSmut 8 weeks later [188]. The results of this phase I study showed that prime/boost ChAd3/MVA-NSmut induced both CD4+ T cell and CD8+ T cell responses directed towards epitopes on all five HCV non-structural proteins, importantly the effect of the MVA-NSmut enhanced the T cell responses and these were detectable at week 70 [188]. Given the promising cellular responses observed in the phase I trial, this approach was tested in patients with chronic HCV infections although this was unable to reverse T cell exhaustion [189], ruling out the use of ChAd3/MVA-NSmut as a therapeutic vaccine. Recently ChAd3/MVA-NSmut was tested in a large phase I/II trial involving 548 high risk individuals was concluded (clinicaltrials.gov identifier: NCT01436357). At the time of writing, this trial has concluded, and data have yet to be published. However, a press release statement from the National Institute of Allergy and Infectious Disease stated that 14 vaccinated individuals became chronically infected with HCV, suggesting that this candidate does not provide protection against HCV infection [190]. Understanding the reasons for this failure will be vital to inform our understanding of vaccine design. Given that the ChAd3/MVA-NSmut candidate exclusively targeted T-cell epitopes, the failure of this vaccine candidate could further emphasize the need for both humoral and cellular immune responses in clearance of acute infections.

Table 1. Summary of recent hepatitis C virus vaccine candidates. Subunit, virus-like particle (VLP), viral vector, peptide and DNA vaccine approaches are listed with the vaccine target, genotype (Gt) and isolate from which the candidate was derived, tested species and the humoral and cellular immune responses were reported.

Vaccine Type	HCV Target	HCV Strain	Tested Species	Antibody Response *	CD4+ T Cell Response †	CD8+ T Cell Response †	Ref.
Subunit							
HCV-1 rE1E2	E1E2	Gt1a HCV-1	humans	homologous and heterologous	yes	N.D	[162,164]
H77 $sE2_{\Delta 123}$	E2core	Gt1a H77	guinea pigs	homologous and heterologous	N.D	N.D	[170]
Virus-Like particles							
core, E1, E2 from Gt1a, 1b, 2a and 3a	core, E1, E2	Gt1a H77, Gt1b BK, Gt2a JFH1, Gt3a	mice, pigs	homologous neutralising antibodies	yes	yes	[181,184]
HBV/HCV-LPs	E1, E2	Gt1a H77	rabbit	homologous, heterologous activity towards Gt1a and 1b, reduced activity towards Gt2a and 3a isolates.	N.D	N.D	[191]
HBV/HCV-LPs	linear E1 and E2 epitopes	not stated	mice	heterologous towards Gt1a, 1b and 2a	N.D	N.D	[192]
murine leukaemia VLP-HCVE1E2	E1, E2	Gt1a H77	mice, macaques	homologous, heterologous towards Gt1b, 2a, 2b and 4c	yes	N.D	[193]
Viral vector							
ChAd3/MVA-Nsmut	NS3, NS4a, NS4b, NS5a, NS5b	Gt1a BK	humans	N/A	yes	yes	[188]
Peptide							
p7	p7	Gt1b J4	mice	N/A	yes	yes	[154]
HCVp6-MAP	E1, E2, NS4b, NS5a, NS5b	Gt4a ED43	mice	homologous, heterologous towards JFH1	yes	yes	[155]
DNA							
pVax-sE1E2-IMX313P	E1, E2	Gt1b	mice	homologous, heterologous towards Gt1a, 1b, 2a, 2b, 3a, 4a, 5, 6	yes	N.D	[158]
DREP-HCV/MVA-HCV	core, E1, E1, p7, NS2, NS3	Gt1a H77	mice	non-neutralising IgG	yes	yes	[156]
pVax-N3-NS5b	NS3, NS4, NS5b	Gt1b, Gt3a	mice	N/A	yes	yes	[157]

* N/A (not applicable) for vaccine candidates that are not designed to elicit HCV-specific B cell responses. † N.D (not determined) in the study.

6. Conclusions

In the 30 years since the discovery of HCV, it has been apparent that this virus is highly complex and presents a major public health challenge. Encouragingly, efforts toward a vaccine continue and investigation into a range of approaches have yielded interesting results. The vast improvements in in vitro analysis of HCV have greatly aided our understanding of how nAbs work, informing rational vaccine design. In this review, we have highlighted the potential advantages of adopting reference panels of patient-derived E1E2 sequences in order to assess vaccine candidates for their potential to induce nAbs capable of targeting circulating HCV strains. Adopting this approach will provide a more rigorous tool for evaluating the nAb response produced by novel HCV vaccine candidates a characteristic that will likely be essential in a successful HCV vaccine.

Author Contributions: Writing—original draft preparation, J.D.D.; review and editing, R.A.U., A.W.T. and J.K.B.; funding acquisition, J.K.B. All authors have read and agreed to the published version of the manuscript.

References

1. Choo, Q.L.; Kuo, G.; Weiner, A.J.; Overby, L.R.; Bradley, D.W.; Houghton, M. Isolation of a cDNA clone derived from a blood-borne non-A, non-B viral hepatitis genome. *Science* **1989**, *244*, 359–362. [CrossRef]
2. Collaborators, H. Global prevalence and genotype distribution of hepatitis C virus infection in 2015: A modelling study. *Lancet Gastroenterol. Hepatol.* **2017**, *2*, 161–176. [CrossRef]
3. Ly, K.N.; Xing, J.; Klevens, R.M.; Jiles, R.B.; Holmberg, S.D. Causes of death and characteristics of decedents with viral hepatitis, United States, 2010. *Clin. Infect. Dis.* **2014**, *58*, 40–49. [CrossRef]
4. Joshi, D.; Pinzani, M.; Carey, I.; Agarwal, K. Recurrent HCV after liver transplantation-mechanisms, assessment and therapy. *Nat. Rev. Gastroenterol. Hepatol.* **2014**, *11*, 710–721. [CrossRef] [PubMed]
5. Mitchell, O.; Gurakar, A. Management of Hepatitis C Post-liver Transplantation: A Comprehensive Review. *J. Clin. Transl. Hepatol.* **2015**, *3*, 140–148. [CrossRef] [PubMed]
6. Liang, T.J.; Ghany, M.G. Current and future therapies for hepatitis C virus infection. *N. Engl. J. Med.* **2013**, *368*, 1907–1917. [CrossRef] [PubMed]
7. Falade-Nwulia, O.; Suarez-Cuervo, C.; Nelson, D.R.; Fried, M.W.; Segal, J.B.; Sulkowski, M.S. Oral Direct-Acting Agent Therapy for Hepatitis C Virus Infection: A Systematic Review. *Ann. Intern. Med.* **2017**, *166*, 637–648. [CrossRef] [PubMed]
8. Chen, Q.; Ayer, T.; Bethea, E.; Kanwal, F.; Wang, X.; Roberts, M.; Zhuo, Y.; Fagiuoli, S.; Petersen, J.; Chhatwal, J. Changes in hepatitis C burden and treatment trends in Europe during the era of direct-acting antivirals: A modelling study. *BMJ Open* **2019**, *9*, e026726. [CrossRef]
9. Rong, L.; Dahari, H.; Ribeiro, R.M.; Perelson, A.S. Rapid emergence of protease inhibitor resistance in hepatitis C virus. *Sci. Transl. Med.* **2010**, *2*, 30–32. [CrossRef]
10. Bagaglio, S.; Uberti-Foppa, C.; Morsica, G. Resistance Mechanisms in Hepatitis C Virus: Implications for Direct-Acting Antiviral Use. *Drugs* **2017**, *77*, 1043–1055. [CrossRef]
11. Raj, V.S.; Hundie, G.B.; Schurch, A.C.; Smits, S.L.; Pas, S.D.; Le Pogam, S.; Janssen, H.L.A.; de Knegt, R.J.; Osterhaus, A.; Najera, I.; et al. Identification of HCV Resistant Variants against Direct Acting Antivirals in Plasma and Liver of Treatment Naive Patients. *Sci. Rep.* **2017**, *7*, 4688. [CrossRef]
12. Sarrazin, C.; Zeuzem, S. Resistance to direct antiviral agents in patients with hepatitis C virus infection. *Gastroenterology* **2010**, *138*, 447–462. [CrossRef]
13. McCown, M.F.; Rajyaguru, S.; Kular, S.; Cammack, N.; Najera, I. GT-1a or GT-1b subtype-specific resistance profiles for hepatitis C virus inhibitors telaprevir and HCV-796. *Antimicrob. Agents Chemother.* **2009**, *53*, 2129–2132. [CrossRef] [PubMed]
14. Svarovskaia, E.S.; Dvory-Sobol, H.; Parkin, N.; Hebner, C.; Gontcharova, V.; Martin, R.; Ouyang, W.; Han, B.; Xu, S.; Ku, K.; et al. Infrequent development of resistance in genotype 1-6 hepatitis C virus-infected subjects treated with sofosbuvir in phase 2 and 3 clinical trials. *Clin. Infect. Dis.* **2014**, *59*, 1666–1674. [CrossRef] [PubMed]
15. Vranjkovic, A.; Deonarine, F.; Kaka, S.; Angel, J.B.; Cooper, C.L.; Crawley, A.M. Direct-Acting Antiviral Treatment of HCV Infection Does Not Resolve the Dysfunction of Circulating CD8(+) T-Cells in Advanced Liver Disease. *Front. Immunol.* **2019**, *10*, 1926. [CrossRef]

16. Conti, F.; Buonfiglioli, F.; Scuteri, A.; Crespi, C.; Bolondi, L.; Caraceni, P.; Foschi, F.G.; Lenzi, M.; Mazzella, G.; Verucchi, G.; et al. Early occurrence and recurrence of hepatocellular carcinoma in HCV-related cirrhosis treated with direct-acting antivirals. *J. Hepatol.* **2016**, *65*, 727–733. [CrossRef]
17. Kanwal, F.; Kramer, J.; Asch, S.M.; Chayanupatkul, M.; Cao, Y.; El-Serag, H.B. Risk of Hepatocellular Cancer in HCV Patients Treated With Direct-Acting Antiviral Agents. *Gastroenterology* **2017**, *153*, 996–1005.e1001. [CrossRef]
18. Major, M.; Gutfraind, A.; Shekhtman, L.; Cui, Q.; Kachko, A.; Cotler, S.J.; Hajarizadeh, B.; Sacks-Davis, R.; Page, K.; Boodram, B.; et al. Modeling of patient virus titers suggests that availability of a vaccine could reduce hepatitis C virus transmission among injecting drug users. *Sci. Transl. Med.* **2018**, *10*. [CrossRef]
19. Micallef, J.M.; Kaldor, J.M.; Dore, G.J. Spontaneous viral clearance following acute hepatitis C infection: A systematic review of longitudinal studies. *J. Viral. Hepat.* **2006**, *13*, 34–41. [CrossRef]
20. Poustchi, H.; Esmaili, S.; Mohamadkhani, A.; Nikmahzar, A.; Pourshams, A.; Sepanlou, S.G.; Merat, S.; Malekzadeh, R. The impact of illicit drug use on spontaneous hepatitis C clearance: Experience from a large cohort population study. *PLoS ONE* **2011**, *6*, e23830. [CrossRef]
21. Mosley, J.W.; Operskalski, E.A.; Tobler, L.H.; Buskell, Z.J.; Andrews, W.W.; Phelps, B.; Dockter, J.; Giachetti, C.; Seeff, L.B.; Busch, M.P. The course of hepatitis C viraemia in transfusion recipients prior to availability of antiviral therapy. *J. Viral. Hepat.* **2008**, *15*, 120–128. [CrossRef] [PubMed]
22. Page, K.; Hahn, J.A.; Evans, J.; Shiboski, S.; Lum, P.; Delwart, E.; Tobler, L.; Andrews, W.; Avanesyan, L.; Cooper, S.; et al. Acute hepatitis C virus infection in young adult injection drug users: A prospective study of incident infection, resolution, and reinfection. *J. Infect. Dis.* **2009**, *200*, 1216–1226. [CrossRef] [PubMed]
23. Osburn, W.O.; Fisher, B.E.; Dowd, K.A.; Urban, G.; Liu, L.; Ray, S.C.; Thomas, D.L.; Cox, A.L. Spontaneous control of primary hepatitis C virus infection and immunity against persistent reinfection. *Gastroenterology* **2010**, *138*, 315–324. [CrossRef]
24. Sacks-Davis, R.; Aitken, C.K.; Higgs, P.; Spelman, T.; Pedrana, A.E.; Bowden, S.; Bharadwaj, M.; Nivarthi, U.K.; Suppiah, V.; George, J.; et al. High rates of hepatitis C virus reinfection and spontaneous clearance of reinfection in people who inject drugs: A prospective cohort study. *PLoS ONE* **2013**, *8*, e80216. [CrossRef] [PubMed]
25. Brown, K.S.; Keogh, M.J.; Owsianka, A.M.; Adair, R.; Patel, A.H.; Arnold, J.N.; Ball, J.K.; Sim, R.B.; Tarr, A.W.; Hickling, T.P. Specific interaction of hepatitis C virus glycoproteins with mannan binding lectin inhibits virus entry. *Protein Cell* **2010**, *1*, 664–674. [CrossRef] [PubMed]
26. Hamed, M.R.; Brown, R.J.; Zothner, C.; Urbanowicz, R.A.; Mason, C.P.; Krarup, A.; McClure, C.P.; Irving, W.L.; Ball, J.K.; Harris, M.; et al. Recombinant human L-ficolin directly neutralizes hepatitis C virus entry. *J. Innate Immun.* **2014**, *6*, 676–684. [CrossRef] [PubMed]
27. Xu, Y.; Zhong, J. Innate immunity against hepatitis C virus. *Curr. Opin. Immunol.* **2016**, *42*, 98–104. [CrossRef]
28. Chigbu, D.I.; Loonawat, R.; Sehgal, M.; Patel, D.; Jain, P. Hepatitis C Virus Infection: Host(-)Virus Interaction and Mechanisms of Viral Persistence. *Cells* **2019**, *8*, 376. [CrossRef]
29. Wong, M.T.; Chen, S.S. Emerging roles of interferon-stimulated genes in the innate immune response to hepatitis C virus infection. *Cell Mol. Immunol.* **2016**, *13*, 11–35. [CrossRef] [PubMed]
30. Schoggins, J.W.; Wilson, S.J.; Panis, M.; Murphy, M.Y.; Jones, C.T.; Bieniasz, P.; Rice, C.M. A diverse range of gene products are effectors of the type I interferon antiviral response. *Nature* **2011**, *472*, 481–485. [CrossRef]
31. Patra, T.; Ray, R.B.; Ray, R. Strategies to Circumvent Host Innate Immune Response by Hepatitis C Virus. *Cells* **2019**, *8*, 274. [CrossRef] [PubMed]
32. Heim, M.H. Innate immunity and HCV. *J. Hepatol.* **2013**, *58*, 564–574. [CrossRef] [PubMed]
33. Thomas, D.L.; Thio, C.L.; Martin, M.P.; Qi, Y.; Ge, D.; O'Huigin, C.; Kidd, J.; Kidd, K.; Khakoo, S.I.; Alexander, G.; et al. Genetic variation in IL28B and spontaneous clearance of hepatitis C virus. *Nature* **2009**, *461*, 798–801. [CrossRef] [PubMed]
34. Ge, D.; Fellay, J.; Thompson, A.J.; Simon, J.S.; Shianna, K.V.; Urban, T.J.; Heinzen, E.L.; Qiu, P.; Bertelsen, A.H.; Muir, A.J.; et al. Genetic variation in IL28B predicts hepatitis C treatment-induced viral clearance. *Nature* **2009**, *461*, 399–401. [CrossRef] [PubMed]
35. Khakoo, S.I.; Thio, C.L.; Martin, M.P.; Brooks, C.R.; Gao, X.; Astemborski, J.; Cheng, J.; Goedert, J.J.; Vlahov, D.; Hilgartner, M.; et al. HLA and NK cell inhibitory receptor genes in resolving hepatitis C virus infection. *Science* **2004**, *305*, 872–874. [CrossRef]

36. Amadei, B.; Urbani, S.; Cazaly, A.; Fisicaro, P.; Zerbini, A.; Ahmed, P.; Missale, G.; Ferrari, C.; Khakoo, S.I. Activation of natural killer cells during acute infection with hepatitis C virus. *Gastroenterology* **2010**, *138*, 1536–1545. [CrossRef]
37. Yoon, J.C.; Yang, C.M.; Song, Y.; Lee, J.M. Natural killer cells in hepatitis C: Current progress. *World J. Gastroenterol.* **2016**, *22*, 1449–1460. [CrossRef]
38. Missale, G.; Bertoni, R.; Lamonaca, V.; Valli, A.; Massari, M.; Mori, C.; Rumi, M.G.; Houghton, M.; Fiaccadori, F.; Ferrari, C. Different clinical behaviors of acute hepatitis C virus infection are associated with different vigor of the anti-viral cell-mediated immune response. *J. Clin. Investig.* **1996**, *98*, 706–714. [CrossRef]
39. Mittrucker, H.W.; Visekruna, A.; Huber, M. Heterogeneity in the differentiation and function of CD8(+) T cells. *Arch. Immunol. Ther. Exp. (Warsz)* **2014**, *62*, 449–458. [CrossRef]
40. Luckheeram, R.V.; Zhou, R.; Verma, A.D.; Xia, B. CD4(+)T cells: Differentiation and functions. *Clin. Dev. Immunol.* **2012**, *2012*, 925135. [CrossRef]
41. Laidlaw, B.J.; Craft, J.E.; Kaech, S.M. The multifaceted role of CD4(+) T cells in CD8(+) T cell memory. *Nat. Rev. Immunol.* **2016**, *16*, 102–111. [CrossRef] [PubMed]
42. Swain, S.L.; McKinstry, K.K.; Strutt, T.M. Expanding roles for CD4(+) T cells in immunity to viruses. *Nat. Rev. Immunol.* **2012**, *12*, 136–148. [CrossRef] [PubMed]
43. Zhang, J.; Liu, W.; Wen, B.; Xie, T.; Tang, P.; Hu, Y.; Huang, L.; Jin, K.; Zhang, P.; Liu, Z.; et al. Circulating CXCR3(+) Tfh cells positively correlate with neutralizing antibody responses in HCV-infected patients. *Sci. Rep.* **2019**, *9*, 10090. [CrossRef] [PubMed]
44. Semmo, N.; Klenerman, P. CD4+ T cell responses in hepatitis C virus infection. *World J. Gastroenterol.* **2007**, *13*, 4831–4838. [CrossRef]
45. Schulze Zur Wiesch, J.; Ciuffreda, D.; Lewis-Ximenez, L.; Kasprowicz, V.; Nolan, B.E.; Streeck, H.; Aneja, J.; Reyor, L.L.; Allen, T.M.; Lohse, A.W.; et al. Broadly directed virus-specific CD4+ T cell responses are primed during acute hepatitis C infection, but rapidly disappear from human blood with viral persistence. *J. Exp. Med.* **2012**, *209*, 61–75. [CrossRef]
46. Ulsenheimer, A.; Gerlach, J.T.; Gruener, N.H.; Jung, M.C.; Schirren, C.A.; Schraut, W.; Zachoval, R.; Pape, G.R.; Diepolder, H.M. Detection of functionally altered hepatitis C virus-specific CD4 T cells in acute and chronic hepatitis C. *Hepatology* **2003**, *37*, 1189–1198. [CrossRef]
47. Dustin, L.B. Innate and Adaptive Immune Responses in Chronic HCV Infection. *Curr. Drug Targets* **2017**, *18*, 826–843. [CrossRef]
48. Grakoui, A.; Shoukry, N.H.; Woollard, D.J.; Han, J.H.; Hanson, H.L.; Ghrayeb, J.; Murthy, K.K.; Rice, C.M.; Walker, C.M. HCV persistence and immune evasion in the absence of memory T cell help. *Science* **2003**, *302*, 659–662. [CrossRef]
49. Shoukry, N.H.; Grakoui, A.; Houghton, M.; Chien, D.Y.; Ghrayeb, J.; Reimann, K.A.; Walker, C.M. Memory CD8+ T cells are required for protection from persistent hepatitis C virus infection. *J. Exp. Med.* **2003**, *197*, 1645–1655. [CrossRef]
50. Farci, P.; Alter, H.J.; Wong, D.C.; Miller, R.H.; Govindarajan, S.; Engle, R.; Shapiro, M.; Purcell, R.H. Prevention of hepatitis C virus infection in chimpanzees after antibody-mediated in vitro neutralization. *Proc. Natl. Acad. Sci. USA* **1994**, *91*, 7792–7796. [CrossRef]
51. Grebely, J.; Prins, M.; Hellard, M.; Cox, A.L.; Osburn, W.O.; Lauer, G.; Page, K.; Lloyd, A.R.; Dore, G.J. Hepatitis C virus clearance, reinfection, and persistence, with insights from studies of injecting drug users: Towards a vaccine. *Lancet Infect. Dis.* **2012**, *12*, 408–414. [CrossRef]
52. Zeremski, M.; Shu, M.A.; Brown, Q.; Wu, Y.; Des Jarlais, D.C.; Busch, M.P.; Talal, A.H.; Edlin, B.R. Hepatitis C virus-specific T-cell immune responses in seronegative injection drug users. *J. Viral. Hepat.* **2009**, *16*, 10–20. [CrossRef] [PubMed]
53. Post, J.J.; Pan, Y.; Freeman, A.J.; Harvey, C.E.; White, P.A.; Palladinetti, P.; Haber, P.S.; Marinos, G.; Levy, M.H.; Kaldor, J.M.; et al. Clearance of hepatitis C viremia associated with cellular immunity in the absence of seroconversion in the hepatitis C incidence and transmission in prisons study cohort. *J. Infect. Dis.* **2004**, *189*, 1846–1855. [CrossRef]
54. Strasak, A.M.; Kim, A.Y.; Lauer, G.M.; de Sousa, P.S.; Ginuino, C.F.; Fernandes, C.A.; Velloso, C.E.; de Almeida, A.J.; de Oliveira, J.M.; Yoshida, C.F.; et al. Antibody dynamics and spontaneous viral clearance in patients with acute hepatitis C infection in Rio de Janeiro, Brazil. *BMC Infect. Dis.* **2011**, *11*, 15. [CrossRef] [PubMed]

55. Pestka, J.M.; Zeisel, M.B.; Bläser, E.; Schürmann, P.; Bartosch, B.; Cosset, F.L.; Patel, A.H.; Meisel, H.; Baumert, J.; Viazov, S.; et al. Rapid induction of virus-neutralizing antibodies and viral clearance in a single-source outbreak of hepatitis C. *Proc. Natl. Acad. Sci. USA* **2007**, *104*, 6025–6030. [CrossRef] [PubMed]
56. Dowd, K.A.; Netski, D.M.; Wang, X.H.; Cox, A.L.; Ray, S.C. Selection pressure from neutralizing antibodies drives sequence evolution during acute infection with hepatitis C virus. *Gastroenterology* **2009**, *136*, 2377–2386. [CrossRef]
57. Osburn, W.O.; Snider, A.E.; Wells, B.L.; Latanich, R.; Bailey, J.R.; Thomas, D.L.; Cox, A.L.; Ray, S.C. Clearance of hepatitis C infection is associated with the early appearance of broad neutralizing antibody responses. *Hepatology* **2014**, *59*, 2140–2151. [CrossRef]
58. Walker, M.R.; Leung, P.; Eltahla, A.A.; Underwood, A.; Abayasingam, A.; Brasher, N.A.; Li, H.; Wu, B.R.; Maher, L.; Luciani, F.; et al. Clearance of hepatitis C virus is associated with early and potent but narrowly-directed, Envelope-specific antibodies. *Sci. Rep.* **2019**, *9*, 13300. [CrossRef]
59. Kinchen, V.J.; Zahid, M.N.; Flyak, A.I.; Soliman, M.G.; Learn, G.H.; Wang, S.; Davidson, E.; Doranz, B.J.; Ray, S.C.; Cox, A.L.; et al. Broadly Neutralizing Antibody Mediated Clearance of Human Hepatitis C Virus Infection. *Cell Host Microbe* **2018**, *24*, 717–730.e715. [CrossRef]
60. Gu, J.; Hardy, J.; Boo, I.; Vietheer, P.; McCaffrey, K.; Alhammad, Y.; Chopra, A.; Gaudieri, S.; Poumbourios, P.; Coulibaly, F.; et al. Escape of Hepatitis C Virus from Epitope I Neutralization Increases Sensitivity of Other Neutralization Epitopes. *J. Virol.* **2018**, *92*. [CrossRef]
61. Hadlock, K.G.; Lanford, R.E.; Perkins, S.; Rowe, J.; Yang, Q.; Levy, S.; Pileri, P.; Abrignani, S.; Foung, S.K. Human monoclonal antibodies that inhibit binding of hepatitis C virus E2 protein to CD81 and recognize conserved conformational epitopes. *J. Virol.* **2000**, *74*, 10407–10416. [CrossRef] [PubMed]
62. Allander, T.; Drakenberg, K.; Beyene, A.; Rosa, D.; Abrignani, S.; Houghton, M.; Widell, A.; Grillner, L.; Persson, M.A. Recombinant human monoclonal antibodies against different conformational epitopes of the E2 envelope glycoprotein of hepatitis C virus that inhibit its interaction with CD81. *J. Gen. Virol.* **2000**, *81*, 2451–2459. [CrossRef] [PubMed]
63. Johansson, D.X.; Voisset, C.; Tarr, A.W.; Aung, M.; Ball, J.K.; Dubuisson, J.; Persson, M.A. Human combinatorial libraries yield rare antibodies that broadly neutralize hepatitis C virus. *Proc. Natl. Acad. Sci. USA* **2007**, *104*, 16269–16274. [CrossRef] [PubMed]
64. Law, M.; Maruyama, T.; Lewis, J.; Giang, E.; Tarr, A.W.; Stamataki, Z.; Gastaminza, P.; Chisari, F.V.; Jones, I.M.; Fox, R.I.; et al. Broadly neutralizing antibodies protect against hepatitis C virus quasispecies challenge. *Nat. Med.* **2008**, *14*, 25–27. [CrossRef] [PubMed]
65. Swann, R.E.; Cowton, V.M.; Robinson, M.W.; Cole, S.J.; Barclay, S.T.; Mills, P.R.; Thomson, E.C.; McLauchlan, J.; Patel, A.H. Broad Anti-Hepatitis C Virus (HCV) Antibody Responses Are Associated with Improved Clinical Disease Parameters in Chronic HCV Infection. *J. Virol.* **2016**, *90*, 4530–4543. [CrossRef]
66. Bjoro, K.; Froland, S.S.; Yun, Z.; Samdal, H.H.; Haaland, T. Hepatitis C infection in patients with primary hypogammaglobulinemia after treatment with contaminated immune globulin. *N. Engl. J. Med.* **1994**, *331*, 1607–1611. [CrossRef]
67. Bailey, J.R.; Flyak, A.I.; Cohen, V.J.; Li, H.; Wasilewski, L.N.; Snider, A.E.; Wang, S.; Learn, G.H.; Kose, N.; Loerinc, L.; et al. Broadly neutralizing antibodies with few somatic mutations and hepatitis C virus clearance. *JCI Insight* **2017**, *2*. [CrossRef]
68. Chan, C.H.; Hadlock, K.G.; Foung, S.K.; Levy, S. V(H)1-69 gene is preferentially used by hepatitis C virus-associated B cell lymphomas and by normal B cells responding to the E2 viral antigen. *Blood* **2001**, *97*, 1023–1026. [CrossRef]
69. Giang, E.; Dorner, M.; Prentoe, J.C.; Dreux, M.; Evans, M.J.; Bukh, J.; Rice, C.M.; Ploss, A.; Burton, D.R.; Law, M. Human broadly neutralizing antibodies to the envelope glycoprotein complex of hepatitis C virus. *Proc. Natl. Acad. Sci. USA* **2012**, *109*, 6205–6210. [CrossRef]
70. Chen, F.; Tzarum, N.; Wilson, I.A.; Law, M. VH1-69 antiviral broadly neutralizing antibodies: Genetics, structures, and relevance to rational vaccine design. *Curr. Opin. Virol.* **2019**, *34*, 149–159. [CrossRef]
71. Merat, S.J.; Bru, C.; van de Berg, D.; Molenkamp, R.; Tarr, A.W.; Koekkoek, S.; Kootstra, N.A.; Prins, M.; Ball, J.K.; Bakker, A.Q.; et al. Cross-genotype AR3-specific neutralizing antibodies confer long-term protection in injecting drug users after HCV clearance. *J. Hepatol.* **2019**, *71*, 14–24. [CrossRef] [PubMed]

72. Flyak, A.I.; Ruiz, S.; Colbert, M.D.; Luong, T.; Crowe, J.E., Jr.; Bailey, J.R.; Bjorkman, P.J. HCV Broadly Neutralizing Antibodies Use a CDRH3 Disulfide Motif to Recognize an E2 Glycoprotein Site that Can Be Targeted for Vaccine Design. *Cell Host Microbe* **2018**, *24*, 703–716.e703. [CrossRef] [PubMed]
73. Tzarum, N.; Giang, E.; Kong, L.; He, L.; Prentoe, J.; Augestad, E.; Hua, Y.; Castillo, S.; Lauer, G.M.; Bukh, J.; et al. Genetic and structural insights into broad neutralization of hepatitis C virus by human VH1-69 antibodies. *Sci. Adv.* **2019**, *5*, eaav1882. [CrossRef] [PubMed]
74. Ball, J.K.; Tarr, A.W.; McKeating, J.A. The past, present and future of neutralizing antibodies for hepatitis C virus. *Antiviral Res.* **2014**, *105*, 100–111. [CrossRef]
75. Vieyres, G.; Thomas, X.; Descamps, V.; Duverlie, G.; Patel, A.H.; Dubuisson, J. Characterization of the envelope glycoproteins associated with infectious hepatitis C virus. *J. Virol.* **2010**, *84*, 10159–10168. [CrossRef]
76. Vieyres, G.; Dubuisson, J.; Pietschmann, T. Incorporation of hepatitis C virus E1 and E2 glycoproteins: The keystones on a peculiar virion. *Viruses* **2014**, *6*, 1149–1187. [CrossRef]
77. Kong, L.; Giang, E.; Nieusma, T.; Kadam, R.U.; Cogburn, K.E.; Hua, Y.; Dai, X.; Stanfield, R.L.; Burton, D.R.; Ward, A.B.; et al. Hepatitis C virus E2 envelope glycoprotein core structure. *Science* **2013**, *342*, 1090–1094. [CrossRef]
78. Khan, A.G.; Whidby, J.; Miller, M.T.; Scarborough, H.; Zatorski, A.V.; Cygan, A.; Price, A.A.; Yost, S.A.; Bohannon, C.D.; Jacob, J.; et al. Structure of the core ectodomain of the hepatitis C virus envelope glycoprotein 2. *Nature* **2014**, *509*, 381–384. [CrossRef]
79. El Omari, K.; Iourin, O.; Kadlec, J.; Sutton, G.; Harlos, K.; Grimes, J.M.; Stuart, D.I. Unexpected structure for the N-terminal domain of hepatitis C virus envelope glycoprotein E1. *Nat. Commun.* **2014**, *5*, 4874. [CrossRef]
80. Kong, L.; Kadam, R.U.; Giang, E.; Ruwona, T.B.; Nieusma, T.; Culhane, J.C.; Stanfield, R.L.; Dawson, P.E.; Wilson, I.A.; Law, M. Structure of Hepatitis C Virus Envelope Glycoprotein E1 Antigenic Site 314–324 in Complex with Antibody IGH526. *J. Mol. Biol.* **2015**, *427*, 2617–2628. [CrossRef]
81. Bartosch, B.; Vitelli, A.; Granier, C.; Goujon, C.; Dubuisson, J.; Pascale, S.; Scarselli, E.; Cortese, R.; Nicosia, A.; Cosset, F.L. Cell entry of hepatitis C virus requires a set of co-receptors that include the CD81 tetraspanin and the SR-B1 scavenger receptor. *J. Biol. Chem.* **2003**, *278*, 41624–41630. [CrossRef]
82. Pileri, P.; Uematsu, Y.; Campagnoli, S.; Galli, G.; Falugi, F.; Petracca, R.; Weiner, A.J.; Houghton, M.; Rosa, D.; Grandi, G.; et al. Binding of hepatitis C virus to CD81. *Science* **1998**, *282*, 938–941. [CrossRef] [PubMed]
83. Scarselli, E.; Ansuini, H.; Cerino, R.; Roccasecca, R.M.; Acali, S.; Filocamo, G.; Traboni, C.; Nicosia, A.; Cortese, R.; Vitelli, A. The human scavenger receptor class B type I is a novel candidate receptor for the hepatitis C virus. *Embo J.* **2002**, *21*, 5017–5025. [CrossRef] [PubMed]
84. Evans, M.J.; von Hahn, T.; Tscherne, D.M.; Syder, A.J.; Panis, M.; Wolk, B.; Hatziioannou, T.; McKeating, J.A.; Bieniasz, P.D.; Rice, C.M. Claudin-1 is a hepatitis C virus co-receptor required for a late step in entry. *Nature* **2007**, *446*, 801–805. [CrossRef] [PubMed]
85. Ploss, A.; Evans, M.J.; Gaysinskaya, V.A.; Panis, M.; You, H.; de Jong, Y.P.; Rice, C.M. Human occludin is a hepatitis C virus entry factor required for infection of mouse cells. *Nature* **2009**, *457*, 882–886. [CrossRef] [PubMed]
86. Liu, S.; Yang, W.; Shen, L.; Turner, J.R.; Coyne, C.B.; Wang, T. Tight junction proteins claudin-1 and occludin control hepatitis C virus entry and are downregulated during infection to prevent superinfection. *J. Virol.* **2009**, *83*, 2011–2014. [CrossRef]
87. Dubuisson, J.; Cosset, F.L. Virology and cell biology of the hepatitis C virus life cycle: An update. *J. Hepatol.* **2014**, *61*, S3–S13. [CrossRef]
88. Tscherne, D.M.; Jones, C.T.; Evans, M.J.; Lindenbach, B.D.; McKeating, J.A.; Rice, C.M. Time- and temperature-dependent activation of hepatitis C virus for low-pH-triggered entry. *J. Virol.* **2006**, *80*, 1734–1741. [CrossRef]
89. Tong, Y.; Lavillette, D.; Li, Q.; Zhong, J. Role of Hepatitis C Virus Envelope Glycoprotein E1 in Virus Entry and Assembly. *Front. Immunol.* **2018**, *9*, 1411. [CrossRef]
90. Drummer, H.E. Challenges to the development of vaccines to hepatitis C virus that elicit neutralizing antibodies. *Front. Microbiol.* **2014**, *5*, 329. [CrossRef]
91. Keck, Z.; Wang, W.; Wang, Y.; Lau, P.; Carlsen, T.H.; Prentoe, J.; Xia, J.; Patel, A.H.; Bukh, J.; Foung, S.K. Cooperativity in virus neutralization by human monoclonal antibodies to two adjacent regions located at the amino terminus of hepatitis C virus E2 glycoprotein. *J. Virol.* **2013**, *87*, 37–51. [CrossRef] [PubMed]

92. Tzarum, N.; Wilson, I.A.; Law, M. The Neutralizing Face of Hepatitis C Virus E2 Envelope Glycoprotein. *Front. Immunol.* **2018**, *9*, 1315. [CrossRef] [PubMed]
93. Cuevas, J.M.; Gonzalez-Candelas, F.; Moya, A.; Sanjuan, R. Effect of ribavirin on the mutation rate and spectrum of hepatitis C virus in vivo. *J. Virol.* **2009**, *83*, 5760–5764. [CrossRef] [PubMed]
94. Echeverria, N.; Moratorio, G.; Cristina, J.; Moreno, P. Hepatitis C virus genetic variability and evolution. *World J. Hepatol.* **2015**, *7*, 831–845. [CrossRef]
95. Smith, D.B.; Bukh, J.; Kuiken, C.; Muerhoff, A.S.; Rice, C.M.; Stapleton, J.T.; Simmonds, P. Expanded classification of hepatitis C virus into 7 genotypes and 67 subtypes: Updated criteria and genotype assignment web resource. *Hepatology* **2014**, *59*, 318–327. [CrossRef]
96. Petruzziello, A.; Marigliano, S.; Loquercio, G.; Cozzolino, A.; Cacciapuoti, C. Global epidemiology of hepatitis C virus infection: An up-date of the distribution and circulation of hepatitis C virus genotypes. *World J. Gastroenterol.* **2016**, *22*, 7824–7840. [CrossRef]
97. Borgia, S.M.; Hedskog, C.; Parhy, B.; Hyland, R.H.; Stamm, L.M.; Brainard, D.M.; Subramanian, M.G.; McHutchison, J.G.; Mo, H.; Svarovskaia, E.; et al. Identification of a Novel Hepatitis C Virus Genotype From Punjab, India: Expanding Classification of Hepatitis C Virus Into 8 Genotypes. *J. Infect. Dis.* **2018**, *218*, 1722–1729. [CrossRef]
98. Forns, X.; Purcell, R.H.; Bukh, J. Quasispecies in viral persistence and pathogenesis of hepatitis C virus. *Trends Microbiol.* **1999**, *7*, 402–410. [CrossRef]
99. Farci, P.; Shimoda, A.; Coiana, A.; Diaz, G.; Peddis, G.; Melpolder, J.C.; Strazzera, A.; Chien, D.Y.; Munoz, S.J.; Balestrieri, A.; et al. The outcome of acute hepatitis C predicted by the evolution of the viral quasispecies. *Science* **2000**, *288*, 339–344. [CrossRef]
100. Liu, L.; Fisher, B.E.; Dowd, K.A.; Astemborski, J.; Cox, A.L.; Ray, S.C. Acceleration of hepatitis C virus envelope evolution in humans is consistent with progressive humoral immune selection during the transition from acute to chronic infection. *J. Virol.* **2010**, *84*, 5067–5077. [CrossRef]
101. Islam, N.; Krajden, M.; Shoveller, J.; Gustafson, P.; Gilbert, M.; Wong, J.; Tyndall, M.W.; Janjua, N.Z. Hepatitis C cross-genotype immunity and implications for vaccine development. *Sci. Rep.* **2017**, *7*, 12326. [CrossRef] [PubMed]
102. Tarr, A.W.; Urbanowicz, R.A.; Hamed, M.R.; Albecka, A.; McClure, C.P.; Brown, R.J.; Irving, W.L.; Dubuisson, J.; Ball, J.K. Hepatitis C patient-derived glycoproteins exhibit marked differences in susceptibility to serum neutralizing antibodies: Genetic subtype defines antigenic but not neutralization serotype. *J. Virol.* **2011**, *85*, 4246–4257. [CrossRef] [PubMed]
103. Luxenburger, H.; Grass, F.; Baermann, J.; Boettler, T.; Marget, M.; Emmerich, F.; Panning, M.; Thimme, R.; Nitschke, K.; Neumann-Haefelin, C. Differential virus-specific CD8(+) T-cell epitope repertoire in hepatitis C virus genotype 1 versus 4. *J. Viral. Hepat.* **2018**, *25*, 779–790. [CrossRef] [PubMed]
104. Von Delft, A.; Humphreys, I.S.; Brown, A.; Pfafferott, K.; Lucas, M.; Klenerman, P.; Lauer, G.M.; Cox, A.L.; Gaudieri, S.; Barnes, E. The broad assessment of HCV genotypes 1 and 3 antigenic targets reveals limited cross-reactivity with implications for vaccine design. *Gut* **2016**, *65*, 112–123. [CrossRef]
105. Bankwitz, D.; Steinmann, E.; Bitzegeio, J.; Ciesek, S.; Friesland, M.; Herrmann, E.; Zeisel, M.B.; Baumert, T.F.; Keck, Z.Y.; Foung, S.K.; et al. Hepatitis C virus hypervariable region 1 modulates receptor interactions, conceals the CD81 binding site, and protects conserved neutralizing epitopes. *J. Virol.* **2010**, *84*, 5751–5763. [CrossRef]
106. Prentoe, J.; Jensen, T.B.; Meuleman, P.; Serre, S.B.; Scheel, T.K.; Leroux-Roels, G.; Gottwein, J.M.; Bukh, J. Hypervariable region 1 differentially impacts viability of hepatitis C virus strains of genotypes 1 to 6 and impairs virus neutralization. *J. Virol.* **2011**, *85*, 2224–2234. [CrossRef]
107. Bazzill, J.D.; Ochyl, L.J.; Giang, E.; Castillo, S.; Law, M.; Moon, J.J. Interrogation of Antigen Display on Individual Vaccine Nanoparticles for Achieving Neutralizing Antibody Responses against Hepatitis C Virus. *Nano. Lett.* **2018**, *18*, 7832–7838. [CrossRef]
108. Lavie, M.; Hanoulle, X.; Dubuisson, J. Glycan Shielding and Modulation of Hepatitis C Virus Neutralizing Antibodies. *Front. Immunol.* **2018**, *9*, 910. [CrossRef]
109. Helle, F.; Goffard, A.; Morel, V.; Duverlie, G.; McKeating, J.; Keck, Z.Y.; Foung, S.; Penin, F.; Dubuisson, J.; Voisset, C. The neutralizing activity of anti-hepatitis C virus antibodies is modulated by specific glycans on the E2 envelope protein. *J. Virol.* **2007**, *81*, 8101–8111. [CrossRef]

110. Helle, F.; Vieyres, G.; Elkrief, L.; Popescu, C.I.; Wychowski, C.; Descamps, V.; Castelain, S.; Roingeard, P.; Duverlie, G.; Dubuisson, J. Role of N-linked glycans in the functions of hepatitis C virus envelope proteins incorporated into infectious virions. *J. Virol.* **2010**, *84*, 11905–11915. [CrossRef]
111. Li, D.; von Schaewen, M.; Wang, X.; Tao, W.; Zhang, Y.; Li, L.; Heller, B.; Hrebikova, G.; Deng, Q.; Ploss, A.; et al. Altered Glycosylation Patterns Increase Immunogenicity of a Subunit Hepatitis C Virus Vaccine, Inducing Neutralizing Antibodies Which Confer Protection in Mice. *J. Virol.* **2016**, *90*, 10486–10498. [CrossRef] [PubMed]
112. Ren, Y.; Min, Y.Q.; Liu, M.; Chi, L.; Zhao, P.; Zhang, X.L. N-glycosylation-mutated HCV envelope glycoprotein complex enhances antigen-presenting activity and cellular and neutralizing antibody responses. *Biochim. Biophys. Acta* **2016**, *1860*, 1764–1775. [CrossRef] [PubMed]
113. Urbanowicz, R.A.; Wang, R.; Schiel, J.E.; Keck, Z.Y.; Kerzic, M.C.; Lau, P.; Rangarajan, S.; Garagusi, K.J.; Tan, L.; Guest, J.D.; et al. Antigenicity and Immunogenicity of Differentially Glycosylated Hepatitis C Virus E2 Envelope Proteins Expressed in Mammalian and Insect Cells. *J. Virol.* **2019**, *93*. [CrossRef] [PubMed]
114. Pantua, H.; Diao, J.; Ultsch, M.; Hazen, M.; Mathieu, M.; McCutcheon, K.; Takeda, K.; Date, S.; Cheung, T.K.; Phung, Q.; et al. Glycan shifting on hepatitis C virus (HCV) E2 glycoprotein is a mechanism for escape from broadly neutralizing antibodies. *J. Mol. Biol.* **2013**, *425*, 1899–1914. [CrossRef]
115. Owsianka, A.; Tarr, A.W.; Juttla, V.S.; Lavillette, D.; Bartosch, B.; Cosset, F.L.; Ball, J.K.; Patel, A.H. Monoclonal antibody AP33 defines a broadly neutralizing epitope on the hepatitis C virus E2 envelope glycoprotein. *J. Virol.* **2005**, *79*, 11095–11104. [CrossRef]
116. Voisset, C.; Op de Beeck, A.; Horellou, P.; Dreux, M.; Gustot, T.; Duverlie, G.; Cosset, F.L.; Vu-Dac, N.; Dubuisson, J. High-density lipoproteins reduce the neutralizing effect of hepatitis C virus (HCV)-infected patient antibodies by promoting HCV entry. *J. Gen. Virol.* **2006**, *87*, 2577–2581. [CrossRef]
117. Dreux, M.; Pietschmann, T.; Granier, C.; Voisset, C.; Ricard-Blum, S.; Mangeot, P.E.; Keck, Z.; Foung, S.; Vu-Dac, N.; Dubuisson, J.; et al. High density lipoprotein inhibits hepatitis C virus-neutralizing antibodies by stimulating cell entry via activation of the scavenger receptor BI. *J. Biol. Chem.* **2006**, *281*, 18285–18295. [CrossRef]
118. Fauvelle, C.; Felmlee, D.J.; Crouchet, E.; Lee, J.; Heydmann, L.; Lefevre, M.; Magri, A.; Hiet, M.S.; Fofana, I.; Habersetzer, F.; et al. Apolipoprotein E Mediates Evasion From Hepatitis C Virus Neutralizing Antibodies. *Gastroenterology* **2016**, *150*, 206–217.e204. [CrossRef]
119. Deng, L.; Jiang, W.; Wang, X.; Merz, A.; Hiet, M.S.; Chen, Y.; Pan, X.; Jiu, Y.; Yang, Y.; Yu, B.; et al. Syntenin regulates hepatitis C virus sensitivity to neutralizing antibody by promoting E2 secretion through exosomes. *J. Hepatol.* **2019**, *71*, 52–61. [CrossRef]
120. Wrensch, F.; Ligat, G.; Heydmann, L.; Schuster, C.; Zeisel, M.B.; Pessaux, P.; Habersetzer, F.; King, B.J.; Tarr, A.W.; Ball, J.K.; et al. Interferon-Induced Transmembrane Proteins Mediate Viral Evasion in Acute and Chronic Hepatitis C Virus Infection. *Hepatology* **2019**, *70*, 1506–1520. [CrossRef]
121. Lohmann, V.; Bartenschlager, R. On the history of hepatitis C virus cell culture systems. *J. Med. Chem.* **2014**, *57*, 1627–1642. [CrossRef] [PubMed]
122. Pietschmann, T.; Kaul, A.; Koutsoudakis, G.; Shavinskaya, A.; Kallis, S.; Steinmann, E.; Abid, K.; Negro, F.; Dreux, M.; Cosset, F.L.; et al. Construction and characterization of infectious intragenotypic and intergenotypic hepatitis C virus chimeras. *Proc. Natl. Acad. Sci. USA* **2006**, *103*, 7408–7413. [CrossRef] [PubMed]
123. Gottwein, J.M.; Scheel, T.K.; Jensen, T.B.; Lademann, J.B.; Prentoe, J.C.; Knudsen, M.L.; Hoegh, A.M.; Bukh, J. Development and characterization of hepatitis C virus genotype 1-7 cell culture systems: Role of CD81 and scavenger receptor class B type I and effect of antiviral drugs. *Hepatology* **2009**, *49*, 364–377. [CrossRef] [PubMed]
124. Carlsen, T.H.; Pedersen, J.; Prentoe, J.C.; Giang, E.; Keck, Z.Y.; Mikkelsen, L.S.; Law, M.; Foung, S.K.; Bukh, J. Breadth of neutralization and synergy of clinically relevant human monoclonal antibodies against HCV genotypes 1a, 1b, 2a, 2b, 2c, and 3a. *Hepatology* **2014**, *60*, 1551–1562. [CrossRef] [PubMed]
125. McClure, C.P.; Urbanowicz, R.A.; King, B.J.; Cano-Crespo, S.; Tarr, A.W.; Ball, J.K. Flexible and rapid construction of viral chimeras applied to hepatitis C virus. *J. Gen. Virol.* **2016**, *97*, 2187–2193. [CrossRef]
126. King, B.; Urbanowicz, R.; Tarr, A.W.; Ball, J.K.; McClure, C.P. InFusion Cloning for the Generation of Biologically Relevant HCV Chimeric Molecular Clones. *Methods Mol. Biol. (Clifton N.J.)* **2019**, *1911*, 93–104.
127. Bartosch, B.; Dubuisson, J.; Cosset, F.L. Infectious hepatitis C virus pseudo-particles containing functional E1-E2 envelope protein complexes. *J. Exp. Med.* **2003**, *197*, 633–642. [CrossRef]

128. Flint, M.; Logvinoff, C.; Rice, C.M.; McKeating, J.A. Characterization of infectious retroviral pseudotype particles bearing hepatitis C virus glycoproteins. *J. Virol.* **2004**, *78*, 6875–6882. [CrossRef]
129. Urbanowicz, R.A.; McClure, C.P.; Brown, R.J.P.; Tsoleridis, T.; Persson, M.A.A.; Krey, T.; Irving, W.L.; Ball, J.K.; Tarr, A.W. A Diverse Panel of Hepatitis C Virus Glycoproteins for Use in Vaccine Research Reveals Extremes of Monoclonal Antibody Neutralization Resistance. *J. Virol.* **2016**, *90*, 3288–3301. [CrossRef]
130. Urbanowicz, R.A.; McClure, C.P.; King, B.; Mason, C.P.; Ball, J.K.; Tarr, A.W. Novel functional hepatitis C virus glycoprotein isolates identified using an optimized viral pseudotype entry assay. *J. Gen. Virol.* **2016**, *97*, 2265–2279. [CrossRef]
131. Bailey, J.R.; Wasilewski, L.N.; Snider, A.E.; El-Diwany, R.; Osburn, W.O.; Keck, Z.; Foung, S.K.; Ray, S.C. Naturally selected hepatitis C virus polymorphisms confer broad neutralizing antibody resistance. *J. Clin. Investig.* **2015**, *125*, 437–447. [CrossRef] [PubMed]
132. Kolykhalov, A.A.; Agapov, E.V.; Blight, K.J.; Mihalik, K.; Feinstone, S.M.; Rice, C.M. Transmission of hepatitis C by intrahepatic inoculation with transcribed RNA. *Science* **1997**, *277*, 570–574. [CrossRef]
133. Feinstone, S.M.; Alter, H.J.; Dienes, H.P.; Shimizu, Y.; Popper, H.; Blackmore, D.; Sly, D.; London, W.T.; Purcell, R.H. Non-A, non-B hepatitis in chimpanzees and marmosets. *J. Infect. Dis.* **1981**, *144*, 588–598. [CrossRef] [PubMed]
134. Yanagi, M.; Purcell, R.H.; Emerson, S.U.; Bukh, J. Transcripts from a single full-length cDNA clone of hepatitis C virus are infectious when directly transfected into the liver of a chimpanzee. *Proc. Natl. Acad. Sci. USA* **1997**, *94*, 8738–8743. [CrossRef]
135. Seaman, M.S.; Janes, H.; Hawkins, N.; Grandpre, L.E.; Devoy, C.; Giri, A.; Coffey, R.T.; Harris, L.; Wood, B.; Daniels, M.G.; et al. Tiered categorization of a diverse panel of HIV-1 Env pseudoviruses for assessment of neutralizing antibodies. *J. Virol.* **2010**, *84*, 1439–1452. [CrossRef]
136. Mercer, D.F.; Schiller, D.E.; Elliott, J.F.; Douglas, D.N.; Hao, C.; Rinfret, A.; Addison, W.R.; Fischer, K.P.; Churchill, T.A.; Lakey, J.R.; et al. Hepatitis C virus replication in mice with chimeric human livers. *Nat. Med.* **2001**, *7*, 927–933. [CrossRef] [PubMed]
137. Meuleman, P.; Libbrecht, L.; De Vos, R.; de Hemptinne, B.; Gevaert, K.; Vandekerckhove, J.; Roskams, T.; Leroux-Roels, G. Morphological and biochemical characterization of a human liver in a uPA-SCID mouse chimera. *Hepatology* **2005**, *41*, 847–856. [CrossRef]
138. Chen, J.; Zhao, Y.; Zhang, C.; Chen, H.; Feng, J.; Chi, X.; Pan, Y.; Du, J.; Guo, M.; Cao, H.; et al. Persistent hepatitis C virus infections and hepatopathological manifestations in immune-competent humanized mice. *Cell Res.* **2014**, *24*, 1050–1066. [CrossRef]
139. Ding, Q.; von Schaewen, M.; Hrebikova, G.; Heller, B.; Sandmann, L.; Plaas, M.; Ploss, A. Mice Expressing Minimally Humanized CD81 and Occludin Genes Support Hepatitis C Virus Uptake In Vivo. *J. Virol.* **2017**, *91*. [CrossRef]
140. Yong, K.S.M.; Her, Z.; Chen, Q. Humanized Mouse Models for the Study of Hepatitis C and Host Interactions. *Cells* **2019**, *8*, 604. [CrossRef]
141. Firth, C.; Bhat, M.; Firth, M.A.; Williams, S.H.; Frye, M.J.; Simmonds, P.; Conte, J.M.; Ng, J.; Garcia, J.; Bhuva, N.P.; et al. Detection of zoonotic pathogens and characterization of novel viruses carried by commensal Rattus norvegicus in New York City. *Mbio* **2014**, *5*, e01933-14. [CrossRef]
142. Trivedi, S.; Murthy, S.; Sharma, H.; Hartlage, A.S.; Kumar, A.; Gadi, S.V.; Simmonds, P.; Chauhan, L.V.; Scheel, T.K.H.; Billerbeck, E.; et al. Viral persistence, liver disease, and host response in a hepatitis C-like virus rat model. *Hepatology* **2018**, *68*, 435–448. [CrossRef] [PubMed]
143. Atcheson, E.; Li, W.; Bliss, C.M.; Chinnakannan, S.; Heim, K.; Sharpe, H.; Hutchings, C.; Dietrich, I.; Nguyen, D.; Kapoor, A.; et al. Use of an outbred rat hepacivirus challenge model for design and evaluation of efficacy of different immunisation strategies for HCV. *Hepatology* **2019**. [CrossRef] [PubMed]
144. Kapoor, A.; Simmonds, P.; Gerold, G.; Qaisar, N.; Jain, K.; Henriquez, J.A.; Firth, C.; Hirschberg, D.L.; Rice, C.M.; Shields, S.; et al. Characterization of a canine homolog of hepatitis C virus. *Proc. Natl. Acad. Sci. USA* **2011**, *108*, 11608–11613. [CrossRef] [PubMed]
145. Burbelo, P.D.; Dubovi, E.J.; Simmonds, P.; Medina, J.L.; Henriquez, J.A.; Mishra, N.; Wagner, J.; Tokarz, R.; Cullen, J.M.; Iadarola, M.J.; et al. Serology-enabled discovery of genetically diverse hepaciviruses in a new host. *J. Virol.* **2012**, *86*, 6171–6178. [CrossRef]
146. Pfaender, S.; Brown, R.J.; Pietschmann, T.; Steinmann, E. Natural reservoirs for homologs of hepatitis C virus. *Emerg. Microbes Infect.* **2014**, *3*, e21. [CrossRef]

147. Pfaender, S.; Cavalleri, J.M.; Walter, S.; Doerrbecker, J.; Campana, B.; Brown, R.J.; Burbelo, P.D.; Postel, A.; Hahn, K.; Anggakusuma; et al. Clinical course of infection and viral tissue tropism of hepatitis C virus-like nonprimate hepaciviruses in horses. *Hepatology* **2015**, *61*, 447–459. [CrossRef]
148. Tegtmeyer, B.; Echelmeyer, J.; Pfankuche, V.M.; Puff, C.; Todt, D.; Fischer, N.; Durham, A.; Feige, K.; Baumgartner, W.; Steinmann, E.; et al. Chronic equine hepacivirus infection in an adult gelding with severe hepatopathy. *Vet. Med. Sci.* **2019**, *5*, 372–378. [CrossRef]
149. Shi, B.; Ma, L.; He, X.; Wang, X.; Wang, P.; Zhou, L.; Yao, X. Comparative analysis of human and mouse immunoglobulin variable heavy regions from IMGT/LIGM-DB with IMGT/HighV-QUEST. *Theor. Biol. Med. Model.* **2014**, *11*, 30. [CrossRef]
150. Manso, T.C.; Groenner-Penna, M.; Minozzo, J.C.; Antunes, B.C.; Ippolito, G.C.; Molina, F.; Felicori, L.F. Next-generation sequencing reveals new insights about gene usage and CDR-H3 composition in the horse antibody repertoire. *Mol. Immunol.* **2019**, *105*, 251–259. [CrossRef]
151. Li, Y.; Pierce, B.G.; Wang, Q.; Keck, Z.Y.; Fuerst, T.R.; Foung, S.K.; Mariuzza, R.A. Structural basis for penetration of the glycan shield of hepatitis C virus E2 glycoprotein by a broadly neutralizing human antibody. *J. Biol. Chem.* **2015**, *290*, 10117–10125. [CrossRef] [PubMed]
152. Keck, Z.Y.; Angus, A.G.; Wang, W.; Lau, P.; Wang, Y.; Gatherer, D.; Patel, A.H.; Foung, S.K. Non-random escape pathways from a broadly neutralizing human monoclonal antibody map to a highly conserved region on the hepatitis C virus E2 glycoprotein encompassing amino acids 412–423. *PLoS Pathog.* **2014**, *10*, e1004297. [CrossRef] [PubMed]
153. Pierce, B.G.; Boucher, E.N.; Piepenbrink, K.H.; Ejemel, M.; Rapp, C.A.; Thomas, W.D., Jr.; Sundberg, E.J.; Weng, Z.; Wang, Y. Structure-Based Design of Hepatitis C Virus Vaccines That Elicit Neutralizing Antibody Responses to a Conserved Epitope. *J. Virol.* **2017**, *91*. [CrossRef] [PubMed]
154. Filskov, J.; Andersen, P.; Agger, E.M.; Bukh, J. HCV p7 as a novel vaccine-target inducing multifunctional CD4(+) and CD8(+) T-cells targeting liver cells expressing the viral antigen. *Sci. Rep.* **2019**, *9*, 14085. [CrossRef] [PubMed]
155. Dawood, R.M.; Moustafa, R.I.; Abdelhafez, T.H.; El-Shenawy, R.; El-Abd, Y.; Bader El Din, N.G.; Dubuisson, J.; El Awady, M.K. A multiepitope peptide vaccine against HCV stimulates neutralizing humoral and persistent cellular responses in mice. *BMC Infect. Dis.* **2019**, *19*, 932. [CrossRef] [PubMed]
156. Marin, M.Q.; Perez, P.; Ljungberg, K.; Sorzano, C.O.S.; Gomez, C.E.; Liljestrom, P.; Esteban, M.; Garcia-Arriaza, J. Potent Anti-hepatitis C Virus (HCV) T Cell Immune Responses Induced in Mice Vaccinated with DNA-Launched RNA Replicons and Modified Vaccinia Virus Ankara-HCV. *J. Virol.* **2019**, *93*. [CrossRef]
157. Wijesundara, D.K.; Gummow, J.; Li, Y.; Yu, W.; Quah, B.J.; Ranasinghe, C.; Torresi, J.; Gowans, E.J.; Grubor-Bauk, B. Induction of Genotype Cross-Reactive, Hepatitis C Virus-Specific, Cell-Mediated Immunity in DNA-Vaccinated Mice. *J. Virol.* **2018**, *92*. [CrossRef]
158. Masavuli, M.G.; Wijesundara, D.K.; Underwood, A.; Christiansen, D.; Earnest-Silveira, L.; Bull, R.; Torresi, J.; Gowans, E.J.; Grubor-Bauk, B. A Hepatitis C Virus DNA Vaccine Encoding a Secreted, Oligomerized Form of Envelope Proteins Is Highly Immunogenic and Elicits Neutralizing Antibodies in Vaccinated Mice. *Front. Immunol.* **2019**, *10*, 1145. [CrossRef]
159. Plotkin, S.A. Vaccines: Past, present and future. *Nat. Med.* **2005**, *11*, S5–S11. [CrossRef]
160. Choo, Q.L.; Kuo, G.; Ralston, R.; Weiner, A.; Chien, D.; Van Nest, G.; Han, J.; Berger, K.; Thudium, K.; Kuo, C.; et al. Vaccination of chimpanzees against infection by the hepatitis C virus. *Proc. Natl. Acad. Sci. USA* **1994**, *91*, 1294–1298. [CrossRef]
161. Houghton, M. Prospects for prophylactic and therapeutic vaccines against the hepatitis C viruses. *Immunol. Rev.* **2011**, *239*, 99–108. [CrossRef] [PubMed]
162. Frey, S.E.; Houghton, M.; Coates, S.; Abrignani, S.; Chien, D.; Rosa, D.; Pileri, P.; Ray, R.; Di Bisceglie, A.M.; Rinella, P.; et al. Safety and immunogenicity of HCV E1E2 vaccine adjuvanted with MF59 administered to healthy adults. *Vaccine* **2010**, *28*, 6367–6373. [CrossRef] [PubMed]
163. Ray, R.; Meyer, K.; Banerjee, A.; Basu, A.; Coates, S.; Abrignani, S.; Houghton, M.; Frey, S.E.; Belshe, R.B. Characterization of antibodies induced by vaccination with hepatitis C virus envelope glycoproteins. *J. Infect. Dis.* **2010**, *202*, 862–866. [CrossRef] [PubMed]
164. Law, J.L.; Chen, C.; Wong, J.; Hockman, D.; Santer, D.M.; Frey, S.E.; Belshe, R.B.; Wakita, T.; Bukh, J.; Jones, C.T.; et al. A hepatitis C virus (HCV) vaccine comprising envelope glycoproteins gpE1/gpE2 derived from a single isolate elicits broad cross-genotype neutralizing antibodies in humans. *PLoS ONE* **2013**, *8*, e59776. [CrossRef] [PubMed]

165. Wong, J.A.; Bhat, R.; Hockman, D.; Logan, M.; Chen, C.; Levin, A.; Frey, S.E.; Belshe, R.B.; Tyrrell, D.L.; Law, J.L.; et al. Recombinant hepatitis C virus envelope glycoprotein vaccine elicits antibodies targeting multiple epitopes on the envelope glycoproteins associated with broad cross-neutralization. *J. Virol.* **2014**, *88*, 14278–14288. [CrossRef] [PubMed]
166. Logan, M.; Law, J.; Wong, J.A.J.; Hockman, D.; Landi, A.; Chen, C.; Crawford, K.; Kundu, J.; Baldwin, L.; Johnson, J.; et al. Native Folding of a Recombinant gpE1/gpE2 Heterodimer Vaccine Antigen from a Precursor Protein Fused with Fc IgG. *J. Virol.* **2017**, *91*. [CrossRef]
167. Ruwona, T.B.; Giang, E.; Nieusma, T.; Law, M. Fine mapping of murine antibody responses to immunization with a novel soluble form of hepatitis C virus envelope glycoprotein complex. *J. Virol.* **2014**, *88*, 10459–10471. [CrossRef]
168. Krapchev, V.B.; Rychlowska, M.; Chmielewska, A.; Zimmer, K.; Patel, A.H.; Bienkowska-Szewczyk, K. Recombinant Flag-tagged E1E2 glycoproteins from three hepatitis C virus genotypes are biologically functional and elicit cross-reactive neutralizing antibodies in mice. *Virology* **2018**, *519*, 33–41. [CrossRef]
169. McCaffrey, K.; Boo, I.; Poumbourios, P.; Drummer, H.E. Expression and characterization of a minimal hepatitis C virus glycoprotein E2 core domain that retains CD81 binding. *J. Virol.* **2007**, *81*, 9584–9590. [CrossRef]
170. Vietheer, P.T.; Boo, I.; Gu, J.; McCaffrey, K.; Edwards, S.; Owczarek, C.; Hardy, M.P.; Fabri, L.; Center, R.J.; Poumbourios, P.; et al. The core domain of hepatitis C virus glycoprotein E2 generates potent cross-neutralizing antibodies in guinea pigs. *Hepatology* **2017**, *65*, 1117–1131. [CrossRef]
171. McCaffrey, K.; Boo, I.; Owczarek, C.M.; Hardy, M.P.; Perugini, M.A.; Fabri, L.; Scotney, P.; Poumbourios, P.; Drummer, H.E. An Optimized Hepatitis C Virus E2 Glycoprotein Core Adopts a Functional Homodimer That Efficiently Blocks Virus Entry. *J. Virol.* **2017**, *91*. [CrossRef] [PubMed]
172. Law, J.L.M.; Logan, M.; Wong, J.; Kundu, J.; Hockman, D.; Landi, A.; Chen, C.; Crawford, K.; Wininger, M.; Johnson, J.; et al. Role of the E2 Hypervariable Region (HVR1) in the Immunogenicity of a Recombinant Hepatitis C Virus Vaccine. *J. Virol.* **2018**, *92*. [CrossRef]
173. Torresi, J. The Rationale for a Preventative HCV Virus-Like Particle (VLP) Vaccine. *Front. Microbiol.* **2017**, *8*, 2163. [CrossRef] [PubMed]
174. Bachmann, M.F.; Jennings, G.T. Vaccine delivery: A matter of size, geometry, kinetics and molecular patterns. *Nat. Rev. Immunol.* **2010**, *10*, 787–796. [CrossRef] [PubMed]
175. Baumert, T.F.; Ito, S.; Wong, D.T.; Liang, T.J. Hepatitis C virus structural proteins assemble into viruslike particles in insect cells. *J. Virol.* **1998**, *72*, 3827–3836. [CrossRef] [PubMed]
176. Baumert, T.F.; Vergalla, J.; Satoi, J.; Thomson, M.; Lechmann, M.; Herion, D.; Greenberg, H.B.; Ito, S.; Liang, T.J. Hepatitis C virus-like particles synthesized in insect cells as a potential vaccine candidate. *Gastroenterology* **1999**, *117*, 1397–1407. [CrossRef]
177. Lechmann, M.; Murata, K.; Satoi, J.; Vergalla, J.; Baumert, T.F.; Liang, T.J. Hepatitis C virus-like particles induce virus-specific humoral and cellular immune responses in mice. *Hepatology* **2001**, *34*, 417–423. [CrossRef]
178. Jeong, S.H.; Qiao, M.; Nascimbeni, M.; Hu, Z.; Rehermann, B.; Murthy, K.; Liang, T.J. Immunization with hepatitis C virus-like particles induces humoral and cellular immune responses in nonhuman primates. *J. Virol.* **2004**, *78*, 6995–7003. [CrossRef]
179. Elmowalid, G.A.; Qiao, M.; Jeong, S.H.; Borg, B.B.; Baumert, T.F.; Sapp, R.K.; Hu, Z.; Murthy, K.; Liang, T.J. Immunization with hepatitis C virus-like particles results in control of hepatitis C virus infection in chimpanzees. *Proc. Natl. Acad. Sci. USA* **2007**, *104*, 8427–8432. [CrossRef]
180. Chua, B.Y.; Johnson, D.; Tan, A.; Earnest-Silveira, L.; Sekiya, T.; Chin, R.; Torresi, J.; Jackson, D.C. Hepatitis C VLPs delivered to dendritic cells by a TLR2 targeting lipopeptide results in enhanced antibody and cell-mediated responses. *PLoS ONE* **2012**, *7*, e47492. [CrossRef]
181. Christiansen, D.; Earnest-Silveira, L.; Chua, B.; Meuleman, P.; Boo, I.; Grubor-Bauk, B.; Jackson, D.C.; Keck, Z.Y.; Foung, S.K.H.; Drummer, H.E.; et al. Immunological responses following administration of a genotype 1a/1b/2/3a quadrivalent HCV VLP vaccine. *Sci. Rep.* **2018**, *8*, 6483. [CrossRef] [PubMed]
182. Earnest-Silveira, L.; Chua, B.; Chin, R.; Christiansen, D.; Johnson, D.; Herrmann, S.; Ralph, S.A.; Vercauteren, K.; Mesalam, A.; Meuleman, P.; et al. Characterization of a hepatitis C virus-like particle vaccine produced in a human hepatocyte-derived cell line. *J. Gen. Virol.* **2016**, *97*, 1865–1876. [CrossRef] [PubMed]
183. Collett, S.; Torresi, J.; Earnest-Silveira, L.; Christiansen, D.; Elbourne, A.; Ramsland, P.A. Probing and pressing surfaces of hepatitis C virus-like particles. *J. Colloid Interface Sci.* **2019**, *545*, 259–268. [CrossRef]

184. Christiansen, D.; Earnest-Silveira, L.; Grubor-Bauk, B.; Wijesundara, D.K.; Boo, I.; Ramsland, P.A.; Vincan, E.; Drummer, H.E.; Gowans, E.J.; Torresi, J. Pre-clinical evaluation of a quadrivalent HCV VLP vaccine in pigs following microneedle delivery. *Sci. Rep.* **2019**, *9*, 9251. [CrossRef]
185. Ura, T.; Okuda, K.; Shimada, M. Developments in Viral Vector-Based Vaccines. *Vaccines* **2014**, *2*, 624–641. [CrossRef] [PubMed]
186. Barnes, E.; Folgori, A.; Capone, S.; Swadling, L.; Aston, S.; Kurioka, A.; Meyer, J.; Huddart, R.; Smith, K.; Townsend, R.; et al. Novel adenovirus-based vaccines induce broad and sustained T cell responses to HCV in man. *Sci. Transl. Med.* **2012**, *4*, 115ra1. [CrossRef] [PubMed]
187. Capone, S.; Zampaglione, I.; Vitelli, A.; Pezzanera, M.; Kierstead, L.; Burns, J.; Ruggeri, L.; Arcuri, M.; Cappelletti, M.; Meola, A.; et al. Modulation of the immune response induced by gene electrotransfer of a hepatitis C virus DNA vaccine in nonhuman primates. *J. Immunol.* **2006**, *177*, 7462–7471. [CrossRef] [PubMed]
188. Swadling, L.; Capone, S.; Antrobus, R.D.; Brown, A.; Richardson, R.; Newell, E.W.; Halliday, J.; Kelly, C.; Bowen, D.; Fergusson, J.; et al. A human vaccine strategy based on chimpanzee adenoviral and MVA vectors that primes, boosts, and sustains functional HCV-specific T cell memory. *Sci. Transl. Med.* **2014**, *6*, 261ra153. [CrossRef]
189. Swadling, L.; Halliday, J.; Kelly, C.; Brown, A.; Capone, S.; Ansari, M.A.; Bonsall, D.; Richardson, R.; Hartnell, F.; Collier, J.; et al. Highly-Immunogenic Virally-Vectored T-cell Vaccines Cannot Overcome Subversion of the T-cell Response by HCV during Chronic Infection. *Vaccines* **2016**, *4*, 27. [CrossRef]
190. Trial Evaluating Experimental Hepatitis C Vaccine Concludes|NIH: National Institute of Allergy and Infectious Diseases. Available online: https://www.niaid.nih.gov/news-events/trial-evaluating-experimental-hepatitis-c-vaccine-concludes (accessed on 29 December 2019).
191. Beaumont, E.; Patient, R.; Hourioux, C.; Dimier-Poisson, I.; Roingeard, P. Chimeric hepatitis B virus/hepatitis C virus envelope proteins elicit broadly neutralizing antibodies and constitute a potential bivalent prophylactic vaccine. *Hepatology* **2013**, *57*, 1303–1313. [CrossRef]
192. Wei, S.; Lei, Y.; Yang, J.; Wang, X.; Shu, F.; Wei, X.; Lin, F.; Li, B.; Cui, Y.; Zhang, H. Neutralization effects of antibody elicited by chimeric HBV S antigen viral-like particles presenting HCV neutralization epitopes. *Vaccine* **2018**, *36*, 2273–2281. [CrossRef] [PubMed]
193. Garrone, P.; Fluckiger, A.C.; Mangeot, P.E.; Gauthier, E.; Dupeyrot-Lacas, P.; Mancip, J.; Cangialosi, A.; Du Chene, I.; LeGrand, R.; Mangeot, I.; et al. A prime-boost strategy using virus-like particles pseudotyped for HCV proteins triggers broadly neutralizing antibodies in macaques. *Sci. Transl. Med.* **2011**, *3*, 94ra71. [CrossRef] [PubMed]

15

Factors that Govern the Induction of Long-Lived Antibody Responses

Bryce Chackerian * and David S. Peabody

Department of Molecular Genetics and Microbiology, University of New Mexico School of Medicine, Albuquerque, NM 87106, USA; dpeabody@salud.unm.edu
* Correspondence: bchackerian@salud.unm.edu

Abstract: The induction of long-lasting, high-titer antibody responses is critical to the efficacy of many vaccines. The ability to produce durable antibody responses is governed by the generation of the terminally differentiated antibody-secreting B cells known as long-lived plasma cells (LLPCs). Once induced, LLPCs likely persist for decades, providing long-term protection against infection. The factors that control the generation of this important class of B cells are beginning to emerge. In particular, antigens with highly dense, multivalent structures are especially effective. Here we describe some pathogens for which the induction of long-lived antibodies is particularly important, and discuss the basis for the extraordinary ability of multivalent antigens to drive differentiation of naïve B cells to LLPCs.

Keywords: long-lived plasma cells; antibodies; multivalency; virus-like particles

---

1. Introduction—B-Cell Responses to Vaccination

Most of the effective vaccines in use today work by inducing humoral immune responses. Activation of naïve B cells by vaccine antigens leads to a series of events which ultimately result in the production of memory B cells and differentiation into two classes of antibody secreting cells, short-lived plasmablasts and long-lived plasma cells (LLPCs). The induction of immunological memory is classically invoked to explain the effectiveness of many vaccines. Memory B cells express the membrane-bound B-cell receptor (BCR) and are primed to respond to antigen exposure. They emerge early from germinal centers and often their immunoglobulin molecules have already undergone isotype switching and some degree of affinity maturation, meaning that they can potentially produce more effective antibodies upon re-stimulation. Memory of vaccination can increase the magnitude of the antibody response and drive the more rapid production of class-switched, high affinity antibodies. Thus, for many pathogens, the existence of memory cells provides a kinetic upperhand that tips the balance from the pathogen to the immune system.

Nevertheless, there are a number of important pathogens for which vaccine-based induction of memory cells alone is insufficient to provide protective immunity. In these cases, protection depends on a pre-existing level of antibodies high enough to entirely prevent the initial infection event, because once one of these agents initiates an infection, it establishes a beachhead which is then partially or completely resistant to antibody effector activity. Consider three common human pathogens, human immunodeficiency virus (HIV), human papillomavirus (HPV), and *Plasmodium*, as examples of diseases in which an effective vaccine is dependent on the ability to induce high-titer and long-lasting antibodies: (i) Once transmitted, HIV quickly traffics to regional lymph nodes and other immune tissues where it can infect T cells and macrophages [1]. The HIV provirus integrates into the genomes of these infected cells, where it establishes a persistent virus reservoir. While anti-retroviral drugs can successfully control active HIV infection, this latent reservoir is refractory to both antiretroviral drugs and anti-HIV antibodies, allowing the virus to reemerge if drugs are discontinued. Thus, antibodies can potentially control infection, but cannot eliminate HIV, so prevention of initial infection is critical. (ii) Similarly, after HPV infects its target cells, basal epithelial cells, the virus remains intracellular and not accessible to antibodies. The HPV lifecycle is intimately tied to the differentiation of basal cells into terminally differentiated epithelial cells [2]. Only when these cells differentiate are HPV virions produced and released. However, HPV-associated cancers do not result from productive infection. HPV can also establish latency in infected cells, and, in some cases, integration or episomal maintenance of the HPV genome can lead to dysregulated expression of the viral oncogenes, E6 and E7 [3]. These HPV-infected basal epithelial cells are the origin of neoplastic lesions that can ultimately progress to invasive tumors. Thus, once HPV infection occurs, antibodies have no value in protecting against cancer [4]. Accordingly, vaccines that elicit HPV-neutralizing antibodies can protect against initial infection, but fail to induce the regression of previously established lesions [5]. (iii) Liver infection by the *Plasmodium* parasite, which causes malaria, occurs within a few hours of feeding by an infected *Anopheles* mosquito. Injected sporozoites rapidly migrate through the bloodstream to the liver where they infect hepatocytes [6]. Once inside hepatocytes, *Plasmodium* is resistant to the effects of anti-sporozoite antibodies, meaning that antibodies only have a brief window to exert their effects. Thus, for these (and many other) pathogens, vaccines can be effective only if they elicit neutralizing antibodies maintained at high levels over time. For these pathogens, vaccine-mediated induction of LLPCs is required.

2. The Molecular Events That Mediate B-Cell Activation and the Role of Multivalency

The activation of B cells and the subsequent downstream events that result in antibody production are consequences of the initial interaction between an antigen and the BCR. The signaling events initiated by this interaction, which are the subject of many excellent reviews [7–9], stimulate B cell proliferation and upregulate MHC Class II and the costimulatory molecules that permit subsequent interactions with T helper cells. B-cell activation is a quantitative phenomenon, in which the degree of activation is dependent on both the affinity of the BCR for its cognate antigen [10,11] and the valency of the antigen. The critical role of antigen valency in B-cell responses was first recognized by Renee and Howard Dintzis at the Johns Hopkins School of Medicine [12–14], who assessed the immunogenicity of a T-cell independent antigen consisting of a polymer (polyacrylamide) displaying a model hapten (dinitrophenol; DNP). The modular nature of this system allowed the dissection of antibody responses as a function of the valency and density of DNP display. They concluded that " ... the fundamental molecular event in the induction of the primary immune response is the linking together by a single antigen molecule of a critical number of separate hapten receptors into a molecularly connected entity", which they termed an immunon [12]. Numerous subsequent studies established this relationship between antigen valency and B-cell responsiveness, particularly in the context of T-cell-independent antibody responses [15,16].

The series of events that begins with the activation of naïve B cells by a T-cell-dependent antigen and ultimately result in differentiation to LLPCs are more complicated than what occurs with a T-cell independent antigen, yet antigen valency and density also play an important role in this process. Multivalent interactions promote BCR clustering and the formation of lipid rafts [17–20]. These, in turn, promote signaling to the B cell and receptor-mediated internalization of the antigen complex [21], steps critical for B cells to present antigen on MHC Class II and receive help from CD4 T cells. Accordingly, multivalency enhances BCR clustering [22], BCR/antigen internalization and antigen presentation [23], as well as the upregulation of costimulatory molecules that are important for subsequent interactions with T helper cells [24]. Thus, these multivalent interactions have a profound effect on early steps in B-cell activation and ultimately influence antibody production and other downstream events.

While the influence of multivalency on the early steps in B-cell activation have been extensively studied, less is known about how these events influence the establishment of germinal centers (GCs) and production of LLPCs. GCs are discrete anatomical sites within B-cell follicles in which B cells proliferate and undergo somatic hypermutation and affinity maturation. It is here that they differentiate to memory cells and LLPCs. In GCs, B cells compete for binding with antigens displayed on follicular dendritic cells, and then present antigens to follicular T helper cells, which in turn provide survival signals to the B cell. Although this process does not require a multivalent antigen, enhanced B-cell crosslinking in GCs leads to increased GC B-cell proliferation and promotes differentiation to plasma cells, particularly in scenarios in which T help is limiting [25]. Thus, it is likely that multivalency can exert its stimulatory effects at multiple steps during the B-cell activation and differentiation process.

3. Immune Responses Elicited by Multivalent Vaccines

The basic immunological studies described above were initiated, in part, to explain the potent immunogenicity of multivalent antigens in a vaccine setting. Many different multivalent display strategies have been employed. They include synthetic nanoparticles [26,27], liposomes [28], micelles [29], and polymers [30]. But one of the most common is to display antigens on platforms based on virus-like particles (VLPs). Many viral proteins have an intrinsic ability, when overexpressed, to self-assemble into VLPs. VLPs lack viral genomes, meaning that they are absolutely non-infectious. VLPs can be derived from diverse viruses, including viruses that infect humans, animals, insects, plants, and bacteria (for recent reviews on this subject, see [31,32] and elsewhere in this Special Issue of *Viruses*). VLPs intrinsically display their own antigens in highly dense, repetitive arrays, and they can also be used as platforms for the high valency display of heterologous antigens. Their multivalency is not the only feature contributing to VLP immunogenicity. Most VLPs have a diameter (between 10 and 100–200 nm) that is optimal for uptake into the lymphatic system. Entry into the lymphatics promotes trafficking to regional lymph nodes, deposition in the subcapsular spaces of the lymph nodes that are key sites for B-cell activation, and interactions with antigen-presenting cells, such as dendritic cells (DCs) [33]. Some VLPs (and some engineered nanoparticles as well) also interact with soluble components of the innate immune system to facilitate this trafficking [34,35]. Moreover, VLPs fall into the size range (<500 nm in diameter) of particulate antigens most readily taken up by DCs [36]. Many VLPs, natural [37] or engineered [38], package adjuvants that can also enhance immunogenicity. Lastly, because they are protein-based, VLPs are naturally a rich source of T helper epitopes (or can be engineered to be so [39]), which are critical for the induction of T-cell-dependent antibody responses. Taken together, these immunological features underlie the use of VLPs as effective stand-alone vaccines (against the virus that they were derived from) and as the basis of vaccine platform technologies to display heterologous antigen targets.

The ability of multivalent display to enhance target antigen immunogenicity is well established. Figures 1 and 2 illustrate the potent immunogenicity conferred by VLP display. In Figure 1, we assessed the immunogenicity of a peptide representing a neo-epitope specific to a mutated version of the epidermal growth factor receptor (EGFRvIII) that is particularly prevalent in glioblastoma multiforme brain cancers and is associated with poor outcomes [40]. The EGFRvIII peptide was chemically conjugated either to Qß bacteriophage VLPs or to a commonly used carrier protein, keyhole limpet hemocyanin (KLH), and then used to immunize mice. After a single dose administered without exogenous adjuvant, we showed that the VLP-based immunogen elicited higher titer anti-peptide IgG antibody responses than the KLH-conjugated antigen, and that these antibody responses were elicited more rapidly (Figure 1), despite using a 5-fold lower dose of the VLP-conjugated material. Using VLPs, anti-peptide IgG was detected as early as one week after immunization. Moreover, remarkably stable levels of antibody are induced using VLP-based immunogens. In a separate study, shown in Figure 2, we longitudinally measured antibody responses in groups of mice immunized with recombinant MS2 bacteriophage VLPs, displaying a broadly neutralizing epitope from the HPV type 16 minor capsid protein (L2; the vaccine is described in [41]). Mice were given one or three doses of vaccine and then were followed for nearly two years after vaccination. Three doses elicited higher antibody titers than a single dose, but this difference became less pronounced over time. Notably, even a single dose gave remarkably stable antibody titers; levels were virtually unchanged for nearly two years after vaccination (essentially the life span of the mouse). This is likely due to the potent induction of LLPCs.

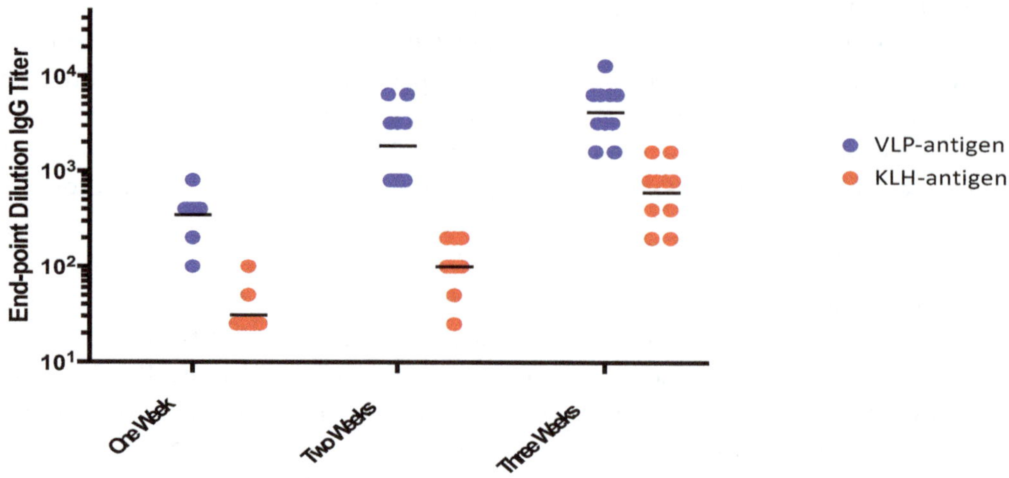

Figure 1. Mice were immunized with a single dose of an EGFRvIII peptide conjugated to Qß VLPs or the same peptide conjugated to keyhole limpet hemocyanin (KLH). Mice were immunized with 5 μg of VLP-EGFRvIII (displaying ~270 EGFvIII peptides per 2520kD VLP) or 25 μg of KLH-EGFRvIII (displaying ~50 EGFvIII peptides per 390 kD molecule of KLH) without exogenous adjuvant. Anti-peptide IgG antibody responses were measured by end-point dilution ELISA, one, two, or three weeks after the immunization. Each dot represents an individual mouse and lines represent the geometric mean of each group.

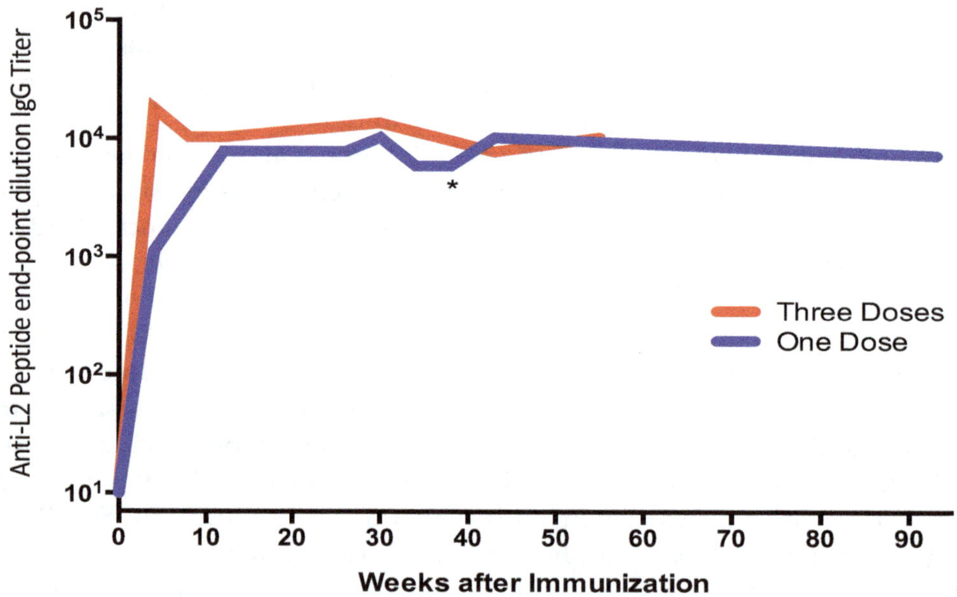

Figure 2. Mice were immunized with one (blue line; immunized at week zero) or three (red line; immunized at weeks zero, four, and eight) doses of 10 μg of recombinant MS2 bacteriophage VLPs displaying a peptide derived from the L2 minor capsid protein of HPV16 without exogenous adjuvant. Anti-peptide IgG antibody responses were measured by end-point dilution ELISA. The line represents the geometric mean of each group (n = 5/group). One of the mice in the "One Dose" group died at week 41 (indicated with an asterisk) for a reason that was unrelated to the vaccine. Antibody levels from the first six months after vaccination in the "One Dose" group were originally reported in Reference [42].

Human clinical data from trials of the VLP-based HPV vaccines Cervarix (GlaxoSmithKline) and Gardasil (Merck) also strongly support the concept that VLPs can efficiently induce LLPCs. A longitudinal study of antibody responses induced by these vaccines [43] revealed that both vaccines induce anti-HPV antibody responses that peak approximately one month after the third dose. After an initial period in which antibody levels decay rapidly (with a half-life of ~3.6 months, probably reflecting the loss of short-lived plasmablasts), these levels stabilize—there was no evidence of a further decline in antibody titers over a 4-year follow-up period. Even a single dose of HPV VLPs elicits exceedingly long-lived antibody responses. A subset of women enrolled in the phase III Costa Rica Vaccine Trial of Cervarix received just a single dose of the vaccine (this was due to various reasons, but most commonly these women discovered that they were pregnant after they received their first dose). Compared to the usual three-dose regimen, a single dose gave lower anti-HPV antibody levels, but the profile of antibody decay in the two groups was quite similar [44]. Antibody levels over the six-year period spanning one to seven years after vaccination were extraordinarily stable; these antibodies were essentially maintained at a constant level during this period. Moreover, no HPV16 or HPV18 infections were detected in this group of women during the observation period [45]. Based on these results, the US National Cancer Institute, in collaboration with a Costa Rican partner, is currently conducting a large randomized, controlled trial (the ESCUDDO study) to assess the immunogenicity and efficacy of a single-dose vaccine regimen.

The longevity of antibody responses elicited by the HPV vaccine parallels the humoral immune responses generated by other multivalent viral vaccines. In a seminal study, Amanna and colleagues longitudinally measured human antibody responses to a diverse panel of vaccine antigens, including viral (i.e., multivalent) vaccines and non-viral (toxoid; monovalent) vaccine antigens [46]. They found that the antibodies elicited by multivalent antigens were extremely durable—for example, antibodies against measles had a calculated half-life of ~3000 years—whereas the half-life of antibodies against the monomeric tetanus and diphtheria toxoid vaccines was much shorter (~11–19 years). Interestingly, there was no relationship between the frequency of vaccine-elicited memory B cells and antibody levels, suggesting that LLPCs were elicited upon the initial exposure to the antigen, and were not due to re-activation of memory cells. Taken together, these data strongly support the idea that multivalent vaccines can elicit long-lasting responses in humans (for a review of these and other human studies, see Reference [47]).

4. The Special Case of Using Multivalent Vaccines to Break B-Cell Tolerance

One of the most striking features of VLP display is its ability to elicit antibody responses against self-antigens. The immune system has erected a set of barriers that normally prevent the induction of autoantibody responses. During the early stages of B-cell development in the bone marrow, central B-cell tolerance mechanisms act to change the specificity (through a process referred to as receptor editing) or eliminate (through apoptosis) a percentage of potentially autoreactive B cells (shown schematically in Figure 3). However, these mechanisms are inefficient, and as a consequence a substantial percentage of naïve B cells that move into the periphery are potentially self-reactive [48,49]. Fortunately, when these self-reactive B cells are exposed to a soluble self-antigen in the periphery in the absence of T help, they undergo a number of changes that establish a state of unresponsiveness to subsequent antigen stimulation, known as anergy. Relative to non-anergic cells, anergic B cells are defined by decreased BCR surface expression, competitive exclusion from lymphoid follicles, and a short half-life [50,51]. Nevertheless, even these B cells are susceptible to activation by multivalent antigens. In a seminal study, Bachmann and colleagues showed that B cells from transgenic mice expressing a soluble form of the vesicular stomatitis virus glycoprotein (VSV-G) responded to vaccination with particulate, ordered forms of VSV-G (such as inactivated virions), but not to immunization with soluble monomeric VSV-G. This study suggested that multivalent antigens could effectively activate anergic B cells. Subsequent studies demonstrated that vaccines consisting of self-antigens arrayed on the surface of the VLPs could effectively induce anti-self antibody responses [52,53], that this ability is critically dependent on the density of the self-antigens displayed on VLPs [54,55], and that these interactions may be mediated by binding to surface-expressed IgD on naïve B cells [56]. These findings have led to the development of vaccine candidates that induce antibodies against self-antigens involved in chronic diseases, including angiotensin II (hypertension) [57], PCSK9 (cardiovascular disease) [58], amyloid-beta and hyper-phosphorylated tau (Alzheimer's Disease) [59,60], and others [61]. Several of these vaccines have been tested in human clinical trials [62].

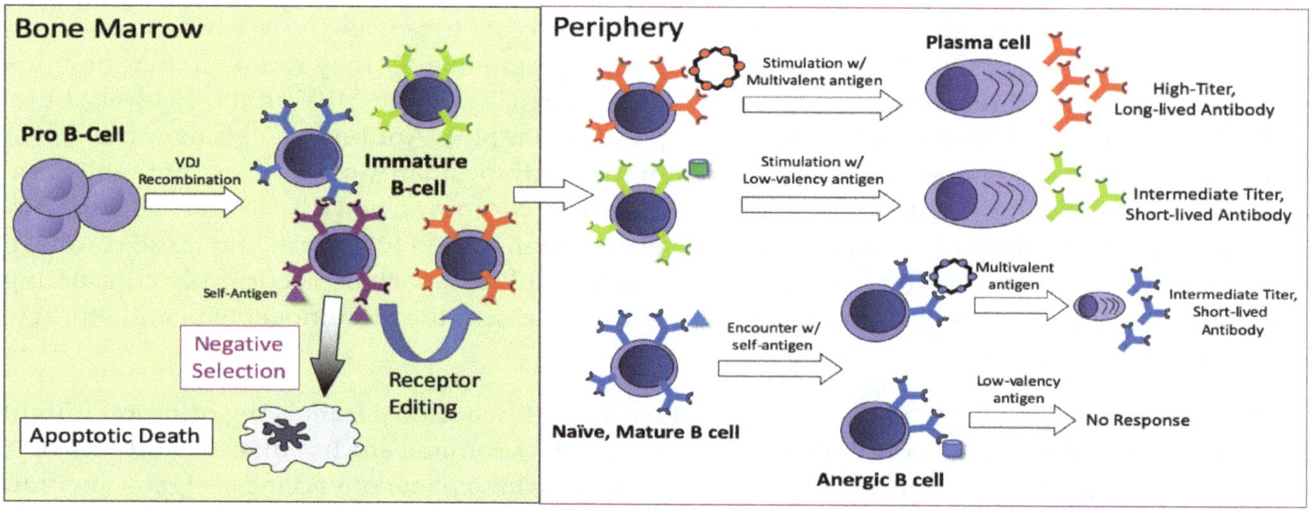

Figure 3. An overview of B-cell development, B-cell tolerance mechanisms, and the outcomes of stimulation with different forms of antigen (self-, low-valency, or multivalent antigen). B-cell responses are dependent on the nature of the antigen and the stage of B-cell development. In the bone marrow, immature B cells that encounter self-antigen either undergo apoptosis or receptor editing, which potentially alters receptor specificity. In the periphery, B cells that encounter multivalent antigens respond strongly, leading to the production of LLPCs that produce large amounts of antibody. Stimulation with low-valency antigens leads to lower titer and less durable antibody responses. If naïve B cells encounter self-antigen they become anergized. Anergic B cells do not respond to stimulation with low-valency antigen, but can be activated by multivalent antigens.

One interesting observation from human clinical trials of VLP-based vaccines targeting amyloid-beta [63] and angiotensin II [64] was that the half-life of the antibodies induced against self-antigens was fairly short, 15–20 weeks. This is in contrast to the durable antibody responses that are observed in vaccination studies using VLPs that target pathogen-derived (foreign) epitopes. Why do VLP-based vaccines that target foreign antigens strongly elicit LLPCs, but generate more transient antibody responses when targeting self-antigens? Studies comparing the reactivity of anergic and non-anergic transgenic B cells may provide an explanation. B cells respond to antigenic stimulation by upregulating a suite of molecules important in activating (i.e., CD86) and receiving help from (CD40) T helper cells. We showed that upregulation of these molecules upon stimulation by VLPs is attenuated in anergic transgenic B cells, relative to non-anergic cells [24]. It is possible that the downregulated expression of the BCR on anergic cells may account for these attenuated responses. Lower levels of BCR are likely to reduce the potential for extensive BCR crosslinking and, consequently, lead to weaker B-cell activation. Alternatively, anergic B cells may have other defects in the signaling pathways involved in B-cell activation. Regardless of the mechanism, these data indicate that reduced B-cell activation has profound downstream consequences. Weaker stimulation results in reduced numbers of LLPCs and less durable antibody responses.

5. Conclusions

VLPs have been exploited as a platform technology to develop vaccines for diverse targets, including specific antigens or epitopes derived from infectious disease targets, self-antigens involved in chronic diseases, and even small molecules, such as drugs of abuse [65]. In general, VLP display is regarded as a method for enhancing the magnitude of an antibody response, similar to how adjuvants can increase the immunogenicity of vaccines. However, as described in this article, and as summarized in Figure 3, the multivalent nature of VLPs also confers special immunostimulatory properties not typically conferred by adjuvants, particularly the ability to elicit durable antibody responses through the induction of LLPCs. For many targets, the induction of long-lived antibody responses is likely to be a key factor in vaccine efficacy. A deeper understanding of the mechanisms whereby multivalent antigens can lead to the induction and maintenance of LLPCs will influence vaccine design and likely lead to improved vaccines in the future.

Author Contributions: B.C., writing—original draft preparation; D.S.P., writing—review and editing; all authors have read and agree to the published version of the manuscript. All authors have read and agreed to the published version of the manuscript.

Acknowledgments: Thanks to Teal Clocksin, Ebenezer Tumban, and Julianne Peabody for generating the data shown in Figures 1 and 2.

References

1. Cicala, C.; Nawaz, F.; Jelicic, K.; Arthos, J.; Fauci, A.S. HIV-1 gp120: A Target for Therapeutics and Vaccine Design. *Curr. Drug Targets* **2016**, *17*, 122–135. [CrossRef] [PubMed]
2. Graham, S.V. Keratinocyte Differentiation-Dependent Human Papillomavirus Gene Regulation. *Viruses* **2017**, *9*, 245. [CrossRef] [PubMed]
3. Mittal, S.; Banks, L. Molecular mechanisms underlying human papillomavirus E6 and E7 oncoprotein-induced cell transformation. *Mutat. Res. Rev. Mutat. Res.* **2017**, *772*, 23–35. [CrossRef]
4. Schiller, J.T.; Lowy, D.R. Understanding and learning from the success of prophylactic human papillomavirus vaccines. *Nat. Rev. Microbiol.* **2012**, *10*, 681–692. [CrossRef]
5. Hildesheim, A.; Herrero, R.; Wacholder, S.; Rodriguez, A.C.; Solomon, D.; Bratti, M.C.; Schiller, J.T.; Gonzalez, P.; Dubin, G.; Porras, C.; et al. Effect of human papillomavirus 16/18 L1 viruslike particle vaccine among young women with preexisting infection: A randomized trial. *JAMA* **2007**, *298*, 743–753. [CrossRef] [PubMed]
6. Sinnis, P.; Zavala, F. The skin: Where malaria infection and the host immune response begin. *Semin. Immunopathol.* **2012**, *34*, 787–792. [CrossRef] [PubMed]
7. Dal Porto, J.M.; Gauld, S.B.; Merrell, K.T.; Mills, D.; Pugh-Bernard, A.E.; Cambier, J. B cell antigen receptor signaling 101. *Mol. Immunol.* **2004**, *41*, 599–613. [CrossRef] [PubMed]
8. Kwak, K.; Akkaya, M.; Pierce, S.K. B cell signaling in context. *Nat. Immunol.* **2019**, *20*, 963–969. [CrossRef]
9. Tolar, P.; Sohn, H.W.; Liu, W.; Pierce, S.K. The molecular assembly and organization of signaling active B-cell receptor oligomers. *Immunol. Rev.* **2009**, *232*, 34–41. [CrossRef]
10. Kouskoff, V.; Famiglietti, S.; Lacaud, G.; Lang, P.; Rider, J.E.; Kay, B.K.; Cambier, J.C.; Nemazee, D. Antigens varying in affinity for the B cell receptor induce differential B lymphocyte responses. *J. Exp. Med.* **1998**, *188*, 1453–1464. [CrossRef]
11. Schwickert, T.A.; Victora, G.D.; Fooksman, D.R.; Kamphorst, A.O.; Mugnier, M.R.; Gitlin, A.D.; Dustin, M.L.; Nussenzweig, M.C. A dynamic T cell-limited checkpoint regulates affinity-dependent B cell entry into the germinal center. *J. Exp. Med.* **2011**, *208*, 1243–1252. [CrossRef] [PubMed]
12. Dintzis, H.M.; Dintzis, R.Z.; Vogelstein, B. Molecular determinants of immunogenicity: The immunon model of immune response. *Proc. Natl. Acad. Sci. USA* **1976**, *73*, 3671–3675. [CrossRef] [PubMed]
13. Dintzis, R.Z.; Middleton, M.H.; Dintzis, H.M. Studies on the immunogenicity and tolerogenicity of T-independent antigens. *J. Immunol.* **1983**, *131*, 2196–2203. [PubMed]
14. Dintzis, R.Z.; Vogelstein, B.; Dintzis, H.M. Specific cellular stimulation in the primary immune response: Experimental test of a quantized model. *Proc. Natl. Acad. Sci. USA* **1982**, *79*, 884–888. [CrossRef] [PubMed]
15. Mond, J.J.; Lees, A.; Snapper, C.M. T cell-independent antigens type 2. *Annu. Rev. Immunol.* **1995**, *13*, 655–692. [CrossRef]
16. Vos, Q.; Lees, A.; Wu, Z.Q.; Snapper, C.M.; Mond, J.J. B-cell activation by T-cell-independent type 2 antigens as an integral part of the humoral immune response to pathogenic microorganisms. *Immunol. Rev.* **2000**, *176*, 154–170.
17. Batista, F.D.; Neuberger, M.S. Affinity dependence of the B cell response to antigen: A threshold, a ceiling, and the importance of off-rate. *Immunity* **1998**, *8*, 751–759. [CrossRef]

18. Cheng, P.C.; Brown, B.K.; Song, W.; Pierce, S.K. Translocation of the B cell antigen receptor into lipid rafts reveals a novel step in signaling. *J. Immunol.* **2001**, *166*, 3693–3701. [CrossRef]
19. Mattila, P.K.; Feest, C.; Depoil, D.; Treanor, B.; Montaner, B.; Otipoby, K.L.; Carter, R.; Justement, L.B.; Bruckbauer, A.; Batista, F.D. The actin and tetraspanin networks organize receptor nanoclusters to regulate B cell receptor-mediated signaling. *Immunity* **2013**, *38*, 461–474. [CrossRef]
20. Pierce, S.K. Lipid rafts and B-cell activation. *Nat. Rev. Immunol.* **2002**, *2*, 96–105. [CrossRef]
21. Gazumyan, A.; Reichlin, A.; Nussenzweig, M.C. Ig beta tyrosine residues contribute to the control of B cell receptor signaling by regulating receptor internalization. *J. Exp. Med.* **2006**, *203*, 1785–1794. [CrossRef]
22. Puffer, E.B.; Pontrello, J.K.; Hollenbeck, J.J.; Kink, J.A.; Kiessling, L.L. Activating B cell signaling with defined multivalent ligands. *ACS Chem. Biol.* **2007**, *2*, 252–262. [CrossRef] [PubMed]
23. Bennett, N.R.; Zwick, D.B.; Courtney, A.H.; Kiessling, L.L. Multivalent Antigens for Promoting B and T Cell Activation. *ACS Chem. Biol.* **2015**, *10*, 1817–1824. [CrossRef] [PubMed]
24. Chackerian, B.; Durfee, M.R.; Schiller, J.T. Virus-like display of a neo-self antigen reverses B cell anergy in a B cell receptor transgenic mouse model. *J. Immunol.* **2008**, *180*, 5816–5825. [CrossRef] [PubMed]
25. Turner, J.S.; Ke, F.; Grigorova, I.L. B Cell Receptor Crosslinking Augments Germinal Center B Cell Selection when T Cell Help Is Limiting. *Cell Rep.* **2018**, *25*, 1395–1403. [CrossRef]
26. Brouwer, P.J.M.; Antanasijevic, A.; Berndsen, Z.; Yasmeen, A.; Fiala, B.; Bijl, T.P.L.; Bontjer, I.; Bale, J.B.; Sheffler, W.; Allen, J.D.; et al. Enhancing and shaping the immunogenicity of native-like HIV-1 envelope trimers with a two-component protein nanoparticle. *Nat. Commun.* **2019**, *10*, 4272. [CrossRef]
27. Havenar-Daughton, C.; Carnathan, D.G.; Boopathy, A.V.; Upadhyay, A.A.; Murrell, B.; Reiss, S.M.; Enemuo, C.A.; Gebru, E.H.; Choe, Y.; Dhadvai, P.; et al. Rapid Germinal Center and Antibody Responses in Non-human Primates after a Single Nanoparticle Vaccine Immunization. *Cell Rep.* **2019**, *29*, 1756–1766. [CrossRef]
28. Dubrovskaya, V.; Tran, K.; Ozorowski, G.; Guenaga, J.; Wilson, R.; Bale, S.; Cottrell, C.A.; Turner, H.L.; Seabright, G.; O'Dell, S.; et al. Vaccination with Glycan-Modified HIV NFL Envelope Trimer-Liposomes Elicits Broadly Neutralizing Antibodies to Multiple Sites of Vulnerability. *Immunity* **2019**, *51*, 915–929. [CrossRef]
29. Moon, J.J.; Suh, H.; Bershteyn, A.; Stephan, M.T.; Liu, H.; Huang, B.; Sohail, M.; Luo, S.; Um, S.H.; Khant, H.; et al. Interbilayer-crosslinked multilamellar vesicles as synthetic vaccines for potent humoral and cellular immune responses. *Nat. Mater.* **2011**, *10*, 243–251. [CrossRef]
30. Zhang, F.; Lu, Y.J.; Malley, R. Multiple antigen-presenting system (MAPS) to induce comprehensive B- and T-cell immunity. *Proc. Natl. Acad. Sci. USA* **2013**, *110*, 13564–13569. [CrossRef]
31. Balke, I.; Zeltins, A. Use of plant viruses and virus-like particles for the creation of novel vaccines. *Adv. Drug Deliv. Rev.* **2019**, *145*, 119–129. [CrossRef] [PubMed]
32. Donaldson, B.; Lateef, Z.; Walker, G.F.; Young, S.L.; Ward, V.K. Virus-like particle vaccines: Immunology and formulation for clinical translation. *Expert Rev. Vaccines* **2018**, *17*, 833–849. [CrossRef] [PubMed]
33. Manolova, V.; Flace, A.; Bauer, M.; Schwarz, K.; Saudan, P.; Bachmann, M.F. Nanoparticles target distinct dendritic cell populations according to their size. *Eur. J. Immunol.* **2008**, *38*, 1404–1413. [CrossRef] [PubMed]
34. Link, A.; Zabel, F.; Schnetzler, Y.; Titz, A.; Brombacher, F.; Bachmann, M.F. Innate immunity mediates follicular transport of particulate but not soluble protein antigen. *J. Immunol.* **2012**, *188*, 3724–3733. [CrossRef] [PubMed]
35. Tokatlian, T.; Read, B.J.; Jones, C.A.; Kulp, D.W.; Menis, S.; Chang, J.Y.H.; Steichen, J.M.; Kumari, S.; Allen, J.D.; Dane, E.L.; et al. Innate immune recognition of glycans targets HIV nanoparticle immunogens to germinal centers. *Science* **2019**, *363*, 649–654. [CrossRef]
36. Foged, C.; Brodin, B.; Frokjaer, S.; Sundblad, A. Particle size and surface charge affect particle uptake by human dendritic cells in an in vitro model. *Int. J. Pharm.* **2005**, *298*, 315–322. [CrossRef]
37. Tumban, E.; Peabody, J.; Peabody, D.S.; Chackerian, B. A universal virus-like particle-based vaccine for human papillomavirus: Longevity of protection and role of endogenous and exogenous adjuvants. *Vaccine* **2013**, *31*, 4647–4654. [CrossRef]
38. Senti, G.; Johansen, P.; Haug, S.; Bull, C.; Gottschaller, C.; Muller, P.; Pfister, T.; Maurer, P.; Bachmann, M.F.; Graf, N.; et al. Use of A-type CpG oligodeoxynucleotides as an adjuvant in allergen-specific immunotherapy in humans: A phase I/IIa clinical trial. *Clin. Exp. Allergy* **2009**, *39*, 562–570. [CrossRef]

39. Zeltins, A.; West, J.; Zabel, F.; El Turabi, A.; Balke, I.; Haas, S.; Maudrich, M.; Storni, F.; Engeroff, P.; Jennings, G.T.; et al. Incorporation of tetanus-epitope into virus-like particles achieves vaccine responses even in older recipients in models of psoriasis, Alzheimer's and cat allergy. *NPJ Vaccines* **2017**, *2*, 30. [CrossRef]
40. Wong, A.J.; Ruppert, J.M.; Bigner, S.H.; Grzeschik, C.H.; Humphrey, P.A.; Bigner, D.S.; Vogelstein, B. Structural alterations of the epidermal growth factor receptor gene in human gliomas. *Proc. Natl. Acad. Sci. USA* **1992**, *89*, 2965–2969. [CrossRef]
41. Tumban, E.; Peabody, J.; Tyler, M.; Peabody, D.S.; Chackerian, B. VLPs displaying a single L2 epitope induce broadly cross-neutralizing antibodies against human papillomavirus. *PLoS ONE* **2012**, *7*, e49751. [CrossRef] [PubMed]
42. Tumban, E.; Muttil, P.; Escobar, C.A.A.; Peabody, J.; Wafula, D.; Peabody, D.S.; Chackerian, B. Preclinical refinements of a broadly protective VLP-based HPV vaccine targeting the minor capsid protein, L2. *Vaccine* **2015**, *33*, 3346–3353. [CrossRef] [PubMed]
43. Einstein, M.H.; Takacs, P.; Chatterjee, A.; Sperling, R.S.; Chakhtoura, N.; Blatter, M.M.; Lalezari, J.; David, M.P.; Lin, L.; Struyf, F.; et al. Comparison of long-term immunogenicity and safety of human papillomavirus (HPV)-16/18 AS04-adjuvanted vaccine and HPV-6/11/16/18 vaccine in healthy women aged 18-45 years: End-of-study analysis of a Phase III randomized trial. *Hum. Vaccin Immunother.* **2014**, *10*, 3435–3445. [CrossRef] [PubMed]
44. Safaeian, M.; Porras, C.; Pan, Y.; Kreimer, A.; Schiller, J.T.; Gonzalez, P.; Lowy, D.R.; Wacholder, S.; Schiffman, M.; Rodriguez, A.C.; et al. Durable antibody responses following one dose of the bivalent human papillomavirus L1 virus-like particle vaccine in the Costa Rica Vaccine Trial. *Cancer Prev. Res.* **2013**, *6*, 1242–1250. [CrossRef] [PubMed]
45. Kreimer, A.R.; Herrero, R.; Sampson, J.N.; Porras, C.; Lowy, D.R.; Schiller, J.T.; Schiffman, M.; Rodriguez, A.C.; Chanock, S.; Jimenez, S.; et al. Evidence for single-dose protection by the bivalent HPV vaccine-Review of the Costa Rica HPV vaccine trial and future research studies. *Vaccine* **2018**, *36*, 4774–4782. [CrossRef] [PubMed]
46. Amanna, I.J.; Carlson, N.E.; Slifka, M.K. Duration of humoral immunity to common viral and vaccine antigens. *N. Engl. J. Med.* **2007**, *357*, 1903–1915. [CrossRef]
47. Slifka, M.K.; Amanna, I.J. Role of Multivalency and Antigenic Threshold in Generating Protective Antibody Responses. *Front. Immunol.* **2019**, *10*, 956. [CrossRef]
48. Merrell, K.T.; Benschop, R.J.; Gauld, S.B.; Aviszus, K.; Decote-Ricardo, D.; Wysocki, L.J.; Cambier, J.C. Identification of anergic B cells within a wild-type repertoire. *Immunity* **2006**, *25*, 953–962. [CrossRef]
49. Wardemann, H.; Yurasov, S.; Schaefer, A.; Young, J.W.; Meffre, E.; Nussenzweig, M.C. Predominant autoantibody production by early human B cell precursors. *Science* **2003**, *301*, 1374–1377. [CrossRef]
50. Cyster, J.G.; Hartley, S.B.; Goodnow, C.C. Competition for follicular niches excludes self-reactive cells from the recirculating B-cell repertoire. *Nature* **1994**, *371*, 389–395. [CrossRef]
51. Fulcher, D.A.; Basten, A. Reduced life span of anergic self-reactive B cells in a double-transgenic model. *J. Exp. Med.* **1994**, *179*, 125–134. [CrossRef] [PubMed]
52. Chackerian, B.; Lowy, D.R.; Schiller, J.T. Induction of autoantibodies to mouse CCR5 with recombinant papillomavirus particles. *Proc. Natl. Acad. Sci. USA* **1999**, *96*, 2373–2378. [CrossRef] [PubMed]
53. Chackerian, B.; Lowy, D.R.; Schiller, J.T. Conjugation of a self-antigen to papillomavirus-like particles allows for efficient induction of protective autoantibodies. *J. Clin. Investig.* **2001**, *108*, 415–423. [CrossRef] [PubMed]
54. Chackerian, B.; Lenz, P.; Lowy, D.R.; Schiller, J.T. Determinants of autoantibody induction by conjugated papillomavirus virus-like particles. *J. Immunol.* **2002**, *169*, 6120–6126. [CrossRef]
55. Jegerlehner, A.; Storni, T.; Lipowsky, G.; Schmid, M.; Pumpens, P.; Bachmann, M.F. Regulation of IgG antibody responses by epitope density and CD21-mediated costimulation. *Eur. J. Immunol.* **2002**, *32*, 3305–3314. [CrossRef]
56. Übelhart, R.; Hug, E.; Bach, M.P.; Wossning, T.; Dühren-von Minden, M.; Horn, A.H.; Tsiantoulas, D.; Kometani, K.; Kurosaki, T.; Binder, C.J.; et al. Responsiveness of B cells is regulated by the hinge region of IgD. *Nat. Immunol.* **2015**, *16*, 534–543. [CrossRef]
57. Maurer, P.; Bachmann, M.F. Immunization against angiotensins for the treatment of hypertension. *Clin. Immunol.* **2010**, *134*, 89–95. [CrossRef]
58. Crossey, E.; Amar, M.J.; Sampson, M.; Peabody, J.; Schiller, J.T.; Chackerian, B.; Remaley, A.T. A cholesterol-lowering VLP vaccine that targets PCSK9. *Vaccine* **2015**, *33*, 5747–5755. [CrossRef]

59. Maphis, N.M.; Peabody, J.; Crossey, E.; Jiang, S.; Ahmad, F.A.J.; Alvarez, M.; Mansoor, S.K.; Yaney, A.; Yang, Y.; Sillerud, L.O.; et al. Qß Virus-like particle-based vaccine induces robust immunity and protects against tauopathy. *NPJ Vaccines* **2019**, *4*, 26. [CrossRef]
60. Vandenberghe, R.; Riviere, M.E.; Caputo, A.; Sovago, J.; Maguire, R.P.; Farlow, M.; Marotta, G.; Sanchez-Valle, R.; Scheltens, P.; Ryan, J.M.; et al. Active Abeta immunotherapy CAD106 in Alzheimer's disease: A phase 2b study. *Alzheimers Dement.* **2017**, *3*, 10–22.
61. Bachmann, M.F.; Whitehead, P. Active immunotherapy for chronic diseases. *Vaccine* **2013**, *31*, 1777–1784. [CrossRef]
62. Mohsen, M.O.; Zha, L.; Cabral-Miranda, G.; Bachmann, M.F. Major findings and recent advances in virus-like particle (VLP)-based vaccines. *Semin. Immunol.* **2017**, *34*, 123–132. [CrossRef] [PubMed]
63. Farlow, M.R.; Andreasen, N.; Riviere, M.E.; Vostiar, I.; Vitaliti, A.; Sovago, J.; Caputo, A.; Winblad, B.; Graf, A. Long-term treatment with active Abeta immunotherapy with CAD106 in mild Alzheimer's disease. *Alzheimers Res. Ther.* **2015**, *7*, 23. [CrossRef] [PubMed]
64. Tissot, A.C.; Maurer, P.; Nussberger, J.; Sabat, R.; Pfister, T.; Ignatenko, S.; Volk, H.D.; Stocker, H.; Müller, P.; Jennings, G.T.; et al. Effect of immunisation against angiotensin II with CYT006-AngQb on ambulatory blood pressure: A double-blind, randomised, placebo-controlled phase IIa study. *Lancet* **2008**, *371*, 821–827. [CrossRef]
65. Maurer, P.; Jennings, G.T.; Willers, J.; Rohner, F.; Lindman, Y.; Roubicek, K.; Renner, W.A.; Müller, P.; Bachmann, M.F. A therapeutic vaccine for nicotine dependence: Preclinical efficacy, and Phase I safety and immunogenicity. *Eur. J. Immunol.* **2005**, *35*, 2031–2040. [CrossRef] [PubMed]

Permissions

All chapters in this book were first published by MDPI; hereby published with permission under the Creative Commons Attribution License or equivalent. Every chapter published in this book has been scrutinized by our experts. Their significance has been extensively debated. The topics covered herein carry significant findings which will fuel the growth of the discipline. They may even be implemented as practical applications or may be referred to as a beginning point for another development.

The contributors of this book come from diverse backgrounds, making this book a truly international effort. This book will bring forth new frontiers with its revolutionizing research information and detailed analysis of the nascent developments around the world.

We would like to thank all the contributing authors for lending their expertise to make the book truly unique. They have played a crucial role in the development of this book. Without their invaluable contributions this book wouldn't have been possible. They have made vital efforts to compile up to date information on the varied aspects of this subject to make this book a valuable addition to the collection of many professionals and students.

This book was conceptualized with the vision of imparting up-to-date information and advanced data in this field. To ensure the same, a matchless editorial board was set up. Every individual on the board went through rigorous rounds of assessment to prove their worth. After which they invested a large part of their time researching and compiling the most relevant data for our readers.

The editorial board has been involved in producing this book since its inception. They have spent rigorous hours researching and exploring the diverse topics which have resulted in the successful publishing of this book. They have passed on their knowledge of decades through this book. To expedite this challenging task, the publisher supported the team at every step. A small team of assistant editors was also appointed to further simplify the editing procedure and attain best results for the readers.

Apart from the editorial board, the designing team has also invested a significant amount of their time in understanding the subject and creating the most relevant covers. They scrutinized every image to scout for the most suitable representation of the subject and create an appropriate cover for the book.

The publishing team has been an ardent support to the editorial, designing and production team. Their endless efforts to recruit the best for this project, has resulted in the accomplishment of this book. They are a veteran in the field of academics and their pool of knowledge is as vast as their experience in printing. Their expertise and guidance has proved useful at every step. Their uncompromising quality standards have made this book an exceptional effort. Their encouragement from time to time has been an inspiration for everyone.

The publisher and the editorial board hope that this book will prove to be a valuable piece of knowledge for researchers, students, practitioners and scholars across the globe.

List of Contributors

Sarah Honjo, Michiaki Masuda and Tomohiro Ishikawa
Department of Microbiology, Dokkyo Medical University School of Medicine, 880 Kita-kobayashi, Mibu-machi, Shimotsuga-gun, Tochigi 321-0293, Japan

Francesco Berlanda Scorza
PATH's Center for Vaccine Innovation and Access, 455 Massachusetts Ave. NW, Suite 1000, Washington, DC 20001, USA

Norbert Pardi
Department of Medicine, University of Pennsylvania, Philadelphia, PA 19104, USA

Ryan A. Langlois
Biochemistry, Molecular Biology, and Biophysics Graduate Program, University of Minnesota, Minneapolis, MN 55455, USA
Center for Immunology, University of Minnesota, Minneapolis, MN 55455, USA
Department of Microbiology and Immunology, University of Minnesota, Minneapolis, MN 55455, USA

Elizabeth J. Fay
Biochemistry, Molecular Biology, and Biophysics Graduate Program, University of Minnesota, Minneapolis, MN 55455, USA
Center for Immunology, University of Minnesota, Minneapolis, MN 55455, USA

Michela Perotti
Faculty of Biomedical Sciences, Institute for Research in Biomedicine, Università della Svizzera Italiana, 6500 Bellinzona, Switzerland
Institute of Microbiology, ETH Zürich, 8093 Zürich, Switzerland

Laurent Perez
Faculty of Biomedical Sciences, Institute for Research in Biomedicine, Università della Svizzera Italiana, 6500 Bellinzona, Switzerland
European Virus Bioinformatics Center, 07743 Jena, Germany

Rashi Yadav and Ebenezer Tumban
Department of Biological Sciences, Michigan Technological University, Houghton, MI 49931, USA

Lukai Zhai
Department of Biological Sciences, Michigan Technological University, Houghton, MI 49931, USA
Van Andel Research Institute, Grand Rapids, MI 49503, USA

Junru Cui, Caitlin M. O'Connell, Connor Hagen, Kim Sawicki, Joan A. Smyth, Paulo H. Verardi, Herbert J. Van Kruiningen and Antonio E. Garmendia
Department of Pathobiology and Veterinary Science, College of Agriculture, Health and Natural Resources, University of Connecticut, Storrs, CT 06269, USA

Da Shi, Xiaobo Wang, Hongyan Shi, Jiyu Zhang, Yuru Han, Jianfei Chen, Xin Zhang, Jianbo Liu, Jialin Zhang, Zhaoyang Ji, Zhaoyang Jing and Li Feng
State Key Laboratory of Veterinary Biotechnology, Harbin Veterinary Research Institute, Chinese Academy of Agricultural Sciences, Xiangfang District, Haping Road 678, Harbin 150069, China

Rodrigo Cañas-Arranz, Patricia de León, María J. Bustos, Elisa Torres and Francisco Sobrino
Centro de Biología Molecular "Severo Ochoa" (CSIC-UAM), 28049 Madrid, Spain

Mar Forner, Sira Defaus and David Andreu
Departament de Ciències Experimentals i de la Salut, Universitat Pompeu Fabra, 08003 Barcelona, Spain

Esther Blanco
Centro de Investigación en Sanidad Animal (CISA-INIA), Valdeolmos, 28130 Madrid, Spain

Elena López-Gil, Sandra Moreno, Javier Ortego, Belén Borrego, Gema Lorenzo and Alejandro Brun
Animal Health Research Centre (CISA), National Institute for Agriculture and Food Research and Technology (INIA), Valdeolmos, 28130 Madrid, Spain

Blanca Chinchilla
Ocular Genomics Institute, Department of Ophthalmology, Massachusetts Eye and Ear Infirmary and Harvard Medical School, Boston, MA 02114, USA

Paloma Encinas, Julio M. Coll, Eduardo Gomez-Casado, Nereida Jiménez de Oya, Estela Escribano-Romero, Ana-Belén Blázquez, Miguel A. Martín-Acebes and Juan-Carlos Saiz
Department of Biotechnology, National Agricultural and Food Research and Technology Institute (INIA), 28040 Madrid, Spain

Javier Mancilla-Ramirez
Escuela Superior de Medicina, Instituto Politécnico Nacional; Hospital de la Mujer, Secretaria de Sauld, Mexico City CP 11340, Mexico

Irene González-Domínguez, Eduard Puente-Massaguer, Laura Cervera and Francesc Gòdia
Departament d'Enginyeria Química Biològica i Ambiental, Universitat Autònoma de Barcelona, Cerdanyola del Vallès, 08193 Barcelona, Spain

Joshua D. Duncan, Richard A. Urbanowicz, Alexander W. Tarr and Jonathan K. Ball
School of Life Sciences, The University of Nottingham, Nottingham NG7 2UH, UK
NIHR Nottingham BRC, Nottingham University Hospitals NHS Trust and the University of Nottingham, Nottingham NG7 2UH, UK
Nottingham Digestive Diseases Centre, School of Medicine, University of Nottingham, Nottingham NG7 2UH, UK

Maria Malm, Timo Vesikari and Vesna Blazevic
Vaccine Research Center, Faculty of Medicine and Health Technology, Tampere University, Biokatu 10, FI-33520 Tampere, Finland

Arturo Cérbulo-Vázquez
Facultad de Medicina, Plan de Estudios Combinados en Medicina (MD, PhD Program), Universidad Nacional Autónoma de México, Mexico City CP 04510, Mexico

Lourdes Arriaga-Pizano, Ilka Boscó-Gárate and Armando Isibasi
Unidad de Investigación Médica en Inmunoquímica, Hospital de Especialidades del Centro Médico Nacional Siglo XXI, Instituto Mexicano del Seguro Social (IMSS), Mexico City CP 06720, Mexico

Gabriela Cruz-Cureño
Escuela Nacional de Ciencias Biológicas, Programa de Inmunología, Instituto Politécnico Nacional, Mexico City CP 11340, Mexico

Eduardo Ferat-Osorio
Servicio de Cirugía Gastrointestinal, Unidad Médica de Alta Especialidad, Hospital de Especialidades Dr Bernardo Sepúlveda Gutiérrez, Centro Médico Nacional Siglo XXI, Instituto Mexicano del Seguro Social (IMSS), Mexico City CP 06720, Mexico

Rodolfo Pastelin-Palacios
Departamento de Biología, Facultad de Química, Universidad Nacional Autónoma de México, Mexico City CP 04510, Mexico

Ricardo Figueroa-Damian
Departamento de Infectología, Instituto Nacional de Perinatología, Mexico City CP 11000, Mexico

Denisse Castro-Eguiluz
Consejo Nacional de Ciencia y Tecnología (CONACYT)-Departamento de Investigación Clínica, Instituto Nacional de Cancerología, Mexico City CP 14080, Mexico

Constantino López-Macías
Unidad de Investigación Médica en Inmunoquímica, Hospital de Especialidades del Centro Médico Nacional Siglo XXI, Instituto Mexicano del Seguro Social (IMSS), Mexico City CP 06720, Mexico
Visiting Professor of Immunology, Nuffield Department of Medicine, University of Oxford, Oxford OX3 7LF, UK
Mexican Translational Immunology Research Group, Federation of Clinical Immunology Societies Centers of Excellence, National Autonomous University of Mexico, Mexico City 04510, Mexico

Bryce Chackerian and David S. Peabody
Department of Molecular Genetics and Microbiology, University of New Mexico School of Medicine, Albuquerque, NM 87106, USA

Index

www.ingramcontent.com/pod-product-compliance
Lightning Source LLC
LaVergne TN
LVHW082152200926
848484LV00008B/2147